PAIN MANAGEMENT IN REHABILITATION

PAIN MANAGEMENT IN REHABILITATION

Editors

Trilok N. Monga, M.D.
Martin Grabois, M.D.

*D*emos

Demos Medical Publishing, 386 Park Avenue South, New York, New York 10016

Library of Congress Cataloging-in-Publication Data

Pain management in rehabilitation / Trilok N. Monga and Martin Grabois, editors
    p. ; cm.
  ISBN 1-888799-63-3 (hardcover : alk paper)
  1. Pain. 2. Chronic pain. 3. Medical rehabilitation.
    [DNLM: 1. Pain—therapy. 2. Pain—diagnosis. 3. Rehabilitation. WL
  704 P144 2002] I. Monga, Trilok N. II. Grabois, Martin.
    RB127 . P332375 2002
    616′.0472—dc21

                                             2001008541

Made in the United States of America

Dedication

This book is dedicated to our wives, Uma and Ellen, for their love, support, and understanding. Further, we would like to dedicate this book to our patients with chronic pain. They have taught and inspired us more than they know.

Acknowledgments

We are fortunate to have some very experienced clinician–scientists who contributed to this project and we are obliged and grateful to all of them for sharing their experience and knowledge. We would like to thank the faculty members of Baylor College of Medicine/University of Texas Houston Physical Medicine and Rehabilitation Alliance for their support in the completion of this project. Last, but not the least, we thank the editors of Demos Publishing for their help, patience, and consideration.

Contents

Preface

Pain is a common symptom of many diseases and is often referred for a physical medicine and rehabilitation consultation. Despite the availability of information on the pathophysiology, assessment, and management of acute musculoskeletal pain, chronic pain still remains an unsolved problem for many patients. Pathophysiology in these patients often remains obscure, assessment difficult, and management frustrating.

These issues become magnified when pain, acute or chronic, complicates a primary disabling disease such as spinal cord injury, cerebrovascular accident, or multiple sclerosis. To date, the physiatric management of these complex syndromes has not been dealt with in a comprehensive fashion, especially with regard to the relationship of pain, functional status, and quality of life in these patients.

Pain Management in Rehabilitation was developed to fill this void. It provides a single source that synthesizes information about the diagnosis and management of various pain syndromes in patients with primary disabling diseases. We seek to discuss pain as it relates to various disease processes from the perspective of both rehabilitation specialists and primary care providers. The assessment and management of pain syndromes are described for some of the most common impairments seen in a rehabilitation setting .

It is our belief that successful management of pain in persons with a primary disabling disease will prevent physiological and functional decline. Moreover, we expect that timely and adequate management of pain will improve not only functional abilities but also psychosocial functioning and will enhance quality of life. This text provides a review of the relevant literature with emphasis on assessment and physiatric management. We have included topics that are not typically addressed in other texts and have excluded topics on neurophysiology of pain and surgical approaches to management of intractable pain, which are adequately covered elsewhere.

We hope that our readers find the information in this book valuable in the care of their patients.

Trilok N. Monga, M.D.
Martin Grabois, M.D.

Contributors

Donna Marie Bloodworth, M.D., Department of Physical Medicine and Rehabilitation, Baylor College of Medicine, Houston, Texas

Victoria A. Brander, M.D., Department of Physical Medicine and Rehabilitation, Northwestern University Medical School; Arthritis Center, Rehabilitation Institute of Chicago, Chicago, Illinois

Barbara S. Douglas, M.D., UMDNJ School of Osteopathic Medicine, Stratford, New Jersey

Alberto Esquenazi, M.D., Moss Regional Amputee Center, Philadelphia, Pennsylvania

Michelle S. Gittler, M.D., Schwab Rehabilitation Hospital and Care Network, Chicago, Illinois

Martin Grabois, M.D., Department of Physical Medicine and Rehabilitation, Baylor College of Medicine, Houston, Texas

Helene Henson, M.D., Department of Physical Medicine and Rehabilitation, Baylor College of Medicine; Veterans Affairs Medical Center, Houston, Texas

Cindy B. Ivanhoe, M.D., Department of Physical Medicine and Rehabilitation, Baylor College of Medicine; Texas Institute for Rehabilitation and Research, Houston, Texas

Deanna M. Janora, M.D., UMDNJ School of Osteopathic Medicine, Stratford, New Jersey

Richard T. Jermyn, D.O., Temple University Hospital, Philadelphia, Pennsylvania

Anthony J. Kerrigan, Ph.D., Department of Physical Medicine and Rehabilitation, Baylor College of Medicine; Veterans Affairs Medical Center, Houston, Texas

Karen J. Kowalske, M.D. Department of Physical Medicine and Rehabilitation, University of Texas; Southwestern Medical Center, Dallas, Texas

Trilok N. Monga, M.D., Department of Physical Medicine and Rehabilitation, Baylor College of Medicine; Veterans Affairs Medical Center, Houston, Texas

Uma Monga, M.D., Department of Radiology, Radiation Oncology Section, Baylor College of Medicine; Veterans Affairs Medical Center, Houston, Texas

P. Michelle Muellner, M.D., Department of Physical Medicine and Rehabilitation, Northwestern University Medical School; Center for Pain Studies, Rehabilitation Institute of Chicago, Chicago, Illinois

Zoraya M. Parrilla, M.D., Mount Sinai Medical Center, New York, New York

Jaywant J. Patil, M.D., Private Practice, Halifax, Nova Scotia, Canada

David S. Rosenblum, M.D., Gaylord Hospital, Wallingford, Connecticut

Michael F. Saffir, M.D. Gaylord Hospital, Wallingford, Connecticut

Gabriel Tan, Ph.D., Department of Anesthesiology, Baylor College of Medicine; Veterans Affairs Medical Center, Houston, Texas

Carlos Vallbona, M.D., Department of Family and Community Medicine, Baylor College of Medicine, Houston, Texas

David J. Weiss, M.D., Schwab Rehabilitation Hospital and Care Network, Chicago, Illinois

Gary Yarkony, M.D., Rehab Medicine Specialists, Elgin, Illinois

Shiela Young, M.A., Private Practice, Houston, Texas

1 Conceptual Model of Pain and Its Management

Martin Grabois, M.D.

Chronic pain is difficult and frustrating to manage, and patients who experience it are often viewed as undesirable (1). This perception is compounded when chronic pain occurs in individuals who have a primary disability. However, specialists in pain management and rehabilitation frequently need to evaluate and treat these individuals. For the patient with a combination of primary disability and chronic pain, a multidisciplinary and comprehensive approach is indicated.

This chapter sets the stage as an introduction to this text to define and characterize pain and discuss the concept of the Multidisciplinary Pain Clinic in terms of evaluation and treatment. Further, the chapter discusses goals, the formulation of treatment plans, and the outcomes that can be expected with appropriate evaluation and treatment.

DEFINITION OF PAIN

The evaluation and treatment of patients with chronic pain that undermines function and quality of life is facilitated by an understanding of the definition of pain and an appreciation of its clinical characteristics.

The definition of pain according to the International Association for the Study of Pain (IASP) is, "an unpleasant sensory and emotional experience, which we primarily associated with tissue damage or describe in terms of such damage, or both" (2). It should be noted that this definition combines the traditional concept that pain reflects a sensory experience but also has an affective and cognitive component (3). These two components, especially the psychosocial factors affect the sensation of pain and its effect on function and quality of life.

The IASP definition also indicates that the relationship between pain and tissue damage is neither uniform nor constant. Based on the findings of the pain assessment, the clinician may infer that the pain is either proportionate or disproportionate to the tissue injury evident on examination (3). Patients with chronic nonmalignant pain syndromes often complain of pain that exceeds demonstrable tissue injury (4).

It is helpful in further understanding pain and its effect on the human body to compare and contrast it with nociception and suffering. *Nociception* is the activity induced in neural pathways by potentially tissue-damaging stimuli (3), whereas *suffering* has been defined as a perceived threat to the patient (5) and may be likened to overall impairment in quality of life (6). Figure 1.1 describes the interrelationship of these concepts: that factors other than nociception itself influences pain and suffering (7). These factors can be major determinants of the pain complaint.

Suffering is a global construct intricately related to the experience of pain (8). Efforts to define suffering have characterized it as a perceived threat to the patient as person (9,10). Suffering may result from numerous aversive perceptions including pain, loss of physical function, social isolation, familial dissolution, psychiatric disturbances, and financial concerns (3).

PAIN CHARACTERISTICS

Pain is best described in a clinical setting by its characteristics. Pain can be defined in terms of temporal aspects, intensity, topography, exacerbating/relieving factors, inferred pathophysiology, syndrome characteristics, and etiology (3). Table 1.1 summarizes these characteristics with their potential descriptions.

Pain can be characterized basically from a temporal point of view as *acute* or *chronic*. The distinction between acute pain and chronic pain is highly salient. Acute pain is defined as pain of recent onset that ends or is anticipated to end during a period of days to weeks (3). When caused by tissue injury, pain of this type has an essential biological function, providing a warning of potential damage and impelling the organism to protect and rest the affected part (11). Acute pain may be accompanied by anxiety and the systemic signs of the sympathetic hyperactivity ("fight to flight") response (12). Pain can be defined by its time course (13). Acute pain is limited to pain of less than thirty days, whereas chronic pain persists for more than six months. *Subacute* pain describes the interval from the end of the first month to the beginning of the seventh month of continued pain. *Recurrent acute* pain defines a pain pattern that persists over an extended period of time but recurs as isolated pain episodes.

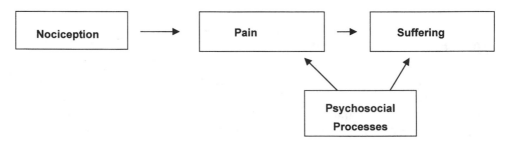

Figure 1.1. Relationship of nociception, pain, and suffering. (Adapted from *Lancet*; from Grabois M. Chronic pain: evaluation and treatment. In: Goodgold J (ed.): *Rehabilitation Medicine*. St. Louis: Mosby-Year Book, 1988.)

Table 1.1. Pain Characteristics

Characteristic	Potential Descriptors
Temporal	Acute vs. recurrent vs. chronic, onset, duration, daily variation, course
Intensity	Pain "on average" pain "at its worst" pain "at its least"
Topography	Focal vs. multifocal; focal vs. referred; superficial vs. deep
Exacerbating/Relieving Factors	Volitional ("incident pain") vs. nonvolitional
Inferred Pathophysiology	Nociceptive pain vs. neuropathic pain vs. psychogenic pain vs. idiopathic pain
Syndrome	Examples: reflex sympathetic dystrophy, thalamic pain, trigeminal neuralgia
Etiology	Examples: trauma (may cause reflex sympathetic dystrophy), stroke (may cause thalamic pain), aberrant arterial loop (may cause trigeminal neuralgia)

(From Portenoy RK, Kanner RM. Definition and assessment of pain. In: Portenoy RK, Kanner RM, (eds.), *Pain Mechanism Theory and Practice*. Philadelphia: FA Davis Co., 1996.)

Subacute pain is possibly the last opportunity for a full restoration of a pain-free existence, much as with acute pain (13). For that reason, subacute pain must be recognized before the pain becomes chronic. Subacute pain is quite similar to acute pain in its etiologic and nociceptive mechanisms (14). By the time pain becomes subacute, the rehabilitative approach used for chronic pain is more appropriate than further acute pain management strategies (13).

Recurrent acute pain is the acute flare-up of peripheral tissue pathology caused by an underlying chronic pathological entity. Unlike chronic or subacute pain, recurrent acute pain implies discrete acute episodes, which return over time (13). The dividing line between recurrent acute and subacute is often a judgment decision by the pain practitioner. Daily pain for several weeks is subacute pain, but several limited pain episodes over many months or years are typical of recurrent acute pain. The importance of recognizing recurrent acute pain is that it may be important to consider a more comprehensive management approach to patients with this type of pain.

Chronic pain syndrome is an abnormal condition in which pain is no longer a symptom of tissue injury, but in which pain and pain behavior become the primary disease processes (15). Chronic pain syndrome is distinct from chronically or intermittently painful disease, in which the patient experiences pain but manifests function and behavior appropriate to the degree of tissue injury. In chronic pain syndrome, subjective and behavioral manifestations of pain persist beyond objective evidence of tissue injury. Chronically painful conditions can lead to chronic pain syndrome, but not all persons with chronically painful conditions

Table 1.2. Differences Between Acute Pain and Chronic Pain

	Chronic Pain	Acute Pain
Temporal Features	Remote, ill-defined onset, unpredictable duration	Recent, well-defined onset; expected to end in days or weeks
Biological Function	Nonapparent	Essential warning; impels rest and avoidance of further harm.
Intensity	Variable	Variable
Associated Effect	Irritability or depression	Anxiety common when severe or cause is unknown
Pain-related Behaviors	May or may not give any indication behaviors of pain	Pain behavior common (e.g., moaning, splinting, rubbing, etc.) when severe or cause is unknown
Associated Features	May have vegetative signs such as lassitude, anorexia, weight loss, insomnia, loss of libido	May have signs of sympathetic hyperactivity when severe
Causes and Examples	Progressive medical disease (e.g., cancer, AIDS); nonprogressive or slowly progressive disease (e.g., osteoarthritis, neuropathic pains); pain determined by psychologic factors	Monophasic (e.g., postoperative, traumatic, burns) or recurrent (e.g., headache, sickle sell disease; hemophilia, inflammatory bowel disease)

(From Portenoy RK, Kanner RM. Definition and assessment of pain. In: Portenoy RK, Kanner RM, (eds.): *Pain Mechanism Theory and Practice*. Philadelphia: FA Davis Co., 1996.)

manifest chronic pain behavior and disability. The difference between acute and chronic pain can further be compared and contrasted in terms of the characteristics noted in Table 1.2.

In chronic pain syndrome, the original causes are often blurred by subsequent complications of multiple procedures, compensation factors, medication dependence, inactivity, and psychosocial behavior changes (16) (see Figure 1.2).

Describing pain intensity and measuring pain is important to appropriate evaluation and treatment as well as evaluating outcomes. Measurement of induced acute pain is easier than measurement of chronic pain (17). In laboratory-induced acute pain there are minimal emotional or cognitive factors, and the quantity of the pain stimulus is easily controlled. In the measurement and assessment of chronic pain, unfortunately, there is no generally accepted laboratory model. A clear linear relationship between the quantity of noxious input and the intensity of pain experience is not apparent in chronic pain. It is difficult to capture what is a personal and private sensory experience. Many times all we have are the patient's words, their recollections of the experience, and the behavior exhibited when they

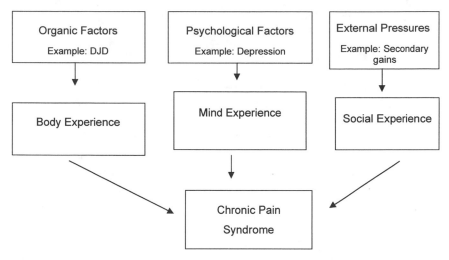

Figure 1.2. Chronic pain syndrome interaction of organic psychological and social factors. (From Grabois M. Chronic pain: Evaluation and treatment. In: Goodgold J, (ed.), *Rehabilitation Medicine.* St. Louis: Mosby-Year Book, 1988.)

have the pain experience (17). In a very real sense all pain is "in the head" and measuring it objectively is difficult. Nevertheless, a pain scale should meet a few basic criteria, including ease of administration and scoring, potential for accurate use by a variety of healthcare professionals, and high interrater reliability and validity (17).

Sternbach (18) noted that pain is a complex experience, and evidence confirming its presence involves several dimensions that depend on changing states and that are continuously influenced by a multitude of extrinsic and intrinsic stimuli. Using the concepts of Sternbach et al. and Fordyce, three components of chronic pain measurement are noted: the subjective, the physiological, and (3) the behavioral. The interaction between these components is dynamic and involves a balanced appraisal of sensory input and the degree to which it is modulated by psychological factors (including other determinants of verbal and overt behavior).

The subjective component of chronic pain management is reflected in rating scales, questionnaires, and diary cards. The visual analog scale (1–10) is the most commonly used rating scale.

Questionnaires have gained wide acceptance, with the McGill Pain Questionnaire being the most popular (19). It evaluates three major classes of work descriptions—sensory, affective, and evaluative—that patients use to specify their subjective pain experience. It has a built-in intensity scale. Multiple reports in the literature have evaluated this method of pain measurement, and it has been used extensively in clinical evaluation and treatment trials. Melzack (20) and others believe it provides a quantity of information that can be treated statistically, and that it is sufficiently sensitive to detect differences in effectiveness among pain relief treatments. Although physiologic techniques such as measurement of cortical evoked potentials, muscle tension, vasodilatation, heart rate, and blood pressure have a firm scientific basis in the measurement of acute pain in the laboratory, they have not been scientifically evaluated in the clinical or chronic pain setting.

Behavioral measurements of pain, as advocated by Fordyce (21), are logical techniques for measuring pain, because people in pain must engage in behavior indicative of their state. Most behavior measurement techniques use three categories of behavior: somatic intervention, impaired functional capacity, and (3) pain complaints. The University of Alabama Behavioral Measurement of Pain Scale is based on ten behaviors such as vocalization and the frequency of intensity of these expressions (22). Although interobserver reliability is good, many trained observers and many observations are needed to obtain accurate and valid information.

Clearly, there is at present no ideal method for evaluating and measuring chronic pain and the effectiveness of treatment techniques (23). Those measurements that reflect subjective, physiologic, and behavioral components using independent and direct monitoring are the most appropriate (17). Reading (24) noted that behavioral indices may assume greater importance as chronicity increases, because the question of how much the patient is able to do rather than how much it hurts may be the more important question in the chronic pain management setting. This is especially true when considering the cost-effectiveness of pain management programs, because functional outcome is often more important to third-party payers than perceived level of pain (24).

Noting exacerbating and relieving factors is also useful in characterizing pain. These factors can suggest an etiology or pathophysiology for the pain and may therefore have diagnostic value (3). For example, pain on weight bearing suggests a structural (nociceptive) musculoskeletal lesion, and allodynia in a region of normal-appearing skin may suggest a neuropathic mechanism. Back pain caused by disc disease is almost invariably relieved by recumbancy, whereas pain associated with vertebral metastasis may be worsened by this maneuver. In some cases, this information can be directly applied in the treatment utilized. Information about the effects of activity or stress, for example, is incorporated into cognitive and behavioral therapies for chronic pain.

The location of pain also has important implications for diagnosis and therapy (3). Pain may be focal, multifocal, or generalized. This distinction is clinically relevant and may indicate or contraindicate specific therapies (3). Pain that is experienced at a site remote from the presumed causative lesion is termed *referred pain* (25).

A constellation of symptoms and signs may define a discrete pain syndrome (2). Recognition of the syndrome may suggest a presumptive etiology for the pain as well as the need for additional evaluation, indicate specific treatments, or allow accurate prognostication (3). Syndrome recognition extends to the constellation of affective and behavioral disturbances that may accompany chronic pain and either suggests a predominating psychologic pathogenesis for the pain or, at least, indicates substantial psychosocial and behavioral dysfunction that must be addressed therapeutically (3).

Definition of the underlying organic process that may be contributing to the pain is central to the comprehensive pain assessment (3). This information may clarify the nature of the disease, indicate prognosis, or suggest the use of specific therapies.

Clinical observation and extrapolation of data from animal models suggest that the presentation and therapeutic response of a pain syndrome may be determined by factors linked to the underlying mechanism of the pain (26,27). According to this scheme, the predominating pathophysiology of pain can be broadly divided into nociceptive, neuropathic, and idiopathic categories (3).

Nociceptive pain is defined as pain that is believed to be commensurate with the presumed degree of ongoing activation of peripheral nociceptors (primary afferent neurons that respond selectively to noxious stimuli) (3). *Neuropathic pain* is defined as pain that is perceived to be sustained by aberrant somatosenory processing by the peripheral or central nervous system (28). Finally, *idiopathic pain* is defined as pain that persists in the absence of an identifiable organic substrate or that is believed to be excessive for the organic process extant. These pathophysiologic constructs have important therapeutic implication (3). The response to opioids, for example, appears to be relatively better during treatment of pains perpetuated in large part by nociception than those pains that are sustained by neuropathic mechanisms (26,29). Nonnociceptive pains are also generally believed to be less responsive than nociceptive pains to techniques that isolate the painful part from the central nervous system; cordotomy, for example has been reported to be far less effective in patients with deafferent pain than in those with pain related to nociceptive lesions (30).

CHRONIC PAIN MANAGEMENT CONCEPTS

Swanson and colleagues (31) remarked that when pain becomes chronic, it increases in complexity and the patient becomes more resistant to treatment. It is widely accepted that continuation of the sequential outpatient–inpatient approach of the medical model is not successful for the typical chronic pain patient (32).

Because chronic pain syndrome is a complex problem with medical and psychosocial aspects, it requires a comprehensive and interdisciplinary approach to evaluation and treatment (32). Chronic pain syndrome should be considered similar in scope to such disabilities as alcoholism, stroke, and spinal cord injury, if the patient is to reach the highest functional goals possible within medical and psychological limitations (33). Pain programs have attempted to accomplish this outcome by an interdisciplinary and comprehensive approach to evaluating and treating patients with chronic pain (34).

Programs for chronic pain management, like those for physical medicine and rehabilitation, are relatively new developments that began during World War II (29). Originated by Alexander and popularized by Bonica (35), these programs have multiplied in recent years and now number in the thousands.

Ideally, a pain clinic should be comprehensive and interdisciplinary and offer a wide range of treatment techniques (34). These clinics, however, differ in their

Table 1.3. IASP Classification of Pain Facilities

Modality-oriented clinic
- Provides specific type of treatment, e.g. nerve blocks, transcutaneous nerve stimulation, acupuncture, biofeedback
- May have one or more healthcare disciplines
- Does not provide an integrated, comprehensive approach

Pain clinic
- Focuses on the diagnosis and management of patients with chronic pain or may specialize in specific diagnoses or pain related to a specific region of the body
- Does not provide comprehensive assessment or treatment; an institution offering appropriate consultative and therapeutic services would qualify but never an isolated solo practitioner

Multidisciplinary pain clinic
- Specializes in the multidisciplinary diagnosis and management of patients with chronic pain or may specialize in specific diagnoses or pain related to a specific region of the body
- Staffed by physicians of different specialties and other healthcare providers
- Differs from a multidisciplinary pain center only because it does not include research and teaching

Multidisciplinary pain center
- Organization of healthcare professionals and basic scientists that includes research, teaching, and patient care in acute and chronic pain
- Typically a component of a medical school or a teaching hospital
- Clinical programs supervised by an appropriately trained and licensed director
- Staffed by a minimum of physician, psychologist, occupational therapists, physical therapist, and registered nurse
- Integrated services are provided and based on interdisciplinary assessment and management
- Offers both inpatient and outpatient programs

(From Fishbain DA. Nonsurgical chronic pain treatment outcome: A review. *International Review of Psychiatry* 2000; 12:170–180.)

staff composition, size, philosophy, and most important, treatment approach. These variations have blurred the distinction between the different types of pain treatment facilities in the minds of physicians and the public (36). Because of this problem, the International Association for the Study of Pain (IASP) developed definitions for four types of pain treatment facilities (Table 1.3) (36).

There is a clear distinction between modality-oriented clinics and pain clinics (37). However, the only difference between multidisciplinary pain clinics and multidisciplinary pain centers (MPC) is the research and teaching conducted at the MPC. These definitions also indicate that MPCs may have larger and more diversified multidisciplinary staffs, including more than one physician specialty. As a consequence, MPCs are likely to offer a wider range of treatments than multidisciplinary pain clinics. Most of the outcome pain facility treatment studies involve MPCs (37).

Pain programs differ in length of stay. Some pain clinics offer three-week programs, others require four to six weeks (38). Because all pain patients do not require four to six weeks of an inpatient program, many are referred to a less costly outpatient program. Some pain clinics utilize a motel residential complex for patients who require isolation from family and work stressors while receiving full-day inpatient treatment, while others, because of the patient's medical status, require a full inpatient program. Many patients, however, are treated in outpatient programs when their medical status justifies it, their insurance carrier authorizes it, and the impact of long-term hospitalization on the patient and her family is deemed harmful to the patient's overall compliance and ultimate success (39).

Pain clinics also differ in their costs. A survey of California-based pain clinics conducted by Casa Colina Hospital revealed that the range of cost for an inpatient program can be from $12,000 on the low end to $34,000 on the high end for a 6- to 8-week major comprehensive pain service. For an outpatient program (half-day, full-day, and single-modality combinations) the cost can range from $2,500 on the low end to $12,500 on the high end (39).

In the traditional organization of a typical pain clinic (Figure 1.3), the director provides overall leadership, while the coordinator is responsible for the day-to day administrative management. The physician who specializes in pain is the patient's case manager. These positions can be held by separate or the same individuals. The clinical team regularly evaluates patients, sets goals, treats patients, and evaluates treatment outcomes (Table 1.4). The team members typically include a physician, psychologist, physical therapist, vocational counselor, occupational therapist, social services counselor, pharmacist, dietitian, and nurse.

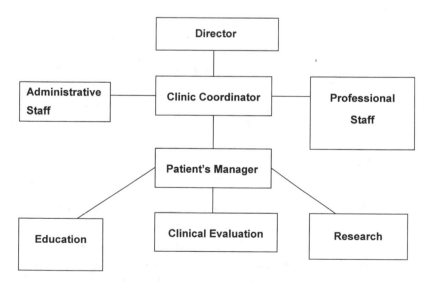

Figure 1.3. Organization of multidisciplinary pain clinic. (From Grabois M. Pain clinics: Role in rehabilitation of patients with chronic pain. *Ann Acad Med Singapore* 1983; 12:428–433.)

Table 1.4. Chronic Pain Management Team

Core Personnel	Consultant Personnel
Attending Physician	Medical Subspecialists (Who are not attending pain physician)
Psychologist	Anesthesiologist
Occupational Therapist	Neurosurgeon
Social Services Counselor	Physiatrist
Rehabilitation Nurse	Psychiatrist
Vocational Counselor	Recreational Therapist
Pharmacist	Biomedical Engineer
Dietitian	

(From Grabois M, McCann MT, Schramm D, Straja A, Smith K. Chronic pain syndromes: Evaluation and treatment. In: Braddom RL, (ed.), *Physical Medicine and Rehabilitation*. Philadelphia:WB Saunders, 1996.)

Some programs use other professionals such as kinesiotherapists, exercise physiologists, and so forth. Other medical subspecialists are usually available on a consultative basis. Core team members such as psychiatrists, anesthesiologists, or physiatrists, if they are not the patient's attending physician, attend regular team conferences that select patients to be accepted for treatment and monitor their progress (34). The physician leads the team and provides overall medical management. The psychosocial–vocational team, consisting of the psychologist, social worker, and vocational counselor, provides leadership in the evaluation and treatment of the behavioral changes that are a result of chronic pain and appropriate vocational intervention (34).

The therapy team members typically consist of nursing, pharmacy, dietary, physical therapy, and occupational therapy personnel, and provide daily therapy to control medication levels, modulate the pain level, and increase patient activity (40). The flow-chart of patient care in a typical pain management program is depicted in Figure 1.4.

Referrals are typically accepted from medical and nonmedical sources. An appropriate history must be supplied, and the patient should complete a pain evaluation form. The most appropriate patients are those chronic pain patients who are motivated to participate in the program, who do not have secondary gain issues that might inhibit improvement, and who accept the concepts and goals of the program (34).

Typically, patients for whom a major comprehensive inpatient residential pain program is recommended are those who exhibit pain for three to six months or more; who are unresponsive to everything the conventional medical model had to offer; whose life (including that of their family) is totally disrupted by pain, depression, and drug-seeking behavior; and who are employment candidates by virtue of the fact that they can benefit from a comprehensive work hardening and full-service vocational restoration program (39).

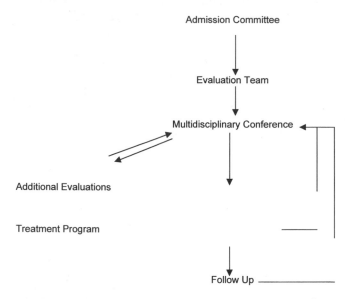

Figure 1.4. Flow chart of processes through typical pain clinic. (From Richards JS, Nepormuceno C, Rilcs M, Sucr Z. Assessing pain behavior: The UAB pain behavior scale. *Pain* 1982; 14:393–398.)

CONCEPTS OF TREATMENT

The cause of the chronic pain syndrome should be determined from a medical and psychosocial point of view and the location of a "pain generator" should be noted. Attempts to decrease or eliminate the pain generators are important and should be carried out first, followed by consideration of other treatment options. Table 1.5 describes a classification for pain patients as well as potential treatment options in patients of chronic pain syndrome.

The goals of treatment in a multidisciplinary program center on concepts of moderating pain, increasing function, and decreasing healthcare utilization (41). These goals can be achieved by modifying medication and invasive procedures, modifying pain and pain behavior, and increasing activity through exercise.

The Fordyce model of behavioral modification is useful in patients with chronic pain syndrome (42). The goal in these patients is not to "cure the pain" but to interrupt the pain behavioral reinforcement cycle by rewarding healthy behavior and setting appropriate goals that the patient must achieve. These goals are to modify medication utilization, modulate the pain response, increase activity, and modify pain behaviors (33).

Medication Management Philosophy

Physicians have a long history of prescribing inappropriate medications, and patients have a long history of using them (Figure 1.5), particularly with respect to narcotic medications. Studies show that patients are usually inadequately treated

Table 1.5. Classification of the Chronic Nonmaligant Pain Patient with Examples and Treatment Strategies

Class	Symptom Treatment Strategies	Objective Findings	Social and Vocational Components	Examples
Ia	High; Multiple approach with emphasis on medication and modalities	High Correlation	High	Rheumatoid arthritis
Ib	High; Medication and modalities approach	High Correlation	Low	Rheumatoid arthritis
IIa	High; Multidisciplinary approach with emphasis on behavior modification	Low Correlation	High	Musculoskeletal or low back pain
IIb	High; Modalities	Low Correlation	Low	Musculoskeletal or low back pain

(From Bloodworth D, Calvillo C, Smith K, Grabois M. Chronic pain syndromes: evaluation and treatment. In: Braddom RL (ed.). *Physical Medicine and Rehabilitation,* 2nd edition. Philadelphia:WB Saunders, 2000.)

for acute pain syndromes, and overtreated for chronic ones (43). In addition, some physicians mistakenly believe that giving medication on an as-needed basis rather than on a scheduled dosage results in less addiction. Physicians also tend to incorrectly label patients who respond to placebo as having a nonorganic type of pain.

Over the years, healthcare professionals have changed their philosophy in utilizing opioid medication in treatment of chronic pain. At one time it was felt that no patients with chronic noncancer pain should be on opioid medication. With enlightened thinking and research, however, it is now felt that the appropriate utilization of opioid medication can be a helpful strategy in patients with chronic pain (44). The American Pain Society and the American Academy of Pain Medicine have developed a position paper for appropriate utilization of opioid medication in patients with chronic pain (45). Many physicians utilize a medication management agreement that delineates the responsibilities of the healthcare team and the patient (46).

When the goal of pharmacologic management of a patient with chronic pain is to moderate or eliminate possible use of narcotics, tranquilizers, and hypnotic medications (17), it usually requires detoxification in an organized treatment program. No new narcotics, tranquilizers, or hypnotic drugs should be prescribed. Once the daily based requirement for the patient is obtained over a few days, a "pain cocktail" approach is used on a time-contingent basis. Figure 1.6 compares the pain cocktail approach with the medication-as-needed method. This cocktail approach of gradual withdrawal can also be used for tranquilizers, hypnotic drugs, and narcotic medications. Kanner (47) believes that judiciously

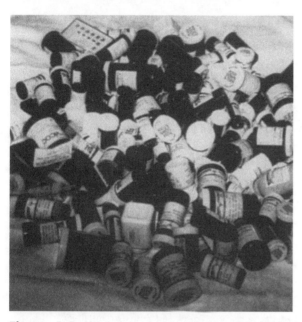

Figure 1.5. Medication usage of chronic pain patient over a one-year period. (From Grabois M, Bloodworth D, Calvillo C, Smith K. Chronic pain syndromes: evaluation and treatment. In: Braddom RL (ed.), *Physical Medicine and Rehabilitation*, 2nd edition. Philadelphia: WB Saunders, 2000.)

Inpatient Days		Pain Cocktail Format
1–6	*Baseline:*	Patient reports preadmission pattern of "one or two of the 50-mg tablets of Demerol [meperidine] two or three times a day, as needed, at home."
		Physician orders to nurse: "May have Demerol, *prn* pain, not to exceed three 50-mg tablets q3h. Carefully record amount taken."
		Analysis of baseline data: Patient averaged 600 mg of Demerol/24 hr, averaging of 3- to 4-hr intervals between requests.
7–9 First cocktail		
	℞ to pharmacist:	Demerol, 1920 mg
		Bevisol, Plebex, or other liquid B complex, 12 mL; cherry syrup qs 240 mL
	Sig:	Pain cocktail, 10 mL po q3h, day and night, not *prn*
	Nursing order:	Pain cocktail, 10 mL po q3h, day and night, not *prn*
		Since the contents of the pain cocktail are not on the label, a copy of the prescription must be kept in a separate pain cocktail book.
10–12		Decrease each daily total by 64 mg, to 1/10 of original amount. A 3-day ℞ is decreased by 64 × 3 or 192 mg.
	℞ to pharmacist:	Demerol, 1728 mg
		Bevisol, Plebex, or other liquid B complex, 12 mL; cherry syrup qs 240 mL
	Sig:	Pain cocktail, 10 mL po q3h, day and night, not *prn*
	Nursing order:	Pain cocktail, 10 mL po q3h, day and night, not *prn*
13–15	*℞ to pharmacist:*	Demerol, 1536 mg
		Bevisol, Plebex, or other liquid B complex, 12 mL; cherry syrup qs 240 mL
	Sig:	Pain cocktail, 10 mL po q3h, day and night, not *prn*
	Nursing order:	Pain cocktail, 10 mL po q3h, day and night, not *prn*
16–18	*℞ to pharmacist:*	Demerol, 1344 mg
		Bevisol, Plebex, or other liquid B complex, 12 mL; cherry syrup qs 240 mL
	Sig:	Pain cocktail, 10 mL po q3h, day and night, not *prn*
	Nursing order:	Pain cocktail, 10 mL po q3h, day and night, not *prn*
19–21	*℞ to pharmacist:*	Demerol, 1152 mg
		Bevisol, Plebex, or other liquid B complex, 12 mL; cherry syrup qs 240 mL
	Sig:	Pain cocktail, 10 mL po q3h, day and night, not *prn*
	Nursing order:	Pain cocktail, 10 mL po q3h, day and night, not *prn*
22–24	*℞ to pharmacist:*	Demerol 960 mg
		Bevisol, Plebex, or other liquid B complex, 12 mL; cherry syrup qs 240 mL
	Sig:	Pain cocktail, 10 mL po q3h, day and night, not *prn*
	Nursing order:	Pain cocktail, 10 mL po q3h, day and night, not *prn*
37–39	*℞ to pharmacist:*	Demerol, 0 mg
		Bevisol, Plebex, or other liquid B complex, 12 mL; cherry syrup qs 240 mL
	Sig:	Pain cocktail, 10 mL po q3h, day and night, not *prn*
	Nursing order:	Pain cocktail, 10 mL po q3h, day and night, not *prn*
(Maintain patient on vehicle for 2–10 days; if all is going well, inform patient and ask if continuation of vehicle is desired.)		

Figure 1.6. Pain cocktail approach: A comparison of as-needed and around-the-clock approaches. (From Bloodworth D, Calvillo O, Smith K, Grabois M: Chronic pain syndromes: Evaluation and Treatment. In: Braddom RL (ed.): *Physical Medicine and Rehabilitation*, 2nd Edition, WB Saunders, Philadelphia 2000.)

used antidepressants, particularly the tricyclic antidepressants, lead to a smoother treatment course for the patient with chronic pain.

Pain Modulation

The complete eradication of chronic pain is rarely achieved and is not the goal of most interventions. The goal is the modification of pain to a more tolerable level. A comprehensive pain management program utilizes an array of modalities to accomplish this goal. Nonpharmacologic methods are usually adjunctive therapies and do not necessarily substitute for pharmacologic interventions (48). Table 1.6 lists commonly used pharmacologic and nonpharmacologic pain-modulating interventions.

Pain modulation techniques take advantage of the body's endogenous pain-modulating abilities first postulated and implied by Melzack and Wall's *gate theory* of pain (49). This theory supports the observation that a direct correlation does not always exist between the extent of organic injury and the expression of pain (50). Melzack and Wall proposed that pain information was modulated at the level of the "target cell" in the substantial gelatinosa, or laminae II and III of the dorsal horn, by afferent information from A delta and C sensory fibers (51). This "gating" effect on the target cell modulates input before it evokes pain perception (33). Since the description of the gate theory, modulation events higher in the neuoraxis and modulation by descending or efferent mechanisms have been proposed. Basbaum and Field (52) proposed that pain modulation occurs at the periaqueductal gray area.

Table 1.6. Pharmacological and Nonpharmacological Pain Interventions

Pharmacological Interventions	Nonpharmacological Interventions
NSAIDs	Behavior modifiers
Antidepressants (TCAs)	Relaxation
Anticonvulsants	Biofeedback
Carbamazepine	Guided visual imagery
Enytion (Dilantin)	Music therapy
Invasive pain modulators	Distraction
Spinal opioids	Hypnosis
Peripheral nerve stimulators	Pain modulators
Dorsal column stimulators	TENS
Epidural and deep brain stimulators	Acupuncture
Invasive pain relievers	Conditioning exercises
Sympathetic nerve blocks	Stretching/flexibility
Epidural anesthetics/steroids	Myofascial release
Root sleeve injections	Spray and stretch
Trigger point injections	

Abbreviations: NSAIDs - nonsteroidal anti-inflammatory drugs; TCAs - tricyclic antidepressants; TENS - transcutaneous electrical nerve stimulation.

(From Bloodworth D, Calvillo C, Smith K, Grabois M. Chronic pain syndromes: evaluation and treatment. In: Braddom RL (ed.): *Physical Medicine and Rehabilitation*, 2nd edition. Philadelphia: WB Saunders, 2000.)

The modulation of pain information and pain perception occurs at multiple sites along the neuroaxis and by afferent and efferent pathways.

The pain modulation network can be activated by the administration of spinal opiates. It can also be activated by electrical stimulation (transcutaneously or percutaneously) to peripheral nerves, or epidurally at the level of the spinal cord or brain (51).

Increasing Activity Level and Function

Therapeutic exercises are intended to improve physical condition and functional capacities. They also indirectly provide pain relief, increase functional activities, and help to achieve a better quality of life (23).

Patients with chronic pain conditions tend to reduce or discontinue their activities because of fear of increased pain or harm. This can result in joint stiffness, decreased endurance, decreased muscle strength, muscle wasting, and a general state of decompensation. The aim of therapeutic exercise for these patients should be reconditioning, improved muscle strength and length, and attainment of optimal joint range of motion.

Appropriate exercises that are specific for pain and general conditioning exercises such as bicycling, walking, and swimming are usually indicated. Fordyce (53) noted that appropriate exercise in a behavior modification program must be relevant to the patient's pain and limitations, and be quantifiable, visible, and accessible. In some patients, however, it is necessary to reduce excessive activity levels by teaching them to pace themselves more appropriately.

Psychosocial Intervention

Recent evidence suggests that the use of psychologic modalities in conjunction with medical interventions and physical therapy increases the effectiveness of the treatment program. A wide variety of interventions is available to improve the psychologic functioning of the chronic pain patient. Psychologic treatments of chronic pain include psychoeducation, psychotherapy, biofeedback and relaxation training, and vocational counseling. Cognitive behavioral approaches to chronic pain rely heavily on skills training and psychoeducational interventions (45,54). Group psychotherapy has been used successfully to enhance the functioning of patients in a pain rehabilitation program (2). Individual (55) and family therapy (19,56) are other interventions frequently used with chronic pain patients to treat underlying psychosocial stresses. Recently a compelling case has been made for including family members and significant others in the evaluation and treatment process (57).

VOCATIONAL REHABILITATION

Vocational counseling is an important component of the psychologic approach to chronic pain. Each patient is evaluated to determine work history, educational background, vocational skills and abilities, and motivation to return to work. The vocational counselor can determine whether past work skills and current aptitudes can be transferred to alternative occupations if necessary. The vocational counselor works with the patient regarding legal rights and obligations, which vary among states (e.g., work's compensation), and helps the patient set realistic vocational goals. They also help the patient to improve overall vocational functioning.

Vocational counseling is used to reduce functional impairment and disability, improve coping strategies, enhance effective use of pain medications, and decrease use of healthcare resources.

EFFECTIVENESS OF PAIN THERAPIES

Although clinical judgment represents a significant contribution to the rationale for current clinical practices it does not replace scientific evidence of efficacy. However, much of the literature pertaining to rehabilitation of chronic pain syndrome consists of retrospective record review surveys or review articles. Although numerous experimental or quasi-experimental studies can be identified, in many cases the inferences that may be drawn from this literature is limited by the lack of control groups, nonequivalent control groups, weak statistical analysis, and other limitations to internal and external validity.

Turk points out that a similar dearth of clinical trials utilizing randomly assigned subjects to control and experimental groups and measuring improvements with double-blind methods plagues virtually every area of pain treatment (65). Double-blind, randomized control trials are the gold standard for determining the dose/response relationship in drug trials, but such methods are virtually impossible to perform in evaluating interventions such as those provided at multidisciplinary pain centers. Only a handful of double-blind, randomized control trials examining any treatment for low back pain could be found despite a review of over 8,000 published papers. Admittedly, there is no perfect study of multidisciplinary pain center treatment outcomes, but the data taken as an aggregate should be summarily dismissed (58,59).

Another important consideration raised by Turk is that most patients being treated in multidisciplinary pain centers represent failures of the conventional healthcare system. These patients have long-standing problems that extend beyond physical pathology and they should be viewed as very poor risks for successful outcomes. Few treatments have been severely criticized, or held to higher standards, than multidisciplinary pain centers. Yet, no other treatment modalities for chronic pain have had as much evidence accumulated to substantiate their efficacy (58,59).

Turk (60) summarized the results of selected studies (61,62,63) and reported the following facts about the efficacy of multidisciplinary pain centers:

- Following treatment at a typical multidisciplinary pain center, the patient reported a reduction in pain ranging from 16 to 60 percent, comparable to the pain reduction reported following surgery. These reductions were reasonably maintained up to five years following treatment.

- More than 65 percent of patients treated at multidisciplinary pain centers discontinued use of opioid medications and were still medication-free one year following discharge from the program. In contrast, patients not treated at such facilities reported an average reduction in medication of only 6 percent one year following treatment.

- On average, 65 percent of patients treated in multidisciplinary pain centers reported increased activity at termination of treatment compared to 35 percent of patients not treated at these facilities who reported increased activity at follow-up.

- The average return-to-work rate following treatment at multidisciplinary pain centers was 67 percent compared to 24 percent for patients not treated at those facilities. Approximately 43 percent more patients were working following treatment at multidisciplinary pain centers than prior to treatment. By contrast, return-to-work following back surgery was as low as 7 percent (7,102 patients) (64,65).

- Patients treated at multidisciplinary pain centers are three to six times less likely to be hospitalized later and have significantly fewer surgeries for pain than those patients not treated at those facilities.

Studies that have investigated the closure rate of disability cases indicate that 64 percent (66) to 89 percent (67) of claims were settled within three months following discharge from multidisciplinary pain centers. This can be compared with 39 percent closure of claims following surgery (68).

Up to 86 percent of pending litigation cases have been reported as being resolved following treatment at multidisciplinary pain center (69,70).

COST-EFFECTIVENESS

The issue of cost-effectiveness also needs clarification. One problem is lack of agreement of how to define cost-effectiveness. Stieg and Turk (71) have defined cost-effectiveness to include the effort on the part of the healthcare practitioners to deliver the best care possible at the lowest possible cost. With regard to pain treatment centers, success was defined as the return of the patient to the role of a productive member of society, implying a significant reduction in disability and medical payments, a good rate of return to work, and low recidivism rates.

In a study by Stieg et al. (72) at the Boulder Memorial Hospital Pain Control Center, in association with the State of Colorado Department of Labor, demonstrated potential savings in medical and disability costs for a group of patients who were treated in an interdisciplinary pain treatment program. Most of these patients were judged to be permanently and totally disabled at the start of treatment. A formula for estimating future cost benefit savings was derived (73).

Turk (60) reviewed and summarized representative data that substantiate the claims of cost-effectiveness of multidisciplinary pain clinics:

- Extrapolating from the meta-analysis conducted by Flor (74), over $27 million would be saved in medical expenditures following treatment at all disciplinary pain centers. For all of the 3,089 patients included in the meta-analysis, treatment result in a net savings of medical expenses of over $9.5 million each year.
- Based on meta-analysis (74), 770 of the 3,089 patients would be expected to have disability claims closed. The average age of these patients was 45 years. Estimating disability payments at $15,000/year (71) would result in over $175 million in savings.
- Thus, the treatment of patients in the studies included by Flor et al. (74) would result in a net savings of over $184 million ($27 million in medical expenditures, $175 million in indemnity expenditures, and $18 million for the cost of multidisciplinary pain center treatment). On average, over $56,000 would be saved for each patient treated. Estimates of the number of people with chronic pain problems suggest that there are 25 to 60 million chronic pain suffers. Extrapolating these findings to the larger population would suggest potential savings in the billions of dollars (59).

CONCLUSIONS

Patients with chronic pain syndrome are typically difficult and frustrating to manage. These patients combine traditional clinical problems with psychosocial, vocational, and behavioral issues. The pain clinic concept, which utilizes a comprehensive, multidisciplinary approach with knowledgeable personnel devoted to treating chronic pain syndrome, is most appropriate for evaluation and treatment of these patients.

The treatment of the patient with chronic pain syndrome should emphasize four components:

- modification of medication;
- modification of pain;
- increase in activity; and
- attention to psychosocial and vocational issues.

With appropriate evaluation and treatment, patients with chronic pain syndrome can achieve reasonable success in improving their quality of life.

REFERENCES

1. Kanfer FH, Karoly P. The psychological self-management: Abiding issues and tentative directions. In: Karoly P, Kanfer FH, eds., *Self-Management and Behavior Change.* Elmsford, New York: Pergamon Press, 1982.
2. Mersky H, Bogduk N, eds., *Classification of Chronic Pain*, 2nd Edition. Seattle: IASP Press, 1994.
3. Portenoy RK, Kanner RM. Definition and Assessment of Pain. In: Portenoy RK and Kanner RM, eds., *Pain Mechanism Theory and Practice.* Philadelphia:FA Davis Co., 1996.

4. Rosomoff HL, Fishbain DA, Goldberg M et al. Physical findings in patients with chronic intractable benign pain of the neck and/or back. *Pain* 1989; 37:279–287.

5. Cassel EJ. The nature of suffering and the goals of medicine. *N Engl J Med* 1982; 306:639–645.

6. Portenoy RK. Issues in the management of neuropathic pain. In: Basbaum A, Besson JM, eds., *Towards a New Pharmacotherapy of Pain*. New York; John Wiley and Sons, 1991.

7. Portenoy RF. Cancer pain: Pathophysiology and syndromes. *Lancet* 1992; 339:1026.

8. Loeser JD. Definition, etiology, and neurological assessment of pain originating in the nervous system following deafferentation. In: Bonica JJ, Lindblom U, Iggo A, eds., *Advances in Pain Research and Therapy*, Vol 5. N.Y.: Raven Press, 1983.

9. Carlsson AM. Assessment of chronic pain. II. Problems in the selection of relevant questionnaire items for classification of pain and evaluation and prediction of therapeutic effects. *Pain* 1984; 18:173–184.

10. Saunders C. The philosophy of terminal care. In: Saunders C, ed., *The Management of Terminal Malignant Disease*. London: Edward Arnold, 1984.

11. Wall PD. On the relation of injury to pain. *Pain* 1979; 6:253–264.

12. Gonzales GR, Elliott KJ, Portenoy RK, et al. The impact of a comprehensive evaluation in the management of cancer pain. *Pain* 1991; 47:141–144.

13. Weiner RS. *Pain Management – A Practical Guide for Clinicians*. 5th Edition, Volume 1. Boca Raton, Fla.:American Academy of Pain Medicine, St. Lucie Press, 1998.

14. Crue BL. The neurophysiology and taxonomy of pain. In: Brena SF, and Chapman SL, eds., *Management of Patients with Chronic Pain*. Jamaica, N.Y.: Spectrum Publications, 1983.

15. Sternbach RA. Psychophysiological pain syndromes. In: Bonica JJ, ed., *The Management of Pain*. Philadelphia: Lea and Febiger, 1990.

16. Bonica JJ. General consideration of chronic pain. In Bonica JJ, ed., *The Management of Pain*. Vol 1. Philadelphia: Lea and Febiger, 1990.

17. Grabois M. Pain clinics: Role in rehabilitation of patients with chronic pain. *Ann Acad Med Singapore* 1983; 12:428–433.

18. Sternback RA. Psychophysiology pain syndromes. In: Bonica JJ, ed., *The Management of Pain*. Philadelphia: Lea and Febiger, 1990.

19. Melzack R. The McGill Pain Questionnaire. In: Melzack R, ed., *Pain Measurement and Assessment*. N.Y.: Raven Press, 1983.

20. Melzack R. Measurement of the dimensions of pain experience. Bram EV, ed., *Pain Measurement in Man: Neurophysiological Correlates of Pain*. N.Y.: Elsevier, 1984.

21. Fordyce WE, Lansky D, Calsyn DA, et al. Pain measurement and pain behavior. *Pain* 1984; 18:53–69.

22. Richards JS, Nepormuceno C, Riles M, Suer Z. Assessing pain behavior: The UAB pain behavior scale. *Pain* 1982; 14:393–398.

23. Bloodworth D, Calvillo C, Smith K, Grabois M. Chronic pain syndromes: evaluation and treatment. In: Braddom RL: *Physical Medicine and Rehabilitation* 2nd edition. Philadelphia: WB Saunders, 2000.

24. Reading AE. Testing pain mechanisms in persons with pain. In: Wall PD, Melzack R, eds., *Textbook of Pain*. N.Y.: Churchill Livingston, 1984.

25. Vecchiet L, Albe–Fessard DA, Lindblom U, eds., *New Trends in Referred Pain and Hyperalgesia*. N.Y.: Elsevier, 1993.

26. Arner S, Myerson BA. Lack of analgesic effect of opioids on neuropathic and idiopathic forms of pain. *Pain* 1988; 33:11–23.

27. Portenoy RK. Mechanism of clinical pain: Observations and speculations. In: Portenoy RK, ed., *Neurologic Clinics*, Vol. 7, No 2. Pain: Mechanism and Syndromes. Philadelphia: WB Saunders, 1989.

28. Portenoy RK. Issues in the management of neuropathic pain. In: Basbhaum A, Bessom JM, eds., *Towards a New Pharmacotherapy of Pain*. N.Y.: John Wiley and Sons, 1991.

29. Portenoy RK, Foley KM, Inturrisi CE. The nature of opioid responsiveness and its impli-cations for neuropathic pain: New hypotheses derived from studies of opioid infusions. *Pain* 1990; 43:273–286.

30. Tasker RD, Dostrowsy JO. Deafferentation and central pain. In: Wall PD, Melzack R, eds., *Textbook on Pain*, 2nd edition. Edinburgh: Churchill Livingstone, 1989.

31. Swanson DW, Floreen AC, Swenson WMP. Programs for managing chronic pain II.: Short term results. *Mayo Clin Proc* 1979; 51:409–411.

32. Greenhott JD, Sternback RA. Conjoint treatment of chronic pain. *Adv Neurol* 1974; 4:595–603.

33. Grabois M. Comprehensive evaluation and management of patients with chronic pain. *Cardiovasc Res Center Bull* 1981; 19:113–117.

34. Grabois M. Chronic pain. Evaluation and Treatment. In: Goodgold J, ed.; *Rehabilitation Medicine*. St. Louis: Mosby-Year Book, 1988.

35. Bonica JJ. Preface. A review of multidisciplinary pain clinics and pain centers. In Gh LKY, ed., *New Approaches to Treatment of Chronic Pain*. National Institute on Drug Abuse Research Monograph 36. Rockville, Md.:1981.

36. Loeser JD. Desirable characteristics for pain treatment facilities: reports of the IASP task force. In: Bond MR, Charlton JE, Woolf CJ, eds., *Proceedings of the 5th World Congress on Pain*. Amsterdam:Elsevier, 1991.

37. Fishbain DA. Nonsurgical chronic pain treatment outcome: A review. *Intern Rev Psychiatry* 200; 12:170–180.

38. Ng LK. New approaches to treatment of chronic pain: a review of multidisciplinary pain clinics and pain centers. NIDA Monograph 36. Rockville, Md.: National Institute of Drug Abuse, 1981.

39. Gottlieb HJ. Multidisciplinary pain clinics, centers and programs.

40. Abelson K, Langley GB, Sheppard H, et al. Transcutaneous electrical nerve stimulation in rheumatoid arthritis. *NZ Med J* 1983; 96:156–161.

41. Sanders SH, Rucker KS, Anderson KO et al. Clinical practice guidelines for chronic non-malignant pain syndrome patients. *J Back Musculoskel Rehab* 1995; 5:15–120.

42. Loeser JD. Pain due to nerve. *Spine* 1985; 10:232–235.

43. Reuler J, Girard D, Nardone D. The chronic pain syndrome: Misconceptions and man-agement. *Ann Intern Med* 1980; 93:588–596.

44. Portenoy RK, Dole V, Joseph H, et al. Pain Management and Chemical Dependence–Evolving Perspectives. *JAMA* 1997; 278(7):591–593.

45. Blanchard EB. The use of temperature biofeedback in the treatment of chronic pain due to causalgia. *J Behav Med* 1979; 4:183–188.

46. Dalessio DJ. Management of the cranial neuralgias and atypical facial pain. *Clin J Pain* 1989; 5:55–59.

47. Kanner R. Psychotrophic drugs in the management of pain. *Curr Concepts Pain* 1983; 1:11.

48. Owens MK. Literature review of nonpharmacologic methods for the treatment of chronic pain. *Holistic Nurs Prac* 1991; 6:24–31.

49. Melzack R, Wall PD. Pain mechanism: A new theory. *Science* 1965; 150:971–979.

50. VanDalfsen RJ, Syrhajala KL. Psychologic strategies in acute pain management. *Crit Care Clin* 1990; 6:421–431.

51. Foley KM. Adjuvant analgesic drugs in cancer pain management. In: Aronoff GE, ed., *Evaluation and Treatment of Chronic Pain*. Baltimore: Urban and Schwartzenberg, 1985.

52. Bashbaum AI, Fields HL. Endogenous pain control mechanism. Review and hypothesis. *Ann Neurol* 1978; 4:452–455.

53. Fordyce W. *Behavioral Methods for Chronic Pain and Illness*. St. Louis: Mosby Year Book, 1976.

54. Hathaway SR, McKinley JC. Minnesota Multiphasic Personality Inventory Manual. New York Psychological Corp., 1976.

55. Turk DC, Melzack R. *Handbook of Pain Assessment*. New York: Guilford, 1992.

56. Blumenthal SM. Vocational rehabilitation with the industrially injured worker. *J Hand Surgery Am* 1987; 12:926–930.

57. Merksey H. Traditional individual psychotherapy and psychopharmacotherapy. In: Holman AD, Turk DC, eds., *Pain Management: A Handbook*. New York: Pergamon Press, 1986.

58. Grabois M, McCann MT, Schramm D, Straja A, Smith K. Chronic pain syndromes: evaluation and treatment. In: Braddom RL, ed.; *Physical Medicine and Rehabilitation*. Philadelphia: WB Saunders, 1996.

59. Grabois M. Pain clinic cost effectiveness and efficacy. In: DeVera JA, Parris W, Erdine S, eds., *Management of Pain A World Perspective* III. Italy: Monduzzi Editore, 1998.

60. Turk DC. Multidisciplinary pain centers: fables, fallacies, and facts. *SPS News* 1995; 6–8.

61. Flor H, Fydrich T, Turk DC. Efficacy of multidisciplinary pain treatment centers: a meta-analytic review. *Pain* 1992; 49:221–230.

62. Cutler RB, Fishbain DA, Rosomoff HL, et al. Does nonsurgical pain center treatment of chronic pain return patients to work? *Spine* 1994; 19(6):643–652.

63. Fishbain DA, Rosomoff HL, Goldberg M, Cutler R, et al. The prediction of return to work to the workplace after multidisciplinary pain center treatment. *Clin J Pain* 1993; 9:3–15.

64. North RB, Campbell JN, James CS, Conover-Walker MK, et al. Failed back surgery syndrome: 5-year follow-up in 102 patients undergoing repeated operation. *Neurosurg* 1991; 28:685–691.

65. North RB, Ewend MG, Lawton MT, et al. Failed back surgery syndrome: 5-year follow-up after spinal cord stimulation implantation. *Neurosurg* 1991; 28:692–699.

66. Painter JR, Seres JL, Newman RI. Assessing benefits of the pain center: Why some patients regress. *Pain* 1980; 8:101–113.

67. Fey SG, Williamson-Kirkland TE, Fraugione R. Vocational restoration in injured workers with chronic pain. *Pain* 1987; Suppl 4:S379.

68. White AWM. The compensation back. *Appl Therapeutic* 1966; 8:871–874.

69. Mayer TG, Gatchel RJ, Kishino N, et al. Objective assessment of spine function following industrial injury: A prospective study with comparison group and one-year follow up. *Spine* 1985; 10:484–493.

70. Mayer TG, Gatchel RJ, et al. Objective assessment of spine function following industrial low back injury. *JAMA* 1985; 258:1763–1767.

71. Stieg RL, Turk DC. Chronic pain syndrome. The necessity of demonstrating the cost benefit treatment. *Pain Management* 1988; 1:58–63.

72. Stieg RL. The cost-effectiveness of pain treatment. Who cares? *Clin Journal of Pain* 1990; 6:301–304.

73. Farrel G, Knowlton S, Taylor M. Second chance: rehabilitating the American worker. Internal Publication of the Northwestern Life Insurance Company, September 1988.

74. Flor H, Fydrich T, Turk DC. Efficacy of multidisciplinary pain treatment centers. A meta-analytic review. *Pain* 1992; 49:221–230.

2

The Evaluation of Pain Complicating Primary Disabling Disease

Donna Marie Bloodworth, M.D.

Pain syndromes complicate many diseases that cause disability. Not uncommonly, more than one pain syndrome may follow a disease process: The literature describes somatic incisional pain, neurogenic phantom pain, and neurogenic neuroma pain following amputation (1). Precisely defined, as well as generalized, pain syndromes exist: For example, *thalamic*, or *central pain syndrome*, characterized by burning hemibody pain and decreased thermal sensory perception on exam, complicates strokes involving the spinothalamic tract (2). More generalized pain syndromes also complicate stroke: A study by Dromerick finds that among stroke inpatients in acute rehabilitation units, musculoskeletal pain is the most common complication, at 31 percent, after urinary tract infection (41 percent) (3). Patients with primary disabling disease may experience acute or chronic types of pain: Three studies on pain associated with multiple sclerosis (MS) note that 53 to 57 percent of patients experience pain (4–6). Moulin (4) explains that 9 percent of patients with MS experience acute pain syndromes, such as trigeminal neuralgia, whereas the remainder of patients experience chronic pain syndromes, such as dysesthetic extremity pain, back pain, painful leg spasms, and abdominal pain. The literature cites many references for pain's complicating primary disabling diseases; these pain syndromes vary in symptomotology, in etiology, and in chronicity.

For the most part, the literature does not distinguish the disabling effects of the complicating pain syndrome from the disabling effects of the primary disease. Archibald notes that MS patients with pain report poorer mental health and more social-role handicap than MS patients with similar disease severity without pain (6). Pentland (7) and Ropper (8) describe the pain syndromes that affect up to three-fourths of Guillian–Barre syndrome (GBS) patients: paresthesias and dysesthesias, low back and radicular pain, meningismus, myalgia and arthralgia, and visceral pain. Anecdotally, the pain syndromes that complicate Guillian–Barre syndrome impose impediments to functional recovery, distinct from the weakness, autonomic dysfunction, and respiratory insufficiency that characterize Guillian–Barre syndrome (7). However, no studies quantify the extent to which the weakness of GBS versus the pain of GBS handicaps and disables patients.

In a converse statement on pain and disability, one author suggests that the relief of pain contributes to improved function. Jones notes that amputee patients, successfully using a prosthesis, report that the loss of a painful limb by amputation was helpful (9). Whether pain relief is an independent or confounded variable is not clear. Although the literature reveals that pain syndromes complicate many primary disabling diseases, the literature hints, but does not conclude, that pain adds additional disability and handicap. Until the literature addresses and quantifies the degree to which pain syndromes add disability and handicap to patients suffering from primary disabling disease, this author recommends that physiatrists query patients about the experience of pain and the degree to which the patient perceives limitation due to pain, and treat significantly disabling pain aggressively.

Requisite to evaluating and treating pain are defining and conceptualizing its complex neuropsychologic phenomena. The definition of *pain,* according to the International Association for the Study of Pain (IASP), is an unpleasant sensation of emotion associated with real or potential tissue damage (10). This definition reveals two components of pain to be evaluated, the patient's subjective report and objective signs of tissue compromise or damage. The patient's pain history details the subjective report of pain, and the physician's examination reveals signs of tissue compromise and injury.

MODELS OF PAIN

There are both models to understand pain and models to evaluate pain (Table 2.1). Fordyce offers a neuropsychologic model of pain, the components of which include nocioception, cognition, suffering, and behavior (11). *Nocioception* occurs at the locale of tissue compromise or injury. The ends of a-delta and c-fibers, nocioceptive transducers, are excited and propagate a neural impulse when tissue is threatened or injured (12). These impulses ascend from the peripheral nervous system's first order nocioceptive afferents to the central nervous system's second-order and subsequent neuronal synapses; then the individual becomes cognizant of tissue injury, or discomfort and pain. Suffering is the emotional burden of the tissue injuring experience. Bonica defines *suffering* as a state of severe distress associated with events that threaten the intactness of the person (13). Behavioral responses to the tissue injuring or threatening experience vary (14).

Table 2.1. Conceptual Models of Pain

Model	Components			
Definition	subjective report	suffering	tissue injury	
Fordyce	nocioception	cognizance	suffering	behavioral response
Temporal	acute	subacute	chronic	
Etiology	somatic (a-delta and c-fiber firing)	neurogenic	psychosomatic	

Interestingly, tissue injury and nocioception do not have to occur concurrently with the experience of pain. Central or thalamic pain syndromes, trigeminal neuraglia, phantom limb pain, and pain of psychologic origin exemplify this incongruence (10,14). Merskey and Bogduk note that the definition of pain avoids tying pain to a stimulus (10). Nocioception is not pain. Nocioception is a physiologic occurrence in which a-delta and c-fibers are stimulated and fire; pain is a psychological state (10). Tissue injury may occur but not be reported as painful, depending on the past pain experiences of the individual, distractions, stoicism, or other factors (14).

Temporal models for pain exist. Pain may be acute, subacute, or chronic. As described by Bonica, acute pain is specific in locale, and occurs as a result of a stimulus or an acute pathophysiologic process and is associated with increases in sympathetic tone and neuroendocrine function (13). Pain serves a useful biologic purpose of warning that something is wrong, tissue is injured or in danger, and that care should be taken (13). The acute pain ends or is anticipated to end during a period of days or weeks. Acute pain is limited to pain duration of less than thirty days, whereas chronic pain persists for more than sixty days. Subacute pain describes the interval from the end of the first month to the beginning of the seventh month of continued pain. By contrast, chronic pain is diffuse and poorly localized, and dull and constant (1,13). Chronic pain occurs remotely from its stimulus or tissue injury, and may be propagated by psychopathologic and environmental factors, such as secondary gain (1,13). Chronic pain is counterproductive; autonomic activity is suppressed or habituated, and the patient is depressed or listless or withdrawn (1,13). The duration of pain from the time of tissue injury, in order for a pain process to be considered chronic, varies in the literature, but Bonica defines *chronic pain* as pain lasting one month beyond the reasonably expected resolution of the tissue injuring process (13). Nocioception and cognizance of pain and appropriate suffering and protective behavior are components of acute pain; however, chronic pain may lack clear sources of nocioception or tissue injury, despite copious subjective reports of pain experience, suffering, and withdrawn behavior.

Not all chronic pain states are behavioral in origin. Physiologic models of chronic pain caused by continual nocioceptive or neurogenic stimulation exist (15). In nocioceptive pain, tissue injury occurs and recurs, inciting a-delta and c-fiber firing (15). Arthritic joint pain, with flares and remissions, is a common example of this model. In neurogenic pain, pain is initiated or caused by a primary lesion or dysfunction in the peripheral or central nervous tissue (15), and the injured tissue is a nerve. In the injured state, the nerve generates painful impulses by a variety of proposed mechanisms. These mechanisms include: neuromal pacemakers in the "nerve scar"; spontaneous dorsal root ganglion firing proximal to the injured nerve tissue; reinnervation of synapses to non-nocioceptive second-order fibers by nocioceptive afferents; and loss of nocioceptive-inhibiting or dampening fibers (15).

In general, patients with acute pain have identifiable tissue injury; a proximate cause of nocioception, with a-delta and c-fiber firing; and the patient manifests proportionate suffering and behavioral adjustment. Patients with chronic pain report suffering and manifest behavioral suppression out of proportion to identifiable tissue injury. Patients with neurogenic pain may experience aberrant nociception subsequent to neural tissue injury, as well as significant pain, suffering, and behavioral alteration. Pain is a complex neuropsychiatric phenomenon. The definition of pain and models of the pain experience provide background to its evaluation.

ASSESSMENT OF PAIN

The assessment of pain (Table 2.2) begins *after* the physician completes a thorough history and physical examination to assess the symptomotology, severity, related impairment, and associated disability and handicap of the primary disease process. The patient's prior functional level, social support, and household accessibility are components of the preliminary history and physical examination. The patient's treatment goals also are solicited.

When a review of systems reveals untreated or significant pain, the physician proceeds with a focused query of the pain complaint. The first step in assessing pain is comparing the complaint to the definition of pain, then quantifying the number of types of pain affecting the patient. Because of anxiety or lack of language sophistication, patients may report discomfort or unpleasant sensations generally as pain. The physician should cull out discomforts as these complaints may have specific treatments, or at least should not be treated with traditional medications for pain relief. Examples include nonpainful numbness, dyspnea, or poor sleep. Next the physician discerns the number and types of pain the patient experiences, because these distinct pain syndromes may have distinct treatments.

Treatment history and efficacy of the specific intervention guide future treatment considerations. Treatment history includes medications, modalities (like thermal, electric, and exercise interventions), and adjuvent treatments such as acupuncture, biofeedback, or relaxation (16). Knowledge about completely, partially, and nonefficacious treatment are all useful in discerning the etiology of the pain and planning future treatment (16). As regards treatment, allergies and medication sensitivity are important. The Clinical Practice Guideline for Acute Pain Management (16) recom-

Table 2.2. Items Included in Pain Evaluation

Physical
Functional
Affective
Cognitive and Behavioral
Economic
Sociocultural

mends inquiring about the patient's attitude toward and use of opioid, anxiolytic, and other medications, and any history of substance abuse.

Similar previous pain experiences, distinct prior pain experiences and their treatment and resolution, and familial history of pain syndromes are pertinent. Also significant in the past medical history is the presence of psychiatric disorders, such as anxiety or depression (16). The physician should note family expectation and beliefs about pain.

Physical examination is tailored to the patient's history. As needed, physical examination includes a complete neurologic exam; a musculoskeletal exam, including examination for tender and trigger points and evaluation of the joints; inspection for traditional signs of tissue injury, including erythema, discoloration, swelling, laxity, crepitus, and deformity; signs of sympathetic hyper- or hypoactivity, such as edema, erythema, and hyperhydrosis, or cyanosis, dryness, and pallor.

The physician can include a special neurologic exam for signs of neurogenic pain in patients with primary nerve injury. *Allodynia* occurs in neurogenic pain and is defined as pain caused by a stimulus that does not normally provoke pain (10). In contrast to *hyperalgesia*, allodynia involves a change in the quality of a sensation from nonpainful to painful. For example a light touch on skin affected by postherpetic neuralgia may feel like burning pain. Allodynia is attributed to "wind-up" of cells in the dorsal horn, which in an inhibited state transduce all sensory information as painful. *Hyperalgesia* refers to an increased response to a stimulus, which is normally painful (10). For example, warm water poured over burned skin feels painfully hot. Hyperalgesia results from the lowered threshold of c-fiber firing caused by humoral factors, such as potassium, bradykinin, and prostaglandins, released because of tissue injury.

ASSESSMENT TOOLS

According to Williams, chronic pain is studied in terms of six variables (Table 2.2):

- physical,
- cognitive and behavioral,
- affective or emotional,
- functional,
- economic,
- and social and cultural (17).

Physical dimensions of pain include its location, spatial distribution, and symptomotology (17). Functional measures include uptime, disability, and productivity; cognitive and behavioral factors include numbers of doctor visits and hospitalizations, drug usage, and verbal and nonverbal behaviors; emotional factors include depression and anxiety (17). Economic factors include costs and lost workdays; and sociocultural factors include independence, productive family involvement, quality of life, and patient goals (17). Not all of these components of chronic pain may ultimately fit a model of pain complicating primary disabling disease.

Clinically reliable and valid measurement tools exist to assess each of the above described six components of the pain experience. White, Doleys, and Turk provide concise and erudite summaries of these assessment tools (14,18,19). These tools have utility primarily in the assessment of disabling chronic pain. Regarding acute pain, Bonica writes that physicians do well in the assessment and treatment of acute pain (20,21). He implies that no tool more sophisticated than a complete history and physical exam and pertinent diagnostic tests is needed for the evaluation of simple pain. A range of tools exists to evaluate the spectrum of pain experiences; familiarity with available tools aids the physician who assesses pain.

The physical descriptors of a pain's intensity and qualities interest the physician. The McGill Pain Questionnaire (MPQ) is a self-report form that includes descriptors of the physical sensation and intensity of the pain, the anatomic location and radiation pattern, the current severity, and the frequency or occurrence (22). The location and pattern of radiation, physical sensation and intensity, frequency, and duration of the pain are initial elements of the pain history. Date of onset, proximate cause, exacerbating and mitigating factors, and activities as related to the pain are additional historical points. This instrument has been extensively used in research and in clinical evaluation and treatment outcome trials.

The Wisconsin Brief Pain Questionnaire consists of seventeen questions and catalogs not only the information captured by the MPQ, but also a history of the pain and its effects on mood and activity (23). The Dartmouth Pain Questionnaire adds to the MPQ and additionally assesses the behavioral effects of pain (24). Examples of the use of these questionnaires to evaluate pain in persons with primary disabilities exist (25). Vermote and colleagues have used the MPQ to assess pain syndromes in patients with MS, and have found that the MPQ differentiates among three pain patterns: paroxysmal pain, persistent pain, and painful tonic spasms (25).

Questionnaires, which catalog historical, descriptive, and functional information about a pain complaint, complement and expand information sought in the basic history and physical examination.

Physiatrists, as specialists, assess function. Simple assessment tools to evaluate the effects of pain on function include time to ambulate a certain distance and diaries of up and down time. Clinical batteries that assess function include the Health Assessment Questionnaire and the Sickness Impact Profile (26). Assessment tools to evaluate cognitive and behavioral effects of pain and affective and depressive effects of pain exist; they may have more utility to psychologists for the assessment of chronic pain. The behavioral and cognitive effects of pain are assessed by clinical tools like the Millon Behavioral Health Inventory (27,28), and the West Haven–Yale Multidimensional Pain Inventory (29). The affective and depressive ramifications of pain are explored by batteries such as the Beck Depression Scale (30). Although these questionnaires and profiles have been shown to have validity in assessing the effect of chronic pain and low back pain on personal physical, cognitive, and emotional function, specific studies in populations with pain complicating primary disabling disease are lacking or sparse.

PRIMARY DISABLING DISEASE AND PAIN

Pain that complicates primary disabling disease may have significance for two reasons: First, if the pain is only mild to moderate, it may not additionally handicap the patient; however, it may negatively impact emotions, sense of well being, and quality of life. Moderate to severe pain may preclude self-care and mobility, creating additional disability and handicap. An assessment strategy from the study of chronic pain, by the researcher Williams, may be useful in assessing pain complicating disabling disease (17) (Table 2.3).

Amyotrophic lateral sclerosis (ALS) provides an example of a primary disabling disease process that is complicated by unpleasant sensations or discomforts, as well as by pain. Dyspnea affects 60 percent of patients suffering with ALS (31). Whereas dyspnea is unpleasant and provokes anxiety and suffering, it does not fit the IASP definition of pain as an unpleasant sensation associated with actual or potential tissue injury. Dyspnea and other unpleasant or disturbing sensory experiences, such as numbness, stiffness, or insomnia, can threaten the sense of well being, inflict anxiety and depression, and impose disability and handicap. Whereas physicians treat dyspnea with narcotics and benzodiazepines, other treatment considerations include supplemental oxygen, nebulizers, and mechanical ventilation. A review of systems may reveal unpleasant sensations or discomforts that the patient experiences; physicians evaluate these reports independent of pain complaints because strategies and tools of evaluation, as well as treatments, differ.

After the physician has separated and addressed discomforts with specific treatments, she must next discern the number of types of pain the patient experiences. Classically, texts describe ALS as a painless disease, except for muscle cramps, which occur early in the disease's course (32). However, Oliver describes three pain syndromes that affect 40 to 64 percent of ALS sufferers and which are associated with the late and terminal phases of ALS: musculoskeletal pain due to stiffness and contracture, skin pain and pressure due to immobility, and painful muscle spasticity (31). Treatments for each pain type are distinct, and respectively include nonsteroidals, joint injections, and positioning for stiffness; narcotic pain relievers and regular turning for pressure relief; and diazepam or quinine for spacticity (31). When a patient complains of pain, the physician distinguishes the number of types and qualities of each pain syndrome, because specific treatments for each type of pain may exist. Postamputation pain provides another example; the amputee patient may experience neuromal pain treated by lidocaine injection, phantom pain treated by tri-

Table 2.3. Assessment of Pain Complicating Primary Disabling Disease

Assess primary disease process
    Traditional history and physical
    Symptoms, severity, related impairments
    Disability and handicap that the patient attributes to the primary disease

    Prior functional level
    Social support
    Household accessibility and assistive devices

    Treatment goals

Assess nonpainful discomfort and unpleasant sensations separately from pain
    (e.g., insomnia, dyspnea, dysphagia, numbness, stiffness)

Assess the number of types of pain syndromes present

For each pain syndrome assess:
    Location and pattern of radiation
    Physical sensation and intensity
    Frequency and duration
    Date of onset and presumed cause
    Exacerbating and mitigating factors or activities

    Treatment history and efficacy of each intervention
        Modalities: Thermal, electrical, exercise
        Medications: NSAIDs, Narcotics, Adjuvent (TCAs, etc.)
        Adjuvent: Acupuncture, biofeedback
    Allergies and medications sensitivities
    Patient and family attitudes toward narcotics, anxiolytics
    History of substance abuse

    Similar past pain experiences
    Past pain experiences and course of resolution
    Psychiatric history

    Inquire about what disability and handicap the patient attributes only to pain
      (e.g., "If I did not hurt I could do....")

Physical Examination
    Neurologic exam
    Musculoskeletal exam
    Orientation and affective assessment
    Exam for traditional signs of tissue injury
    Exam for pseudomotor and vasomotor instability or other sympathetic signs
    Special sensory exam for allodynia, hyperalgesia, dysesthesia, paresthesia

In the follow-up phase
    Review interim diagnostic testing
    Review treatment interventions (medication, modalities, etc.) for adverse reactions,
      efficacy
    Assess the need for medication adjustment or additions

Assess the need for further diagnostics

cyclic antidepressants, or somatic stump pain treated by traditional pain medications (1).

PAIN, PRIMARY DISEASE, AND FUNCTIONAL CAPACITY

There is limited literature regarding primary disease, pain, and its effects on functional ability at a personal level or functional capacity at an occupational level. When querying primary disease and functional capacity, the available literature focuses on physiologic exercise tolerance (33–35) or personal care ability (36–38). The literature cites some studies of primary disease, pain, and effects on function (39,40). These studies focus on endpoints of personal ability or social dependence. Nydevik studied a population of severely impaired stroke victims, in long-term care facilities over twelve months, and found that pain further increased dependence (39). Helm interviewed 107 lower-limb amputees about functional ability and social dependence, and found that increased age paralleled decreased physical ability and social dependence whereas postoperative pain and higher levels of amputation paralleled reduced functional ability but not social dependence (40). Helm did not study the endpoint, return to occupation (40), and social dependence is not defined (40). The occupational status of this group with primary disability and of the subset of patients with pain is not discussed.

The perception or experience of chronic pain or chronic low back pain may affect functional capacity for occupation, or occupational participation. Pain, in particular widespread or poorly characterized pain, does adversely affect working capacity (41). Andersson studied persons with chronic pain and found that, in comparison to persons with localized chronic pain, persons with widespread chronic pain had a worse prognosis regarding the duration of pain and working capacity (41). Persons with widespread pain were significantly more likely to experience work absenteeism, sick leave, or disability caused by pain (41). When selecting patients to participate in treatment programs, disability exaggeration in chronic low back pain patients does not predict success or failure in a multidisciplinary program for chronic pain, nor does it predict return or lack of return to employment at one or two years (42). By contrast, Kaplan demonstrated that persons with chronic pain who perceived that they were more impaired performed more poorly on functional capacity evaluation (43). No literature describing the functional capacity or work status of persons with primary disability plus pain was found.

CONCLUSIONS

A dearth of literature exists on the effect of pain, distinct from the effect of a primary disease process, on function, effect, cognition, and behavior. However, the literature includes many examples of primary diseases that are complicated by subsequent pain syndromes. At least anecdotally, these pain syndromes themselves may disable and handicap. When the physician encounters untreated or significant pain, knowledge of acute and chronic pain assessment and measurement, as well as familiarity with models and theories of pain perception, provide a template for assessing secondary pain syndromes. A comprehensive history characterizing the pain and its pertinent historical features; a physical exam to identify tissue injury, sympathetic, and neurogenic signs; and diligent and timely follow-up of interventions serve the patient and the physician well.

REFERENCES

1. Walsh NE, Dumitru D, Ramamurthy S, Schoenfeld LS. Treatment of the patient with chronic pain. In DeLisa JA, Gans BM (eds). *Rehabilitation Medicine: Principles and Practice*. Philadelphia: JB Lippincott Company, 1993, pp. 973–995.
2. Leijon G, Boivie J, Johannson I. Central post-stroke pain: neurological symptoms and pain characteristics. *Pain* 1989;36:13–25.
3. Dromerick A, Reding M. Medical and neurologic complications of stroke during inpatient rehabilitation. *Stroke* 1994;25(2):358–361.
4. Moulin DE, Foley KM, Ebers GC. Pain syndromes in multiple sclerosis. *Neurol* 1988;38(12):1830–1834.
5. Indaco A, Iachetta C, Nappi C, Socci L, Carrieri PB. Chronic and acute pain syndromes in patients with multiple sclerosis. *Acta Neurol* 1994;16(3):97–102.
6. Archibald CJ, McGrath PJ, Ritvo PG, Fisk JD, Bhan V, Maxner CE, Murray TJ. Pain prevalence, severity and impact in a clinical sample of multiple sclerosis patients. *Pain* 1994;58(1):89–93.
7. Pentland B, Donald SM. Pain in the Guillian–Barre Syndrome: a clinical review. *Pain* 1994;59:159–164.
8. Ropper AH, Shanani BT. Pain in Guillian–Barre Syndrome. *Arch Neurol* 41: 1984; 511–514.
9. Jones L, Hall M, Schuld W. Ability or disability? A study of the functional outcome of 65 consecutive lower limb amputees treated at the Royal South Sydney Hospital. *Disabil Rehabil* 1993;15 (4):184–188.
10. Task Force on Taxonomy of the International Association for the Study of Pain. Merskey H, Bogduk N, eds., *Classification of Chronic Pain: Descriptions of Chronic Pain Syndrome and Definitions of Pain Terms*. Seattle: IASP Press, 1994. pp. 210–213.
11. Fordyce WE, Brena SF DeLatuer B Holcomb RJ Loeser JD. Relationship of patient semantic pain descriptors to physician diagnostic judgments, activity level measures and MMPI. *Pain* 1978;5: 292–303.
12. Bonica JJ. Anatomic and physiologic basis of nociception and pain. In Bonica JJ, ed., *The Management of Pain*. Malvern, Pa.: Lea and Febiger, 1990, pp.28–94.
13. Bonica JJ. Definitions and taxonomy of pain. In Bonica JJ, ed., *The Management of Pain*. Malvern, Pa.: Lea and Febiger, 1990, pp.18–27.
14. White P. Pain measurement. In Warfield C, ed., *Principles and Practice of Pain Management*. New York: McGraw-Hill, 1993, pp. 27–42.
15. Loeser JD. Pain due to nerve injury. *Spine* 10: 232–235, 1985.
16. *Clinical Practice Guideline: Acute Pain Management*. Operative and medical procedures and trauma. Process of pain assessment and reassessment. U.S. Department of Health and Human Services, 1992, pp.7–14.
17. Williams RCV. Toward a set of reliable and valid measures for chronic pain assessment and outcome research. *Pain* 1988;35:239–251.

18. Doleys DM, Murray JB, Klapow JC, Coleton MI. Psychological Assessment. In Ashburn MA, Rice LJ, eds., *The Management of Pain*. New York: Churchill Livingstone, 1998, pp. 27–50.

19. Turk DC, Melzack. *Handbook of Pain Assessment*. New York: Guilford, 1992.

20. Bonica JJ. History of pain concepts and therapies. In Bonica JJ, ed., *The Management of Pain*. Malvern, Pa.: Lea and Febiger, 1990, pp. 2–17.

21. *Clinical Practice Guideline: Acute Pain Management*. Operative and medical procedures and trauma. Introduction. U.S. Department of Health and Human Services, 1992, pp. 3–6.

22. Melzack R. The McGill pain questionnaire: major properties and scoring methods. *Pain* 1975;1:277–299.

23. Daut RL, Cleeland CS, Flannary RC. Development of the Wisconsin Brief Pain Questionnaire to assess pain in cancer and other diseases. *Pain* 1983;17:197–210.

24. Corson LJ, Schneirder MJ. The Dartmouth Pain Questionnaire: an adjunct to the McGill Pain Questionnaire. *Pain* 1984;19:59–69.

25. Vermote R, Ketelaer P, Carton H. Pain in multiple sclerosis patients. A prospective study using the McGill Pain Questionnaire. *Clin Neurol Neurosurg* 1986;88(2):87–93.

26. Berger M, Bobbitt FA, Carter WB, Gibson BS. The Sickness Impact Profile: Development and final revision of a health status measure. *Med Care* 1981;19: 787–805.

27. Milon T, Green C, Meagher R. *Milon Behavioral Health Inventory Manual*, 3rd edition. Minneapolis, Minn.: National Computer Systems, 1981.

28. Gatchel RJ, Mayer TG, Capra P. Milon Behavioral Health Inventory: Its ability in predicting physical function in patients with low back pain. *Arch Phys Med Rehabil* 1986;67: 878–882.

29. Kerns RS, Turk DC, Rudy TE. The West Haven–Yale Multidimensional Pain Inventory. *Pain* 1985;23: 345–356.

30. Beck AT, Ward CH, Mendelson M, Mock J, Erbaugh J. An inventory for measuring pain. *Arch Gen Psych* 1961;4:561–571.

31. Oliver D Terminal care. In Williams AC, ed., *Motor Neuron Disease*. New York: Chapman and Hall Medical, 1994, pp. 281–296.

32. Smith RA, Gillie E, Licht J. Palliative treatment of motor neuron disease. In Vinken PJ, Bruyn GW, Klawans HL, eds., *Diseases of the Motor System*. New York: Elsevier, 1991, pp. 467–468.

33. Ong KC , Benedicto JP, Chan AH, Tan YS, Ong YY. Cardiopulmonary exercise testing in heart transplant candidates. *Ann Acad Med Singapore*. 2000;29(4): 442–446.

34. Metra M, Faggiano P, D'Aloia A, Nodari S, Gualeni A, Raccagni D, DeiCas L. Use of cardiopulmonary exercise testing with hemodynamic monitoring in the assessment of ambulatory patients with chronic heart failure. *J AM Coll Cardiol* 1999;33(4):943–50.

35. Farstad T, Brockmeier F, Bratlid D. Cardiopulmonary function in premature infants with bronchopulmonary dysplasia: A Follow up. *Eur J Pediatr* 1995;154(10) 853–8.

36. Rostagno C, Galanti G, Comeglio M, Bodddi V, Olivo G, Gastone G. Comparison of different methods of functional evaluation in patients with chronic heart failure. *Eur J Heart Fail* 2000;2(3) :273–280.

37. Wyser C, Stulz P, Soler M, Tamm M, Muller Barnd J, Habicht J, Perruchoud AP, Bolliger CT. Prospective evaluation of an algorithm for the functional assessment of lung transplant candidates. *Am J Respir Crit Care Med* 1999;159(5 pt1):1450–1456.

38. Cahalin LP, Mathier MA, Semigran MJ, Dec GW, DiSalvo TG. The six-minute walk test predicts peak oxygen uptake and survival in patients with heart failure. *Chest* 1996;11(2):325–32.

39. Nydevik I, Eller B, Larsen L, Milton A, Wall B, Hulter-Asberg K. Functional status of stroke patients in long-term care—a basis for the development of rehabilitation and care. *Scand J Caring Sci* 1993;7(2): 85–91.

40. Helm P, Engle T, Holm A, Kristiansen VB, Rosendahl S. Function after lower limb amputation. *Acta Orthop Scand* 57(2):154–7.

41. Andersson HI, Ejlertsson G, Rosenberg C. Characteristics of subjects with chronic pain, in relation to location and widespread pain report. Prospective study of symptoms, clinical findings and blood tests in subgroups of a geographically defined population. *Scand J Rheumatol* 1996;25(3):146–54.

42. Hazard RG, Bendix A, Fenwick JW. Disability exaggeration as a predictor of functional restoration outcomes for patients with chronic low-back pain. *Spine* 1991;16(9):1062–1067.

43. Kaplan GM, Wurtele SK, Gillis D. Maximal effort during functional capacity evaluations: An examination of psychological factors. *Arch Phys Med Rehabil* 1996;77(2):161–164.

3

Psychosocial and Vocational Issues in Pain Rehabilitation

Gabriel Tan, Ph.D.
Sharon Young, M.A.

In the preface to *Psychological Approaches to Pain Management*, the editors note that "...it has become equally evident that numerous psychosocial factors frequently occur secondary to a trauma or disease. These psychosocial factors must be evaluated and treated...in order to ensure therapeutic success. Moreover, research has suggested that the social and familial context in which pain persists also plays a central role in the maintenance of disability" (1).

Although acute pain is frequently experienced by patients going through rehabilitation of various medical conditions, it is chronic, persistent pain that is likely to profoundly affect psychosocial and vocational adjustment. Nevertheless, the role of acute pain should not be underestimated. Pain, whether acute or chronic, promotes self-absorption, anxiety, fear, sleep deprivation, and helplessness—a sense of one's body being out of control (2). Inadequately treated acute pain can result in abnormal physiologic and psychologic responses that can lead to medical complications, lasting psychologic difficulties, chronic pain syndromes, and even death (3). The influences of psychologic factors on the evolution of acute to chronic pain with respect to attributional style has been discussed elsewhere (4).

Regardless of its source, chronic pain is more than a physical symptom. Its continuous presence creates widespread manifestations of suffering, including demoralization and affective disturbance; preoccupation with pain; limitation of personal, social, and work activities; increased use of medications and of health-care services; and a generalized adoption of the sick role (5). Recent research has provided a strong support toward the notion that regardless of the medical conditions and trauma that originally caused and were associated with the pain, a common set of psychosocial effects and issues is involved (6–10). Similarly, chronic pain may be classified with a consistent set of criteria regardless of the anatomic site of pain (11).

To understand the psychosocial and vocational impact of chronic pain, it is imperative not to lose sight of the fact that individuals respond differently to the same noxious stimuli and, therefore, that the same lesion or medical condition may lead to widely differing self-reported pain experience and psychosocial effects. A great deal of research has been directed towards identifying cognitive factors that contribute to pain and disability (12). Many studies have consistently shown that patients' attitudes, beliefs, and expectancies about their pain and medical condition, about themselves and their coping resources, and about the healthcare system affect their reports of pain and its impact on their lives (13–15). For example, pain severity ratings by cancer patients could be predicted not only by their use of analgesics and their affective state but also by their interpretations of pain (16). Patients who attributed their pain to a worsening of their underlying disease experienced more pain than patients with more benign interpretations, despite the same level of disease progression. In a study of patients with low back pain, 83 percent of these patients reported they were unable to complete a movement sequence that included leg lifts and lateral bends because of anticipated pain; only 5 percent were unable to perform the activities because of actual lack of ability (17). Another study found that patients' beliefs about their pain and disability were significantly related to actual measures of disability, but not to the physicians' ratings of disease severity (18). Beliefs about controllability appear to be a central issue in the experience of pain and its effect. Perception that pain is uncontrollable led to report of more intense pain (19). The relationship between perceived controllability and pain experience has been demonstrated in a variety of pain syndromes including migraine headaches (20), chronic low back pain, and rheumatoid arthritis (RA) (13). The latter study also showed that situation-specific and general cognitive variables explained 32 and 60 percent of the variance in pain and disability, respectively. The addition of disease-related variables improved the predictions only marginally.

Other cognitive variables including self-efficacy, cognitive errors such as "catastrophizing," "over-generalization," "personalization," and selective abstraction have been shown to greatly influence pain experience, pain behavior, disability, successful vocational rehabilitation, and outcome of pain treatment. For a detailed discussion, please refer to Gatchel and Turk (1, pages 17–20).

Depression is a major psychosocial issue with patients suffering from chronic pain. Research suggests that anywhere from 40 to 50 percent of chronic pain patients suffer from depression. In the majority of cases, depression appears to be patients' reaction to their plight (21). There is also evidence that patients' appraisal of the impact of the pain on their lives and their ability to exert any control over the pain and their lives mediated this pain–depression relationship. Those patients who felt they could carry on their life activities despite their pain and could maintain some control over their pain and life were less likely to be depressed (22, 23).

Less widely known but equally important is the role of anger in chronic pain. For instance, anger and hostility explained 33 percent of the variance in pain severity among spinal cord injured patients (24). It has also been found that internalization of angry feelings accounted for a significant proportion of variances in measures of pain intensity, perceived life interference, and frequency of pain behavior (24).

PSYCHOSOCIAL FACTORS, PAIN, AND PHYSICAL FUNCTION

Psychosocial factors may act indirectly on pain and disability by reducing physical activity and consequently reducing muscle flexibility, muscle tone, strength, and physical endurance. Fear of re-injury, fear of loss of disability compensation, and job dissatisfaction can also influence the return to work (1). Psychosocial factors such as cognitive appraisals and affective arousal may directly influence the physiology of pain by increasing sympathetic nervous system arousal (25), thus producing endogenous opioids (26) and elevating levels of muscle tension (27).

PSYCHOSOCIAL FACTORS, PAIN, AND VOCATIONAL FUNCTION

Return to work is an important goal of rehabilitation medicine. Supporting this objective is a preponderance of evidence indicating better adjustment, both physical and psychosocial, for employed versus work-disabled pain patients (28–30). These studies also showed a strong association between prolonged disability and poor functioning. Longitudinal studies have shown that return to work may be accompanied by improved physical function, reduction in pain intensity, and a decrease in emotional distress (31,32). To better understand how employment-related factors affect the emotional status of chronic pain patients, Jahoda has proposed a model that explains the negative psychological consequences of unemployment that results from relative deprivations of income, structured and purposeful activity social contact, status, and identity (33). Using this model, a path analysis indicates that pain severity has a direct association with both emotional distress and employment status. In addition, employment status was only indirectly related to emotional distress; this relationship was mediated by levels of reported financial strain and structured purposeful time use (34). Research on prediction of return to workplace after pain treatment and rehabilitation has not led to consistent findings. In reviewing 164 multidisciplinary outcome studies on chronic pain patients' return to work, Fisbain, Rosomoff, and Goldberg (35) concluded that "it is unclear which variables or set of variables predict return to the workplace after multidisciplinary pain center treatment"(p. 178).

ARTHRITIC PAIN: PSYCHOSOCIAL ISSUES AND DISABILITY

Pain associated with arthritis is the primary reason that arthritis patients seek medical attention. A survey of a heterogeneous sample of arthritic patients found that 66 percent of patients with rheumatoid arthritis and 75 percent of patients with degenerative joint disease ranked pain as the most important symptom to be treated (36). One form of arthritis, rheumatoid arthritis (RA), has received the most attention from researchers in terms of its psychosocial and vocational impact.

Arthritic pain among RA patients is closely intertwined with depression. Several reviews have yielded variable results, but overall findings support that 21 to 34% of RA patients suffer from depression (37). This rate is similar to the prevalence of depression found in other severe and chronic illnesses (38).

Depression in RA appears to relate more closely to socioeconomic and cognitive factors than to disease activity and severity (39–44), but RA flares could also exacerbate depression (45).

A significant relationship between pain and depression among RA patients has been well established, although the causal direction is still being debated (37,46,47). Several longitudinal studies using structural equations modeling have attempted to unravel this puzzle. One such study examined 242 RA patients over a two-year interval and found that prior pain (and the interaction of high levels of pain and high levels of sleep problems) was associated with subsequent depression (48). Another study examining 243 RA patients over six weeks of data collection provided some support for a causal model in which pain was hypothesized to predict subsequent depression (49). In contrast, support for a model in which depression exerted more influence over pain rather than vice versa has also been found (50).

A relationship has been found between pain, depression, and disability among RA patients. For instance, RA patients who are unable to maintain gainful employment report higher levels of pain and depression (51).

In addition to depression, several other psychosocial factors have been found to relate to pain among RA patients. Among these are conflict about pain with significant others and a recent history of major life stressors (52). The Nuprin Pain Report, a national pain survey of 1,254 persons over age 18 commissioned by the Bristol-Meyers Company, found that individuals with a high internal locus of control regarding health matters reported significantly less pain than those with low internal locus of control. The greatest pain management challenges occurred in patients who were middle-aged, living on limited incomes, and experiencing major stresses in everyday life (42). These high-risk RA pain patients were also prone to worrying, felt isolated, and lacked social support.

Although less well studied, the psychosocial impact of osteoarthritis (OA) is also receiving increased attention from the research community. In addition to disease-related variables such as degeneration of cartilage and bone, muscle weakness and limitations in joint motion, anxiety, coping style, attentional focus on symptoms, and possibly depression have been found to significantly affect pain and disability among OA patients (53). A study involving seniors aged 55 to 74 years living in the community revealed that those with more chronic and severe pain in the hip and/or knee had relatively higher levels of physical as well as psychosocial disability, compared to a reference group without any signs of OA (54). A subsequent publication from the same survey concluded that physical, and especially psychological, disability are mediators in the relationship between pain chronicity and quality of life. Furthermore, seeking social support as a coping style is a more important predictor of the self-reported quality of life than either pain chronicity or physical disability (55).

This review so far attests to the complex nature of the relationships between pain in arthritic patients and psychosocial variables. Few studies have directly examined the vocational issues among arthritic patients. Less direct measures, such as disability and functional status, were more likely to be included in the research.

In a national survey, 31 percent of RA patients reported varying degrees of limitations with ADL (56). Almost 60 percent had to discontinue employment within 10 years of disease onset. Although both physical functioning and psychological variables make significant contributions to an RA patient's disability, workplace factors and social responsibilities were also important (57).

A majority of the studies to date appears to conclude that arthritic pain and psychosocial variables are significantly and highly correlated, although the direction of causality remains controversial. One study found that, whereas arthritis severity ratings predicated only 13 percent of the pain variance, psychological factors predicated an additional 41 percent of the variance (40).

Several recent studies have attempted to integrate and elucidate the complex relationship between the disease of arthritis, arthritic pain, psychosocial variables, and disability under the purview of a biopsychosocial model. One such longitudinal study (58) using path analysis revealed that pain and helplessness were significant mediators of the relationship between disease activity and future disability in RA. Figure 3.1 further elucidates the relationships between the variables studied. A limitation of this model is that the research was done with a relatively small sample of male veterans suffering from RA, therefore, generalization to all arthritic patients would require replication with females and with other arthritic patients. Another limitation of much of the research to date has been the fact that most studies have utilized adult subjects.

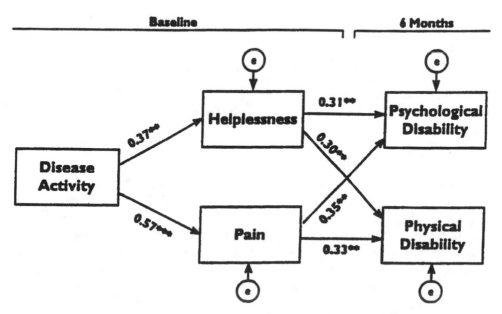

Figure 3.1. Pain and helplessness as mediators between disease activity and future disability in rheumatoid arthritis. Reprinted with permission from Arthritis Care & Research © American College of Rheumatology.

Juvenile RA has been relatively neglected. It has been suggested that pain in juvenile chronic arthritis has been underestimated because children do not verbalize their pain adequately and they tend to rate pain lower than adults on existing pain rating scales (59). A more detailed discussion of the psychosocial aspects of pediatric pain is provided in a separate section of this chapter.

In reviewing the literature on coping with arthritic pain, Buckelew and Parker (60) concluded that patient education focusing on the medical aspects of RA is helpful in producing an increase in knowledge about arthritis. Cognitive-behavioral interventions and self-help groups, on the other hand, have been shown to improve coping for RA patients (61). Among highly adherent patients, cognitive-behavioral interventions have led to pain reduction. However, long-term maintenance of treatment gains have not been consistently demonstrated and future research must focus on issues of relapse prevention and maintenance (61). It has also been noted that because arthritis is a progressive disease, arthritic patients would require ongoing interventions to adapt to changes in the disease progression as well (62).

Several forms of biofeedback have also been shown to be helpful for RA patients (27). EMG biofeedback has resulted in long-lasting reduction in rheumatic back pain. A combination of thermal biofeedback and cognitive-behavioral procedures for pain management have resulted in immediate improvements in pain rating, pain behavior, and rheumatoid factor titer (63). Affect arousal in psychotherapy appears to reduce depression and increase beta-endorphin production among RA patients. Parker and Wright (46) showed that stress management intervention is capable of producing important clinical benefits for patients with RA. In general, there is an accumulating body of evidence that supports the use of psychologically based treatment for patients with arthritis.

BURN PAIN: PSYCHOSOCIAL AND VOCATIONAL ISSUES

Being severely burned is usually a frightening, physically and psychologically devastating experience. Treatment during hospitalization is painful, eliciting dependency and helplessness for the burn patient. This pain is best viewed as a conditioned response in which patients generally experience episodes of severe pain inflicted by necessary treatments (debridement, dressing changes, and immobilization) superimposed on low intensity background pain.

Choinierè (64) points out that whereas patients' pain is greater during treatment than at rest, pain severity rarely diminishes over the course of treatment. In point of fact, Choinierè posits that burn pain generally intensifies during the intermediate and late phases of treatment. Explanations for this include return of sensation, increasing apprehension and anticipatory anxiety, exhaustion caused by sleep deprivation and recurrent pain experience, and the operant conditioning of the pain response.

A close association exists between pain and the anxiety generated by severe tissue damage, as well as the primary role anxiety plays in burn patients' recovery; this has been well documented by Wall (65). Burn patients experience anxiety about past, present, and future. Anxiety about the past includes events surrounding the injury itself and possible guilt. Present anxiety about treatment tends to revolve around painfulness, dependency, and helplessness. Anxiety about the future involves the patient's potential for future survival, ability to sustain protracted recurrent suffering, disfigurement, ability to continue employment, and the capacity to retrieve a sense of efficacy and resourcefulness (66–72).

Choinierè (64) points out that inadequate analgesic pain management elevates anticipatory anxiety. Anticipatory anxiety predisposes the burn patient to increased state anxiety. State anxiety, as measured by State-Trait Anxiety Inventory (STAI), increases pain experience for burn patients, both procedural and at rest (73). Thus a vicious cycle ensues in which the fear and anticipatory anxiety about procedures such as dressing changes exacerbate pain perception during procedures, thus ultimately lowering the patient's pain threshold. Psychosocial outcomes include social withdrawal, severe anxiety, depression, hostility and hostile dependency (alienating support systems), aggressive behavior, and regression, thus rendering wound treatment and adequate pain management difficult. Successful recognition and handling of anger is essential for the burn patient; failure to address this during inpatient treatment often results in lasting psychopathological sequelae (64). According to Andreasen, these changes can and do impact patients' coping styles over time, given the length of treatment (66). Conservation withdrawal and regression are common. In some cases posttraumatic stress syndrome features complicate psychosocial adjustment and significantly impede efforts at vocational rehabilitation (74).

The potential development of helplessness and decline in perceived self efficacy derive from the severe anxiety, fear, depression, and acute grief reactions that occur in the face of extended hospitalization and recurrent painful treatments over protracted periods. Burn patients in pain also undergo psychological regression as a function of helplessness, dependency, and fear of dying (75). Fear of dying can be exacerbated by the anxiety that these patients experience because of separation from close family and friends (76).

The relationship between burn patient and treating professional is crucial to successful treatment (76). A key ingredient to establishing and maintaining rapport with the burn patient is addressing pain status and the adequacy of analgesia. According to Blumenfeld and Schoeps (77), the absence of this is perceived by patients as insensitive and impedes pain control and the assessment of other issues such as psychologic reaction to injury, altered body image, prior pain experience, anxiety, depression, guilt, fear, or neuropsychologic impairment. These issues require careful assessment before designing treatment and rehabilitation (77).

The professional treatment team can provide psychologic support, education, analgesic and anti-anxiolytic medication, and surgical and physical therapeutic approaches to improving appearance. Empathetic psychotherapy that is geared toward enhancing a sense of control and encourages the patient to take as active as possible a role in treatment and rehabilitation results in a better prognosis.

Involvement of strong social supports in treatment, such as those provided by a spouse or parent, can enhance pain treatment. Tempereau, Grossman, and Brones

(78) found that the psychosocial impact of disfigurement and disability is modulated by the inclusion of family members into later aspects of patient care (such as dressing changes). Blumenfield and Schoeps (77) point out that requests for pain medication diminish during family visits.

In addition to the physical injury itself, a patient's pain is influenced by emotional and subjective variables. Pain impulses can be modulated via medication, memories (i.e., prior pain experience), and emotion. The severity of pain for burn patients can leave patients sleep-deprived, fatigued, and disoriented, all of which interfere with the energy, attention, and discipline required for many psychological interventions. Pain severity and its effects necessitate a combination of analgesic medication and psychotherapeutic techniques to achieve adequate pain control (77,79). Psychologic procedures are designed to enhance a patient's perceived self-control and diminish the anxiety, depression, and impaired perceived self-efficacy that facilitates rehabilitation efforts. Most notably, pain experience is enhanced by feelings of isolation, fear, and anxiety that derive from a sense of loss of control.

Psychologic interventions can modify the impact of stress for burn patients. Patterson (80), Meichenbaum (81), and others point out that some interventions, when introduced early, can improve coping; these include hypnotherapy, relaxation training, biofeedback, behavior modification (e.g., operant methods and desensitization strategies), and cognitive behavioral strategies such as stress inoculation training, guided imagery, distraction, and direct coping skills training (68,82–84).

Despite the limitations imposed by small sample sizes, studies, such as those of Meichenbaum (81) and Patterson (80)—are promising for many of these interventions. Although generalizability has only been demonstrated thus far for hypnotherapy (83), behavior modification, and stress reduction procedures, burn patients derive significant improvement from all of these therapeutic procedures.

Coping with both the social and vocational disorder that results from physical handicaps and disfigurement is a critical consideration in the rehabilitation of burn patients. In addition to the frequent experience of excruciating pain, these patients are confronted with physical handicaps such as impairment of motion, itching, recurrent tumor and infection, scar contracture, and limitations caused by loss of vision, limbs, or digits. Bernstein (85) points out that disfigurement is a burn patient's primary presenting concern affecting psychosocial and vocational rehabilitation. Disfigured patients can become socially isolated, demoralized, and experience loss of their social network. Facial disfigurement can result in the patient losing his affective signaling system (85). Changes imposed by severe burns poses a threat to the basic unity of the patient's body image or body schema: how he thinks he looks, how he wants to look, and his interpersonal context (86).

Relative effectiveness of psychosocial and vocational rehabilitation of burn patients requires solid rapport between patient and treatment team, adequate analgesic management, inclusion of social supports, and motivation in the patient. Patient energy and effort requirements necessitate a mental health professional's involvement in treatment. This professional can provide the opportunity for a patient to resolve conflicts and learn skills for coping with the pain and stress caused by burn injury. Rehabilitation of the burn patient rests both on the Aristotelian idea that the aim of human beings is action and on the importance of relationship. In general, patients who can be helped to appraise the multitude of physical and psychological stressors as a challenge rather than a threat tend to cope better (87). Those who acquire pain stress management skills experience less psychiatric comorbidity.

PAIN IN CANCER: PSYCHOSOCIAL AND VOCATIONAL IMPACTS

For cancer patients, pain is a subjective, multidimensional experience that affects the quality of their life. Cancer pain involves nociceptive, physical experience, as well as personality, affect, cognition, behavior, and social relationships. A considerable body of scientific knowledge supports the view that cancer pain is multidimensional. Despite empirical evidence that psychosocial variables play a substantial role in coping and quality of life, relatively few studies delineate the degree to which these factors exert their influence. Holland and Roland (88) point out that coping with anxieties (e.g., fear of death), pain, disfigurement, disability, financial hardships, and disruption of relationships do exert an influence on pain behavior, but this relationship varies widely among individuals and is modulated by both premorbid functioning and the meaning of the disease in the lifespan of the patient. The social isolation caused by disfigurement is a central variable requiring professional attention (89).

Quality of life is a major issue for cancer patients. It is operationally defined here as the sense of physical and psychological well-being across the multiple functional domains of a cancer patient's life. Physical well being is affected by pain and impacts the individual's ability to accomplish activities of daily living, work, mobility, body image, and the patient's appraisal of the attention-capturing signals of pain, all of which impact self-esteem, body image, and the ability to maintain the balance of family and vocational pursuits. Psychologic well-being can be impaired when pain negatively impacts coping skills; this increases the likelihood of occurrence of affective disturbances such as anxiety disorders and depression. Social support networks, family stability, and financial status also can be compromised by cancer pain (90).

Although pain accounts for a substantial amount of the variance in the psychosocial and vocational functioning of cancer patients, it is difficult to isolate pain when assessing quality of life. There are many areas of functioning that negatively impact cancer patients (88,91). Many instruments that measure this do not include an assessment of pain, and many of the measures of pain intensity and quality do not address the relationship between pain and its effects on quality of life for this group of patients. However, pain is only one of a number of distressing symptoms.

Many studies found that pain is a prevalent symptom for cancer patients (88,90,91). These authors indicate that pain is a significant factor for 30 to 50 percent of patients receiving surgery, radiation, and/or chemotherapy. Portenoy and Hagen (90) found pain prevalence greater than 90 percent in some groups of cancer patients in advanced stages of the disease.

Pain severity affects quality of psychosocial and vocational functioning. Patients with perceptions of pain as mild to moderate in intensity generally experienced little interference in functioning. By contrast, those patients who perceive their pain as being of equal or greater than anticipated intensity experience disproportionately greater interference in their functioning (88). Decline is minimal when pain intensity is low, but increases rapidly when intensity increases. It follows then, that interference with physical, psychologic, and social functioning occurs only when pain intensity is substantially elevated. Rather than increasing anxiety and diminishing cooperation, accurate information about anticipated pain levels permits cancer patients to prepare to cope, thus increasing their perceived sense of control. Because perceived control decreases pain experience, accurately informed patients are able to cope more effectively with less psychologic comorbidity.

Although it is generally assumed that the relationship between pain severity and quality of life is inverse, patient perceptions and cognitions about pain can influence the intensity of pain experience and the degree of consequent distress. Ventafridda et al. (92) found that patients treated by an interdisciplinary team in a continuing care program that dealt with psychosocial issues and coping had a better quality of life than those managed by family at home.

It is important to note that perception of the degree of pain experienced is exacerbated by negative mood states such as depression. Patients with pain and fatigue, pain and confusional state, and pain and physical disability tend to have increased pain experience (93,94).

The relationship between pain severity and psychosocial and vocational functioning does not appear to be linear. In a large survey examining the relationship between pain intensity and quality of life, Daut and Cleeland (95) found that there tends to be an inverse relationship between pain intensity and degree of interference in psychosocial and vocational functioning. Meta-analytic studies indicate a complex relationship between psychologic distress and pain experience in this patient population. Fishman (89) found that perceived relief of pain, rather than pain intensity, is a significant intervening variable. Depression and activity levels are found to be more related to the perception of pain relief than pain intensity per se (96).

Another aspect of pain that affects many cancer patients is the extent to which it is chronic. Relevant factors include duration, course (improving or ameliorating), expectation of increase or decrease, and temporal expectation of improvement. The perceived meaning of pain impacts the intensity of the pain experience and is hypothesized to affect quality of life. This is especially cogent as it applies to the meaning conveyed (i.e., signaling the progression of the disease).

Adequate management of the cancer patient combines comfort and function to minimize disruption in psychosocial and vocational functioning. This requires a combination of anticancer therapy and cancer pain management. Levy (97) posits that both share profit from prevention, early detection, specific therapy, adequate dose intensity, combinations of treatment modalities, and psychosocial support. He asserts that effective control of cancer pain is easily achievable with an inter-disciplinary team approach.

Psychologic variables that affect coping with cancer pain are psychologic har-diness, learned resourcefulness, locus of control, and the nature of attributions (i.e., internal versus external) that patients make, all of which influence pain behavior. Some of these are modifiable traits and some are acquirable skills. In any case, psychologic variables must be taken into account in planning pain management strategies for each patient depending on whether the target is a time-limited aversive procedure (e.g., bone marrow aspiration), recurrent, or chronic cancer pain. Cognitive informational style—monitoring versus blunt-ing—is an important variable to take into account when examining indications for treatment (98). In other words, knowledge about whether the patient's cop-ing style is to seek information or to avoid it can provide key information to directing optimum patient management. Some examples of psychologic treat-ment options are relaxation training alone, relaxation and imagery, hypnosis, or distraction strategies.

As noted above, according to Lazarus and Folkman (87), perceived control moderates pain experience and enhances coping. The combined use of Patient Control Anesthesias (PCAs) and cognitive and behavioral therapies reduces pain experience and thus the suffering it causes. These procedures enhance perceived control and efficacy. Enhanced efficacy in turn has a positive effect on activity level, self-esteem, social interaction, and the ability to maintain normalcy to the greatest extent possible.

Some patients can become distressed when their pain is alleviated. This tends to occur when (*a*) patients are motivated by secondary gain (e.g., they are able to secure family support only when they suffer), (*b*) patients' denial depends on a focus on pain symptomatology versus disease, and (*c*) patients are inappropriately fearful of addiction to analgesic or opioids (99).

Pain in patients with some types of cancer has a particular impact on quality of life. According to Stonnington (100), for patients born with bone tumors, pain and quality of life can also become associated with other factors such as impair-ment, disability, and handicap. Restriction of activity or function caused by the patient's impairment (e.g., inability to ambulate) can lead to muscle atrophy and deconditioning, as well as further pain when the patient attempts to use those deconditioned muscles.

In summary, contemporary clinical issues relating to managing the patient with cancer pain strongly emphasize cognitive-behavioral, psychosocial, and pharma-cologic strategies in concert. Each intervention, best planned and executed by an interdisciplinary team, offers unique contributions that benefit patient care. A bet-ter understanding of the disease (for patients and their support systems), knowing what to expect, and having a range of coping strategies in confronting and adjust-ing to the pain while preserving balance in the various domains of their lives con-stitute important factors that help cancer patients deal with the psychosocial and vocational issues confronting them.

PAIN IN SPINAL CORD INJURY: PSYCHOSOCIAL AND VOCATIONAL IMPACT

Depression, decline in quality of life, and other psychosocial changes following spinal cord injury (SCI) have been well documented (101), as has the vocational impact of SCI (102). Psychosocial and vocational issues may often interact to compound post-SCI adjustment. For instance, depression may severely compromise job performance, while loss of employment may contribute to a sense of worthlessness.

The prevalence of moderate to severe chronic pain among SCI patients varies widely, from 27 to 77 percent depending on the study being referenced (103). Although there is no consensus concerning the clinical and functional significance of such pain for SCI patients, several studies have shown that distress caused by pain is over and above that associated with the spinal cord injury itself (104).

Older age has been associated with increased prevalence of pain (104). Anger and negative cognition, less acceptance of disability status, and punishing response from significant others appear to lead to greater pain severity (101). Although only recently depicted in the literature as an area of concern, the psychosocial impact of chronic pain on SCI patients has increasingly become a significant additional challenge to their management. When surveyed, SCI patients with chronic pain were found to be more psychosocially impaired than those without chronic pain (105). Pain in SCI is believed to cause more severe disability than the paralysis resulting from the SCI (103).

Pain and depression appear to develop over time following SCI injury. For instance, pain and depression were shown to be independent of each other on admission to an inpatient treatment facility. However, as the course of hospitalization continued, a strong relationship seemed to evolve, with pain having a greater impact on depression than vice versa (106).

Psychosocial difficulties of SCI patients with pain include anxiety, fatigue, loneliness, depression, drug abuse, and social and family problems (107). Several studies have shown that psychosocial variables predict subjective pain severity and compromised activities of daily living (ADL) better than any medical or demographic factors (108). The association of chronic pain with psychosocial impairment appears to hold up even after controlling for the correlation of pain with other medical problems and higher levels of injury (109).

In reviewing the literature on depression following SCI, Boekamp et al. (110) proposed using the diathesis–stress model to identify SCI patients at increased risk for depression. These authors suggest that social support and recent stressors should be routinely assessed to identify patients at high risk for depression. Fostering independence, encouraging patients to develop new sources of self-esteem, and encouraging family members to mutually provide a supportive environment should be among the focus of intervention.

Several investigators (111,112) have advocated a biopsychosocial treatment approach to SCI pain and associated psychosocial issues using a multidisciplinary team format with patient self-management as the goal of intervention. Cairns (106) indicates that reducing pain has a greater effect on reducing depression than vice versa. This approach would suggest that interventions aimed at treating psychosocial problems such as depression would be more successful if there is a concurrent effort to treat the pain symptoms.

Very little has been published concerning the vocational impact of pain in SCI patients although several studies have examined the vocational impact of SCI itself (101,102,113).

PAIN AND SEXUAL FUNCTIONING

An often overlooked and neglected area of psychosocial issues in rehabilitation has been the effects of chronic pain and other physical and psychologic compromises exerted on the patient's sexual functioning. A recent study by Monga et al. (114) found that only 20 percent of chronic pain patients consider their current sexual life to be adequate. Furthermore, it was found that patients who reported symptoms of depression and distress had more sexual problems. The most powerful predictor of sexual functioning was found to be control appraisal, that is, how much control patients perceive they have over their pain and their life. Previous studies (115–117) have found similar but lower rates of sexual problems.

In another recent study, Tan et al. (118) investigated the relationship between sexual functioning, age, and depression. Using the method of structural equation modeling, these authors found that age and sexual functioning were inversely correlated as expected. For chronic pain patients, however, depression adversely affected satisfaction but not their drive or interest in or frequency of sexual activities.

The effect of pain on sexual functioning with other rehabilitation populations has not been systematically researched. An exception was the study of sexuality in head and neck cancer patients (119), which found a higher rate of satisfaction with sexual functioning as compared to the chronic pain patients (49 versus 20 percent). However, the effect of pain was not partialled out from that attributable to the cancer itself.

The role of psychosocial factors on sexual dysfunction among the rehabilitation population has been described by Tan and Bostick (120). Stressing that the sexual concerns of this population do not differ significantly from the general population, these authors argued that psychosocial and sexual functioning are so highly intertwined that any attempt to address psychosocial rehabilitation must include issues related to sexual functioning. Elements of a comprehensive program aimed at addressing these issues were presented for the rehabilitation population.

SPECIAL ISSUES IN PEDIATRIC REHABILITATION

Although much research is available on pediatric pain management and coping, little long-term longitudinal data is available on children's psychosocial and educational functioning following painful illness or treatment. Emerging new conceptualizations of pain, integrated with current knowledge of child development, suggest new approaches for those clinicians working with children facing pain and fear in rehabilitation settings.

Current conceptualizations of pain and recent research with children in stressful medical situations suggest that it is usually most helpful to maximize the child's active involvement in her own care to increase both the perception and the reality of control (79). To do this, the child's developmental status must be considered. A child's appraisal of pain and her coping vs. catastrophizing responses to it are determined in large part by her cognitive developmental status. The child's level of social development and the interactional contexts in which pain often occurs also determine her experience of pain. The child's distress and the clinician's response are multidimensionally influenced by physiologic, cognitive, social, and cultural factors (121,122). This model dictates that children in pain are best served by a collaborative approach between patient and provider, in which the child is an essential and active participant in her own care.

Depending on their cognitive-developmental maturation, children may manifest their pain experience through behavior rather than verbalization. Behaviors that seem maladaptive and out of control, such as crying and complaining, may in fact represent organized and appropriate coping behavior on the part of the child who appraises a situation as threatening. Thus, the child may perceive that her only resource for coping with a situational threat is a parent who will rescue her if a sufficient level of distress is communicated (79). A two-factor model that separates the intensity of pain from its negative affective characteristics (e.g., suffering) may be helpful. Visual analog scales may be used by the skilled clinician to assess these factors separately in children as young as seven years of age. Prior to this age, global self-report of pain is generally practical with children as young as four (123). It is the affective, more than the sensory component of pain, that appears to be substantially influenced by the pain's perceived meaning (124,125) including its perceived controllability (79,126). Pain and psychosocial distress are closely intertwined among children going through rehabilitation for their medical conditions, perhaps more so than for their adult counterparts.

Additionally, systemic levels of interventions are recommended to augment traditional individual approaches. A child's coping with pain is heavily influenced by the stressors and challenges posed by school, peers, and family, and is affected powerfully by the interpersonal interactions that take place between adults and children in these situations. Treatment focus should move beyond exclusive attention to the young patient, to attend to the modification of interactional patterns involving the child and others in those settings(127).

Informed clinical practice therefore requires that children's pain and coping be understood within an interactional and a developmental context. Folkman and Lazarus' appraisal-based model of coping (87) provides a useful basis for this conceptualization.

Research suggests that engaging children as active participants in their treatment enhances control perceptions and reduces trauma sequelae and adjustment problems. Kavanaugh (128) has reported that providing children with information and maximizing their opportunities to predict and control painful procedures has significant positive effects on their adjustment when undergoing treatment for severe burns. Tarnowski and his colleagues (129) investigated self-mediated debridement in a single-subject design with a severely burned 12-year-old. The child was allowed to debride himself in the hydrotherapy tank under the supervision of a physical therapist. Although this took longer than therapist-administered debridement, it was verified that the debridement was completed thoroughly and no other complications were noted. A clinically significant reduction in observed behavioral distress was reported, and the self-mediated approach was greatly preferred by the child. This is a compelling example of the potential for this approach.

OTHER REHABILITATION PATIENT POPULATIONS

Traumatic brain injury and its psychosocial and vocational sequelae have been widely researched (130–132). Although not entirely understood, psychiatric symptoms creating difficulties in psychosocial and vocational functioning are believed to be caused by both neurologic changes, exacerbation of premorbid psychological difficulties (133), and exposure to overwhelming stress, including catastrophic traumatic events (particularly those involving loss of gross or fine motor functioning) (134). Posttraumatic stress disorder (PTSD) is the most prevalent. When untreated or overlooked, these psychosocial sequelae can seriously impede rehabilitation efforts (134–136). Adverse, long-term impact on employment and productivity has been documented (131,137).

Pain symptoms such as chronic headaches and musculoskeletal pain are common sequelae of TBI. Unfortunately, there has been no study testing the effect of pain (as opposed to the trauma itself) on the patient's psychosocial and vocational functioning.

Pain is a common complaint following a stroke. Poststroke pain can be either centrally mediated, peripheral in nature, or secondary to overall medical condition (138). However, there has been no known published study examining the psychosocial and vocational impact of poststroke pain.

Similarly, postamputation pain is quite common and phantom limb pain has received increasing attention in rehab medicine (139). However, very little has been published on how such a pain influences psychosocial and vocational rehabilitation. One study (140) comparing postamputation pain with musculoskeletal pain found that amputees who reported significant pain (34 percent of the amputees group) showed a higher level of overall disability than patients with chronic musculoskeletal pain. This group also showed significantly greater disability than those amputees who reported only low-level pain. The authors conclude that, contrary to common perception, 25 percent of the patients showed no significant evidence of psychopathology. Mild anxiety and depression were present in slightly more than 50 percent of the subjects in this study.

Peripheral neuropathies can cause severe debilitating pain and cases of compulsive targeted self-injurious behavior have been reported (140). Unfortunately, the psychosocial and vocational impact of pain associated with these conditions has not been researched.

Sixty-four percent of patients attending a multiple sclerosis (MS) clinic reported pain symptoms at some time during the course of the disease (141). This

survey also found that female MS respondents were more likely to report pain
and significantly higher levels of pain intensity than their male counterparts;
among those with pain complaint, 49 percent reported difficulty performing their
job, 44 percent reported difficulty sleeping, 34 percent reported turmoil in their
interpersonal relationship, and 4 percent stated they have never been pain free.
Other studies found that the suicidal risk for MS patients was higher than the
general population (142); MS patients with pain showed poorer mental health
and more social-role conflict (143) and a greater number of initial symptoms
than those without pain (144).

GUIDELINES ON INTERVENTIONS

Interventions targeted at eliminating or reducing the adverse effects of psychosocial and vocational issues through rehabilitation have been previously discussed
within each of the rehabilitation populations included in this chapter.
Interventions can aim at:

- increasing patient's ability to cope with pain;
- reducing or reversing the adverse effects of psychosocial problems such as
  depression; or
- a combination of the above.

In a review article on coping with chronic pain, Jensen et al. (12), conclude
that there is good evidence to support the statement that "patients who believe
they can control their pain, who avoid catastrophizing about their condition, and
who believe they are not severely disabled appear to function better than those
who do not" (pp 1). Although the role played by coping strategies is less clear
because of methodologic problems with many of the studies reviewed, what is
clear from the authors' review is that coping strategies appear to be associated
with adjustment to chronic pain. For example, studies have linked active coping
strategies with adaptive outcome measures, whereas passive coping strategies
have been linked with maladaptive outcome measures such as increased pain and
depression (145–147). Similarly, behavioral coping strategies such as guarding,
and cognitive coping strategies such as catastrophizing, have been associated
with increased disability and depression respectively (148). The cognitive-behavioral approaches to pain management and management of psychosocial problems
have been cited throughout this chapter.

In *Psychosocial Factors in Pain* (149), Turk and Gatchel delineated three critical elements to successful pain management: acceptance of treatment, motivation
for self-management, and treatment adherence (150). A relapse-prevention model
to address the problem of long-term maintenance can be integrated within a cognitive-behavioral treatment program (151). Turk and Gatchel (149) also contains
many chapters of specific interest to clinicians involved in the rehabilitation of
patients with chronic pain covering, for instance, prevention with special reference to chronic musculoskeletal disorders, back pain, and cancer pain.

CONCLUSIONS

It should be clear by now that successful rehabilitation must address both pain and its psychosocial and vocational issues. Addressing one and not the other is likely to compromise the likelihood of success. A recent finding that perceived control over the *effects* of pain in one's life and perceived control over life in general were more strongly associated with adaptive functioning than the perceptions of control over pain itself further testify to the importance of addressing the psychosocial aspects of pain (152). Tan et al. (153) provide some guidelines for clinically managing chronic pain. Referral to and the involvement of a multidisciplinary pain management program or team should be considered when routine pain management treatment fails to get positive results.

In addition to cognitive behavioral approaches, hypnosis, biofeedback, operant conditioning, relaxation training, and various psychotherapies and support groups have been successfully utilized in the treatment of chronic pain and related psychosocial problems (1). The effective treatment of depression, perhaps the most prevalent psychosocial problem related to chronic pain, is widely available in the form of antidepressant medications, psychotherapy, or a combination of both. Newer and promising treatment procedures in the management of chronic pain and related psychosocial problems such as electroencephalogram (EEG) biofeedback (154), and an individualized stepped-care approach for managing pain in primary care (151) should be integrated into a broader framework that addresses the psychosocial and vocational issues in rehabilitation.

REFERENCES

1. Gatchel RJ, Turk DC: *Psychological Approaches to Pain Management.* New York: Guilford Press, 1996.
2. Chapman CR, Cox GB. Anxiety, pain, and depression surrounding elective surgery: A multivariate comparison of abdominal surgery patients with kidney donors and recipients. *J Psychosomatic Res*, 1977; 21(7).
3. Sarafino EP. *Health Psychology: Biopsychosocial Interactions*, 3rd ed. New York: Wiley, 1998.
4. Jones SE. Effect of psychological processes on chronic pain. *Br J Nurs*, 1993; 2: 463–464, 466–467.
5. Parsons T. Definitions of health and illness in the light of American values and social structure. In Jaco, EJ ed., *Patients, Physicians, and Illness.* New York: Springer-Verlag, 1958, p. 3–29.
6. Jamison RN, et al. Cognitive-behavioral classification of chronic pain: Replication and extension of empirically-derived patient profiles. *Pain*, 1994; 57: 233–239.
7. Talo S. *Psychological Assessment of Function in Chronic Low Back Pain Patients.* Turku, Finland: Social Insurance Institute, 1992.
8. Turk DC, Rudy TE. Toward an empirically derived taxonomy of chronic pain patients: Integration of psychological assessment data. *J Consulting Clin Psychol*, 1988; 56: 233–238.
9. Turk DC, Rudy TE. Robustness of an empirically derived taxonomy of chronic pain patients. *Pain*, 1990; 43: 27–36.
10. Walter L, Brannon LA. A cluster analysis of the Multidimensional Pain Inventory. *Headache*, 1991; 31: 476–479.

11. Von Korff M, Dworkin S, LeResche L. Graded chronic pain status: An epidemiologic evaluation. *Pain*, 1990; 40: 279–291.
12. Jensen MP, Turner JA, Romano JM. Coping with chronic pain: A critical review of the literature. *Pain*, 1991; 47: 249–283.
13. Flor H, Turk DC. Chronic back pain and rheumatoid arthritis: Predicting pain and disability from cognitive variables. *J Behavioral Med*, 1988; 11: 251–265.
14. Jensen MP, Turner JA, Romano JM. Correlates of improvement in multidisciplinary treatment of chronic pain. *J Consulting Clin Psychol*, 1994; 62: 172–179.
15. Tota-Fawcette ME, et al. Predictors of response to pain management treatment: The role of family environment and changes in cognitive processes. *Clin J Pain*, 1993; 9: 115–123.
16. Spiegel D, Bloom JR. Pain in metastatic breast cancer. *Cancer*, 1983; 52: 341–345.
17. Council JR, et al. Expectancies and functional impairment in chronic low back pain. *Pain*, 1988; 33: 323–331.
18. Slater MA, et al. Pain and impairment beliefs in chronic low back pain: Validation of the Pain and Impairment Relationship Scale (PAIRS). *Pain*, 1991; 44: 51–56.
19. Leventhal H, Everhart D. Emotion, pain and physical illness. In Izard, CE, ed., *Emotion and psychopathology*. New York: Plenum 1979; p. 263–299.
20. Mizener D, Thomas M, Billings R. Cognitive changes of migraineurs receiving biofeedback training. *Headache*, 1988; 28: 339–343.
21. Turk DC, Salovey P. Chronic pain as a variant of depressive disease: A critical reappraisal. *J Nervous Mental Dis*, 1984; 172: 398–404.
22. Turk DC, Okifuji A, Scharff L. Assessment of older women with chronic pain. *J Women and Aging*, 1994; 6: 25–42.
23. Turk DC, Okifuji A, Scharff L. Chronic pain and depression: Role of perceived impact and perceived control in different age cohorts. *Pain*, 1995; 61: 93–102.
24. Kerns RD, Rosenberg R, Jacob MC. Anger expression and chronic pain. *J Behavioral Med*, 1994; 17: 57–68.
25. Bandura A, et al. Catecholamine secretion as a function of perceived coping self-efficacy. *J Consulting Clin Psychol*, 1985; 53: 406–414.
26. Bandura A, et al. Perceived self-efficacy and pain control: Opioid and nonopioid mechanisms. *J Personality Soc Psychol*, 1987; 53: 563–571.
27. Flor H, et al. Symptom-specific psycho-physiological responses in chronic pain patients. *Psychophysiology*, 1992; 29: 452–460.
28. Costello R, Schoenfeld L, Ramamurthy S. Sociodemographic and clinical correlates of P-A-I-N. *J Psychosomatic Res*, 1989; 33: 315–321.
29. Jackson T, Iezzi A, Lafreniere K. Differential effects of employment status on chronic pain and healthy comparison groups. *International J Behavioral Med*, 1996; 3: 359–371.
30. Sandstrom J. Clinical and social factors in rehabilitation of patients with chronic low back pain. *Scand J Rehab Med*, 1986; 18: 35–43.
31. Cairns D, Mooney V, Crane P. Spinal pain rehabilitation: inpatient and outpatient treatment results and development of predictors for outcome. *Spine*, 1984; 9: 91–95.
32. Tollison C. Comprehensive treatment approach for lower back workers' compensation injuries. *J Occupat Rehab*, 1991; 1: 281–287.
33. Jahoda M. *Employment and Unemployment: A Social-Psychological Analysis*. Cambridge: Cambridge University, 1982.
34. Jackson T, et al. Relations of employment status to emotional distress among chronic pain patients: A path analysis. *Clin J Pain*, 1998; 14: 55–60.
35. Fisbain DA, et al. The prediction of return to the workplace after multidisciplinary pain center treatment. *Clin J Pain*, 1993; 9: 3–15.
36. McKenna F, Wright V. Pain and rheumatoid arthritis. *Ann Rheum Dis*, 1985; 44: 805.
37. Creed F, Murphy S, Jayson MV. Measurement of psychiatric disorder in rheumatoid arthritis. *J Psychosomatic Res*, 1990; 34: 79–87.

38. Frank RG, Beck NC, Parker JC. Depression in rheumatoid arthritis. *J Rheumatology*, 1988; 15: 920–925.

39. Hawley DJ, Wolfe F. Anxiety and depression patients with rheumatoid arthritis: A prospective study of 400 patients. *J Rheumatology*, 1988; 15: 932–941.

40. Lichtenberg PA, Swensen CH, MW S. Further investigation of the role of personality lifestyle and arthritic severity in predicting pain. *J Psychosomatic Res*, 1986; 30: 327–337.

41. Lichtenberg PA, Skehan MW, Swensen CH. The role of personality, recent life stress, and arthritic severity in predicting pain. *J Psychosomatic Res*, 1984; 28: 231–236.

42. Parker JC, et al. Pain in rheumatoid arthritis: relationship to demographic, medical, and psychological factors. *J Rheumatology*, 1988; 15: 433–437.

43. Smith TW, et al. Cognitive distortion in rheumatoid arthritis: relation to depression and disability. *J Consulting Clin Psychol*, 1988; 56: 412–416.

44. Smith TW, Peck JR, Ward JR. Helplessness and depression in rheumatoid arthritis. *Health Psychology*, 1990; 9: 377–389.

45. Affleck G, et al. Attributional processes in rheumatoid arthritis patients. *Arthritis and Rheumatism*, 1987; 30: 927–931.

46. Parker JC, Wright GE. The implications of depression for pain and disability in rheumatoid arthritis. *Arthritis Care and Research*, 1995; 8: 279–283.

47. Romano JM, Turner JA. Chronic pain and depression: Does the evidence support a relationship? *Psychol Bull*, 1985; 97: 18–34.

48. Nicassio PM, Wallston KA. Longitudinal relationships among pain, sleep problems, and depression in rheumatoid arthritis. *J Abnormal Psychol*, 1992; 101: 514–520.

49. Brown GK. A causal analysis of chronic pain and depression. *J Abnormal Psychol*, 1990; 99: 127–137.

50. Parker JC, et al. Psychological factors, immunologic activation, and disease activity in rheumatoid arthritis. *Arthritis Care and Research*, 1992; 5: 196–201.

51. Fifield J, Reisine ST, Grady K. Work disability and the experience of pain and depression in rheumatoid arthritis. *Soc Sci Med*, 1992; 33: 5.

52. Fawcett JA. Depression in painful chronic disorders: the role of pain and conflict about pain. *J Pain and Symptom Mgmt*, 1994; 9: 520–526.

53. Dekker J, et al. Pain and disability in osteoarthritis: A review of bio-behavioral mechanisms. *J Behavioral Med*, 1992; 15: 189–214.

54. Hopman-Rock M, et al. Physical and psychosocial disability in elderly subjects in relation to pain in the hip and/or knee. *J Rheumatology*, 1996; 23: 1037–1044.

55. Hopman-Rock M, Kraaimaat FW, Bijlsma JW. Quality of life in elderly subjects with pain in the hip or knee. *Quality of Life Research*, 1997; 6: 67–76.

56. Felts W, Yelin E. The economic impact of the rheumatic diseases in the United States. *J Rheumatology*, 1988; 16: 867–884.

57. Reisine ST, et al. Work disability among women with rheumatoid arthritis. *Arthritis and Rheumatism*, 1989; 32: 538–543.

58. Schoenfeld-Smith K, et al. A biopsychosocial model of disability in rheumatoid arthritis. *Arthritis Care and Research*, 1996; 9: 368–375.

59. Truckenbrodt H. Pain in juvenile chronic arthritis: Consequences for the musculoskeletal system. *Clin Experimental Rheumatol*, 1993; 11: 59–63.

60. Buckelew SP, Parker JC. Coping with arthritis pain: A review of the literature. *Arthritis Care and Research*, 1989; 2: 136–145.

61. Keefe FJ, Van Horn Y. Cognitive-behavioral treatment of rheumatoid arthritis pain: maintaining treatment gains. *Arthritis Care and Research*, 1993; 6: 213–222.

62. Bradley LA. Behavioral interventions for managing chronic pain. Comment. *Bull Rheumatol Dis*, 1994; 43: 2–5.

63. Bradley LA, et al. Effects of psychological therapy on pain behavior of rheumatoid arthritis patients. Treatment outcome and six-month follow-up. *Arthritis and Rheumatism*, 1987; 30: 1105–1114.

64. Choiniere M. Pain of Burns. In Wall, PD, Melzack, R, eds., *Textbook of Pain*. London: Churchill Livingstone, 1994, p. 523–537.

65. Wall PD. On the relationship of injury to pain. *Pain*, 1979; 6: 253–264.

66. Andreasen NJC, et al. Management of emotional reactions in seriously burned adults. *N Eng J Med*, 1972; 286: 65–69.

67. Konigova R. The psychological problems of burned patients. The Rudy Hermans Lecture, 1991; 18: 189–199.

68. Osgood PF, Szyfelbein SK. Management of burn pain in children. *Pediat Clin N Am*, 1989; 36: 1991–1013.

69. Rosenbaum M. *Learned Resourcefulness*. 1990.

70. Steiner H, Clark WR. Psychiatric complications of burned adults: A classification. *J Trauma*, 1977; 17: 134–143.

71. Watkins PN, et al. Psychological stages in adaptation following burn injury: A method for facilitating psychological recovery of burn victims. *J Burn Care and Rehab*, 1988; 9: 376–384.

72. Watkins PN, et al. The role of the psychiatrist in the team treatment of the adult patient with burns. *J Burn Care and Rehab*, 1992; 13: 19–27.

73. Charlton JE, et al. Factors affecting pain in burned patients—A preliminary report. *Postgraduate Medical Journal*, 1983; 59: 604–607.

74. Blakeney P, Herndon D. Long-term psychological adjustment following burn injury. *J Burn Care and Rehab*. 1988; 9: 661–665.

75. Schoenberg B, et al. *Loss and Grief: Psychological Management in Medical Practice*. New York: Columbia University Press, 1970.

76. Tarnowski KJ. Behavioral aspects of pediatric burns. In Roberts MC, Peterson L, eds., *Issues in Clinical Child Psychology*. New York: Plenum, 1994.

77. Blumenfeld M, Schoeps MM. *Psychological Care of the Burn and Trauma Patient*. Baltimore: Williams & Wilkins, 1993.

78. Tempereau C, Grossman RA, Brones. Psychological regression and marital status: Determinants in psychiatric management of burn victims. *J Burn Care and Rehab*, 1987; 8: 286–291.

79. Bush JP, Harkins SW. Conceptual foundations: Pain and child development. In Bush JP, Harkins SW, eds., *Children in Pain: Clinical and Research Issues from a Developmental Perspective*. New York: Springer-Verlag, p. 1–30, 1991.

80. Patterson DR. Burn pain. In Barber J, ed., *Hypnosis and Suggestion in the Treatment of Pain*. New York: W. W. Norton & Co., p. 267–302, 1996.

81. Meichenbaum D, Turk D. The cognitive behavioral management of anxiety, anger, and pain. In Davidson PO, ed., *The Behavioral Management of Anxiety, Depression, and Pain*. New York: Brunner/Mazel, 1976.

82. Freund PR, Marvin JA. Post burn pain. In Bonica JJ, ed., *The Management of Pain*. Philadelphia: Lea & Febiger, 1990.

83. Patterson DR. Practical applications of psychological techniques in controlling burn pain. *J Burn Care and Rehab*, 1992; 13: 13–18.

84. McGrath P. *Pain in Children*. New York: Guilford Press, 1990.

85. Bernstein NR, O'Connell K, Chekel D. Patterns of burn adjustment. *J Burn Care and Rehab*, 1992; 13: 4–12.

86. Partridge J. *Changing Faces*. Vol. London: Plenum Press, 1991.

87. Lazarus RS, Folkman S. *Stress, Appraisal, and Coping*. New York: Springer, 1984.

88. Holland JC, Rowland J, eds. *Handbook of Psycho-Oncology: Psychological Care of the Patient with Cancer*. New York: Oxford University Press, 1989.

89. Fishman B. The treatment of suffering in patients with cancer pain: Cognitive behavioral approaches. In Foley KM, Bonica JJ, Ventafridda V, eds., *Second Annual Congress on Cancer Pain: Advances in Pain Research and Therapy*. New York: Raven Press, 1990, p. 301–316.

90. Portenoy RK, Hagen NA. Breakthrough pain: Definition, prevalence, and characteristics. *Pain*, 1990; 41: 273–281.

91. Ahles TA, Blanchard EB, Ruckdeschel JC. The multidimensional nature of cancer related pain. *Pain*, 1983; 17: 277–288.

92. Ventafridda V, et al. A validation study of the WHO method for cancer pain relief. *Cancer*, 1987; 59: 851–856.

93. Bukberg J, Penman D, Holland J. Depression in hospitalized cancer patients. *Psychosomatic Med*, 1984; 43: 199–222.

94. Derogatis LR, et al. The prevalence of psychiatric disorders among cancer patients. *JAMA*, 1983; 249: 741–757.

95. Daut RL, Cleeland CS. The prevalence and severity of pain in cancer. *Cancer*, 1982; 1913–1918.

96. Saltzburg D, et al. The relationship of pain and depression to suicidal ideation in cancer patients. ASCO Annual Meeting 1989, ASCO: San Francisco.

97. Levy MH. Effective integration of pain management into comprehensive cancer care. *Postgraduate Medical Journal*, 1991; 67: 35–43.

98. Miller SM. To see or not to see: Cognitive informational styles in the coping process. In Rosenbaum M, ed., *Learned Resourcefulness: On Coping Skills, Self-control, and Adaptive Behavior.* New York: Springer Publishing, 1990, p. 95–126.

99. Breitbart W, Passik SD, Rosenfeld BD. Psychiatric and psychosocial aspects of cancer pain. In Wall PD, Melzack R, eds., *Textbook of Pain.* Edinburgh: Churchill Livingstone, 1995, p. 825–860.

100. Stonnington HH. Diagnosis and treatment of bone tumors: A team approach. In Stonnington HH, ed., *Rehabilitation.* Thorofare N.J.: Slack, Inc., 1983.

101. Krause JS. Adjustment after spinal cord injury: A 9–year longitudinal study. *Arch Physical Med Rehab*, 1997; 78: 651–657.

102. Fiedler I, Indermuehle D. Barriers to employment in spinal cord injury. S Ueda, R Nakamura, S Ishigami, eds., The 8th World Congress of the International Rehabilitation Medicine Association. Monduzzi Editore, 1997, p. 807–12.

103. Britell WW, Mariano AJ. Chronic pain in spinal cord injury. In *Physical Medicine and Rehabilitation: State of the Art Reviews*, 1991.

104. Anke AG, Stenehjem AE, Stanghelle JK. Pain and life quality within 2 years of spinal cord injury. *Paraplegia*, 1995; 33: 555–559.

105. Morrison GE, et al. Post stroke pain: Treatment in a community hospital. *Arch Physical Med Rehab*, 1989; 69: 203–209.

106. Cairns DM, Adkins RH, Scott MD. Pain and depression in acute traumatic spinal cord injury: Origins of chronic problematic pain? *Arch Physical Med Rehab*, 1996; 77: 329–335.

107. Britell WW, et al. Problem survey in SCI outpatient clinic population: A case of multi-faceted, ongoing care. *Arch Physical Med Rehab*, 1986; 67: 654.

108. Richards JS. Chronic pain and spinal cord injury: Review and comment. *Clin J Pain.* 1992. p. 119–122.

109. Mariano A, Britell CW, Umlauf R. Chronic pain and the psychosocial functioning of spinal cord injured patients (paper presentation). Society of Rehabilitative Medicine, 1989.

110. Boekamp JR, Overholser JC, Schubert DS. Depression following a spinal cord injury. *Internat J Psychiatry Med*, 1996; 26: 329–349.

111. Mariano AJ. Chronic pain and spinal cord injury. *Clin J Pain*, 1992; 8: 87–92.

112. Umlauf RL. Psychological interventions for chronic pain following spinal cord injury. *Clin J Pain*, 1992; 8: 111–118.

113. DeVito MJ, et al. Employment after spinal cord injury. *Arch Physical Med Rehab*, 1987; 68: 494–498.

114. Monga TN, et al. Sexuality and sexual adjustment of patients with chronic pain. *Disability and Rehabilitation*, 1998; 20: 317–329.

115. Maruta T, Osborne D. Sexual activity in chronic pain patients. *Psychosomatics*, 1978; 20: 241–248.
116. Osborne D, Maruta T. Sexual adjustment and chronic back pain. *Medical Aspects of Human Sex*, 1980; 14: 94–113.
117. Sjogren K, Fugl-Meyer AR. Chronic back pain and sexuality. *International Rehabilitation Medicine*, 1981; 3: 19–25.
118. Tan G, et al. Sexual functioning, age, and depression revisited. *Sexuality and Disability*, 1998; 16: 77–86.
119. Monga U, et al. Sexuality in head and neck cancer patient. *Arch Physical Med Rehab*, 1997; 78: 298–304.
120. Tan G, Bostick R. Sexual dysfunction among those with disabling conditions; psychological determinants and interventions. In Monga TN, ed., *Sexuality and Disability, State of the Arts Review in Physical Medicine and Rehabilitation*. Philadelphia: Henley and Belfus, 1995.
121. Lipton J, Marbach J. Ethnicity and pain experience. *Scientific Medicine*, 1984; 19: 1279–1297.
122. Reid VJ, Bush JP. Ethnic factors influencing pain expression: Implications for clinical assessment. In Miller TW, ed., *Chronic Pain*. Madison, Conn.: International Universities Press, 1990.
123. Zeltzer LK, et al. A psychobiological approach to pediatric pain: Part 1 history, physiology, and assessment strategies. *Curr Problems Pediatr*, 1997; 26: 225–253.
124. Price DD, Harkins SW, Baker C. Sensory affective relationships among different types of clinical and experimental pain. *Pain*, 1987; 28: 297–307.
125. Siegel LJ, Smith KE. Children's strategies for dealing with pain. *Pediatrician*, 1989; 16: 110–118.
126. Rudolph KD, Dennig MD, Weisz SL. Discriminants and consequences of children's coping in the medical setting: Conceptualization, review, and critique. *Psychol Bull*, 1995; 118: 328–357.
127. Gilman JB, L. ML. Pediatric pain management: Professional and pragmatic issues. In Bush JP, Harkins SW, eds., *Children in Pain: Clinical and Research Issues from a Developmental Perspective*. New York: Springer-Verlag, 1991, p. 117–148.
128. Kavanaugh C. Psychological intervention with the severely burned child: Report of an experimental comparison of two approaches and their effects on psychological sequelae. *J Psychiatry*, 1983; 22: 145–156.
129. Tarnowski KJ, et al. Pediatric burn injury: Self versus therapist mediated debridement. *Pediatr Psychol*, 1987; 12: 567–579.
130. McAllister TW. Mild traumatic brain injury and post-concussive syndrome. In Silver JM, Yudofsky SC, Hales RE, eds., *Neuropsychiatry of Traumatic Brain Injury*. Washington, D.C.: American Psychiatric Press, 1994, p. 81–132.
131. Satz P, et al. Neuropsychological, psychosocial, and vocational correlates of Glasgow Outcome Scale at six months post-injury: A study of moderate to severe traumatic brain injury patients. *Brain Injury*, 1998; 12: 555–567.
132. Sherer M, et al. Characteristics of impaired awareness after traumatic brain injury. *J International Neuropsychol Soc*, 1998; 4: 380–387.
133. Tate RL. It is not only the kind of injury that matters, but the kind of head: The contribution of premorbid and psychosocial factors to rehabilitation outcomes after severe traumatic brain injury. *Neuropsychol Rehab*, 1998; 8: 1–18.
134. Bryant RA. Relationship between acute stress disorder and posttraumatic stress disorder following mild traumatic brain injury. *American J Psychiatry*, 1998; 155: 625–629.
135. Ohry A, Rattok J, Solomon Z. Post traumatic stress disorder in brain injury. *Brain Injury*, 1996; 10: 687–695.
136. Hickling EJ, et al. Traumatic brain injury and posttraumatic stress disorder: A preliminary investigation of neuropsychological test results in PTSD secondary to motor vehicle accidents. *Brain Injury*, 1998; 12: 265–274.

137. Sander AM, et al. A multicenter longitudinal investigation of return to work and community integration following brain injury. *J Head Trauma Rehab*, 1996; 11: 70–84.

138. Garrison RP. Mediation of post stroke pain. *American J Psychiatry*, 1998; 155: 233–246.

139. Sherman RA, et al. Phantom pain: A lesson in the necessity for careful clinical research on chronic pain problems. *J Rehab Res Dev*, 1988; 25: vii-x.

140. Marshall M, Helmes E, Deathe AB. A comparison of psychosocial functioning and personality in amputee and chronic pain populations. *Clin J Pain*, 1992; 8: 351–357.

141. Warnell P. The pain experience of a multiple sclerosis population: A descriptive study. *Axone*, 1991; 13: 26–28.

142. Stenager EN, Stenager E. Suicide and patients with neurologic diseases: Methodologic problems. *Arch Neurology*, 1992; 49: 1296–1303.

143. Archibald CJ, et al. Pain prevalence, severity and impact in a clinic sample of multiple sclerosis patients. *Pain*, 1994; 58: 89–93.

144. Sullivan MJ, et al. Depression before and after diagnosis of multiple sclerosis. *Multiple Sclerosis*, 1995; 1: 104–108.

145. Broome ME, et al. Children's medical fears, coping behaviors, and pain perceptions during a lumbar puncture. *Oncol Nurs Soc*, 1990; 17: 361–367.

146. Holmes JA, Stevenson CA. Differential effects of avoidant and attentional coping strategies on adaptation to chronic and recent-onset pain. *Health Psychology*, 1990; 9: 577–584.

147. Snow-Turek AL, Norris MP, Tan G. Active and passive coping dimensions in chronic pain patients (poster presentation). Texas Psychological Association Annual Convention, Houston, Tex., 1994.

148. Tan G, Jensen MP, Robinson-Whelan S, Thornby JI, Monga TN. Coping with chronic pain: A comparison of two measures. *Pain*, 2001; 90: 127–133.

149. Gatchel RJ, Turk DC, eds. *Psychosocial Factors in Pain*, New York: Guilford Press, 1999.

150. Turk DC, Gatchel RJ. Psychosocial factors and pain: revolution and evolution. In Gatchel RJ, Turk DC, eds., *Psychosocial Factors in Pain*, New York: Guilford Press, 1999.

151. Von Korff M. Pain management in primary care: An individualized stepped-care approach. In Gatchel RJ, Turk DC, eds., *Psychosocial Factors in Pain*. New York: The Guilford Press, 1999.

152. Tan G, Jensen MP, Robinson-Whelan S, Thornby JI, Monga TN. Measuring control appraisals in chronic pain. *Pain*, 2002 (in press).

153. Tan G, Lim P, Maymi L. Managing chronic pain: A continuing dilemma for modern medicine. *Federal Practitioner*, 1997; 14: 11–22.

154. Melzack R, Perry C. Self-regulation of pain: The use of alpha feedback and hypnotic training for the control of pain. *Experimental Neurology*, 1975; 46: 452–469.

4 Pain Syndromes Following Spinal Cord Injury

Gary M. Yarkony, M.D.
Michelle S. Gittler, M.D.
David J. Weiss, M.D.

Pain in its various forms is a uniform accompaniment of traumatic spinal cord injury (SCI) and has been reported to occur in 100 percent of persons with this condition (1). Following SCI and throughout the life of the injured person, the type of pain experienced may vary (2). At the time of injury there is pain associated with the initial trauma and other associated injuries. At that time there may be pain associated with complications such as those occurring in the gastrointestinal, genitourinary, and musculoskeletal systems. Pain occurs following surgery and therapy. As the person enters the rehabilitation phase, central pain, also known as *dysesthetic* or *phantom pain*, may become more prominent. Musculoskeletal pain occurs as body parts are stressed to compensate for weaknesses in paralyzed areas. As the aging process occurs, musculoskeletal pain increases as degenerative changes take their toll. Because of the numerous etiologies of pain in SCI and the limited understanding of central pain, relieving pain is a perplexing problem for the injured person as well as for his physicians and therapists.

This chapter provides guidelines for the clinical approach to a person with traumatic SCI complaining of pain and focuses on the complex problem of central pain.

CLASSIFICATION

Numerous classifications have been proposed to describe pain after traumatic SCI. The system described by Donovan et al. (3) is commonly used.

Radicular pain is not specific to SCI (Table 4.1). It may be present from the day of injury or be obscured by concurrent SCI. It may occur in waves and be described as burning or aching. The distribution may be segmental, and only partial sensory function may be present in the affected roots.

Visceral pain is a burning type of pain that is probably a variant of central pain; it occurs in the abdominal or pelvic area. Although it is not caused by intraabdominal pathology, it must be considered and investigated as the clinical situation warrants.

Table 4.1. Classification of Pain in Spinal Cord Injury

Radicular – Cauda Equina
Central
Visceral
Musculoskeletal
Psychogenic

(Based on Donovan, *Paraplegia* 20: 139-146, 1982.)

Musculoskeletal pain can occur in SCI as it does in the general population. Although the medical treatment does not always differ from that of uninjured persons, medical equipment considerations and attendant care responsibilities may play a part in the treatment plan to diminish the mechanical stress that causes musculoskeletal complications.

Psychogenic or *supratentorial pain* may occur concomitantly with other pain syndromes or by itself. It is largely a diagnosis made when all other pain has been ruled out and the pattern of pain is not consistent with other syndromes. Psychological care is an important part of psychogenic pain management.

Central pain or *spinal cord pain* is the main focus of this chapter. Central pain is often described as shooting (4), stabbing, burning, or tingling, or a feeling of pressure and pounding. It usually occurs in the first year, but there is no limit to its onset post-injury. Fortunately, it generally decreases with time. It may be exacerbated by psychological factors or it may cause increased stress (5). The pain may be exacerbated by those complications of SCI that create noxious stimuli such as bowel, bladder, skin, and other complications. It commonly occurs in the legs, trunk, buttocks, and upper extremities. It occurs with all etiologies and at all levels of SCI but is especially common after gunshot wounds.

CLINICAL APPROACH

Because of the many possible etiologies of pain after SCI a comprehensive evaluation is required. The cause of the pain should not be ascribed to the injury of the spinal cord (central or dysesthetic pain) without a careful evaluation. This, of course, begins with a detailed history and physical examination. The differential diagnosis should not only consider the five broad classifications of pain particular to SCI, but must consider sources of pain that occur in the general population.

Pain may be caused by complications such as *heterotopic ossification* (6) or *posttraumatic (syringomyelia) cystic myelopathy* (7). Heterotopic ossification can cause localized pain and loss of range of motion. It can also cause peripheral nerve entrapments or a presentation that mimics deep venous thrombosis. Posttraumatic cystic myelopathy, although rare, is a particularly devastating problem because it may cause further sensory and motor loss in a person who is already severely disabled. It can occur between two months to years after SCI. The pain is often described as dull and aching in the head and upper arms, and it may be aggravated by coughing, sneezing, or straining.

Visceral pain is particularly difficult to assess because it may be central in origin or as a result of an intra-abdominal complication. The differential diagnosis may consider usual urinary tract infections, bowel impactions, and genitourinary stones. Pancreatitis, cholelithiasis, gastrointestinal bleeding or obstruction, superior mesenteric syndrome, and other rarer intra-abdominal complications may occur as well (8).

If the physician's evaluation determines that the pain is central in nature, the impact on the individual must be considered, because treatment options may have significant side effects. Consideration should be given to the degree of pain and the impact of the proposed treatment. If the pain is not functionally limiting or interfering with sleep or other activities, treatment may not be necessary. In these instances an explanation of the pain process and reassurance that there is no significant medical complication occurring may be all that is needed.

CENTRAL PAIN

To date, the exact mechanism of how central pain is generated has not been well defined. As a result, there is an historical debate over this mechanism. A *hard-wired system* is the traditional thinking behind how a noxious stimulus is processed. It is thought that nociceptor afferents only synapse in the dorsal horns of the spinal cord. These neurons then blindly activate various supraspinal sites, giving rise to pain. From this physiologic basis arose the first theories on central pain in spinal cord injuries.

Holmes (9) microscopically examined the spinal cords of deceased spinal cord–injured patients who had had central pain. He found mild changes that consisted of edema and minute hemorrhages. From these findings, he reasoned that any impulses that crossed these mildly abnormal sensory segments weren't interrupted, but were modified to become irritative afferents. This theory was challenged in 1947 by Davis and Martin (10), who performed cordotomies on eighteen patients for the relief of central SCI pain. The diffuse burning pain of which these eighteen patients complained was not relieved with this lateral pathway sectioning; hence the researchers reasoned that the autonomic nervous system was the carrier mechanism of central pain. Davis hypothesized that the skin and muscles of spinal cord injured patients underwent physiochemical changes that triggered any distal stimulus to conduct through sympathetic fibers. These stimuli then entered the spinal cord through a wide distribution of proximal sympathetic ganglia to reach the thalamus and cortex as pain impulses.

In 1951, Pollock (11) performed an experiment to test Davis' theory. Fifty SCI patients with complete injuries and central pain were studied. The experiment involved anesthetizing each patient below and above the level of the injury. The results of the study showed that patients who were anesthetized below the level of injury did not experience relief from their pain, whereas anesthetic given just proximal to the lesion resulted in a resolution of both dysesthetic and phantom sensations. Pollock concluded that central pain originates in the distal end of the spinal cord segment just proximal to the level of injury.

Botterell (12) first hypothesized that the brain played a significant role in developing central SCI pain. After treating thirty-four patients with central pain both conservatively and surgically (with spinal thalamic tractotomies), he postulated that the origin of pain must be related to the escape of thalamic control. This loss of control over the thalamus was caused by the interruption of ascending spinal pathways and their inhibitory effect on normal noxious or non-noxious afferent impulses. Thus, any and all stimuli caused the thalamic pain centers to be activated and, ironically, central pain became independent of peripheral inputs. Porter and associates (13) agreed with Botterell. They believed that SCI central pain was caused by a second-order neuron. This conclusion was based on findings in thirty-four traumatic cauda equina injured patients who previously had poor results from posterior rhizotomies as a treatment for their pain. They noted substantial improvement in pain levels after cordotomies. Their theory was that peripheral stimuli could not depolarize a second-neuron cell system and pain could not be generated.

Another "hard-wire" theory includes ephaptic spread of ascending or descending impulses within the damaged spinal cord segment, spontaneous activity that is generated at the site of injury, and somatic rearrangement (14,15).

During the past two decades, advances into the transmission of nociceptive stimuli has revealed a system more complicated than that of the hard-wired analogy. We now know that an elaborate system of checks and balances exert bidirectional control at many levels on pain stimulus generation. One of the most comprehensive theories to apply this line of thinking to SCI central pain was proposed by Melzack and Loeser (16). They described five paraplegic patients in whom an entire section of spinal cord was removed. This was done under the assumption that a few remaining pain signal fibers escaped trauma or that the abnormalities in denervated cord segments caused the pain. No previous aggressive interventions, which included various sympathetic blocks, dorsal column stimulator implants, and cordotomies, had given significant pain relief to these patients. What the researchers found was that total cordectomies also gave minimal pain relief. Thus, Melzack and Loeser reasoned that peripheral input into the spinal cord, up to a level of total transection, was not the cause of pain. They conceptualized a central modulating mechanism in which pain is generated when the number of nerve impulses per unit time from somatic projection systems to pain areas in the central nervous system exceeded a critical or suprathreshold level. This derivative of the *gate control theory* of Melzack and Wall is called the *central pattern generating mechanism* (17). This theory states that pools of pain generating neurons that become central pattern generators are located at multiple levels within the spinal cord, brainstem, and brain. Under normal circumstances, these centers generate pain signals that are enhanced, decreased, or turned off by multiple central or peripheral inputs. These modulators include somatic, visceral, and autonomic inputs as well as the neural mechanisms that underlie personality and emotion. If this system of checks and balances is disturbed by an SCI, unchecked abnormal bursting occurs and pain is generated. Therefore, once the abnormal central pattern generating processes are underway, the peripheral contributions may be less important. These peripheral signals may be modulators, but their removal may not stop pain once it is established.

Beric (18) confirmed, to a certain extent, Melzack's theory by undertaking quantitative sensory and neurophysiologic testing on thirteen SCI patients with central pain. His tests revealed relative preservation of dorsal column functions in the absence of spinal thalamic systems. He hypothesized that the main underlying mechanism of dysesthesia in SCI patients is misinterpretation of residual peripheral input.

In 1994, Tasker (19) reaffirmed what Melzack and Loeser had hypothesized sixteen years earlier by stating that either aberrant electrical activity within deafferented central sensory nuclei or hyperactivity within reticulothalamic pathways was the most likely explanation for neural injury pain. He went on to reason that, once established, the pain persists independently of peripheral stimuli. Pagni (20) and Segatore (21) have listed various proposed mechanisms of central nervous injury pain. These include:

- loss of "downstream" inhibition,
- realignment of structural and synaptic connections,
- altered electrochemical activity in dorsal form and rostral sites,
- deafferentation,
- activation of secondary nociceptive pathways,
- release of excitatory pathways,
- irritation of the sympathetic system, and
- hypothalamic origins.

These authors conclude that a unique pathogenetic mechanism does not exist, but rather that a multifactorial cause of central SCI pain exists.

Over the last ten years, the possible biochemical mechanisms of central pain in SCI patients has been studied. Much like structural mechanisms, there is no agreement in the literature on the exact neurochemical basis of central pain after SCI. Eide (22) studied whether blocking central n-methyl-d-aspartate (NMDA) receptors with ketimine would affect central dysesthetic pain after traumatic SCI. He found a marked reduction in continuous and evoked pain in all nine of his studied patients. Thus, he concluded that central dysesthetic pain is dependent on NMDA-abnormal hyperactivity at the spinal and thalamic levels.

Other neurochemicals that are thought to play a role in central SCI pain include gamma amino-butyric acid (GABA), 5-hydroxytryptamine, noradrenaline, and the sodium/potasium channel. Blocking sodium/potasium channels with mexiletine reduced tactile allodynia in animals with ischemic SCIs (23), but did not decrease dysesthetic pain in humans (24). Just the opposite scenario was found with GABA receptors. Central pain was reduced in two patients by activating GABA receptors (25), whereas baclofen, a GABA agonist, failed to decrease allodynia in rats with ischemic SCI (26). Finally, in a controlled study, Davidoff

(27) found that inhibiting the uptake of 5-hydroxytryptamine using trazodone failed to relieve central pain after SCI.

Although there is no one explicitly accepted mechanism to explain the pathophysiology of central pain to date, there are accepted concepts on which to base future theories. It is accepted that there are many structural and biochemical changes at many levels, both peripherally and centrally, and that no single pathway or biochemical can be blocked or removed to resolve pain. It is also clear that we are at the nidus of our knowledge when it comes to SCI and pain.

MUSCULOSKELETAL PAIN

Musculoskeletal pain is one of the most common impairments causing a decreased ability to perform functional activities in the population of the United States (28). Persons with SCI are particularly at risk for musculoskeletal pain, because they use muscle groups in the upper extremities to compensate for lower extremity weakness and have abnormal postures and gait patterns caused by weakness and spasticity. They often have sustained traumatic injuries or fractures to other joints, thus resulting in secondary degenerative joint disease. Insensate joints may develop Charcot's arthropathy. This may also occur as a complication of post-traumatic cystic myelopathy (29).

The shoulder joint is particularly prone to developing tendonitis, bursitis, and osteoarthritis (30,31), with a reported incidence rate of 30 to 70 percent. Initial postinjury pain may be caused by the initial trauma. Lack of range of motion and poor positioning may lead to joint contracture (32). Stress from transfers may contribute as well.

Wheelchair users' shoulder was originally described by Nichols (31). Prolonged use of the upper extremities for wheelchair propulsion and transfers results in degenerative changes. Tendonitis, bursitis, and muscle strains occur; myofascial pain, with trigger points, may be present in the shoulders and neck. Rotator cuff tears are common, because high pressures occur in the shoulder joint during transfers (33).

Compression neuropathies are common after SCI. *Carpal tunnel syndrome* occurs following stress on the wrist as functional activities put excessive pressure on the hands and wrists (34,35). Ulnar neuropathy at the wrists and elbows may occur as well, caused by mechanical forces or improper positioning. Orthotic management and assessment of functional skills by an occupational therapist will assist in the overall therapeutic plan. These interventions should be directed toward diminished stress on the joints during functional activities. This may entail the prescription of equipment to decrease future potential injury such as power wheelchairs and transfer aids.

Degenerative changes occur in the spine and lower extremities (36). Osteoarthritis occurs commonly in the hips and sacroiliac joints. These changes can result in pain and interfere with functions. Some affected individuals will be asymptomatic because of sensory loss. Fractures secondary to osteoporosis and falls or other trauma commonly occur as well (37,38).

Chronic pain can have a significant impact on the life of a person with SCI (39). Interference with sleep has a significant impact on mood and affect. Some people will not be able to work and many will have to stop work. For others, activities of daily living and participation in community activities will be limited. Medications to treat pain may have side effects that limit cognitive function or cause drowsiness, further impairing functional skills.

TREATMENT OF PAIN IN SCI

Unfortunately, "phantom body pain in paraplegic patients (remains) the most mysterious of all pain phenomena (16)." Although multiple theories regarding the mechanisms of pain in the SCI patient exist, we have not yet arrived at a specific treatment for this perplexing problem.

Some of the most complex variables having a clear relationship or association with chronic pain in persons with SCI include depression and psychosocial impairment (40,41). Perceived stress and subjective well-being are also found to have a relationship with pain and SCI (39). Thus, the effective treatment of pain must include attention to subjective factors (anxiety, fatigue, loneliness, depression, and other psychosocial problems). The reader is referred to a comprehensive literature on chronic pain in the general population to understand the multiple approaches to this component of pain syndromes. This section focuses on interventions other than psychosocial counseling in the management of pain syndromes in SCI.

Modalities

Physical modalities are commonly employed in attempts at modulating pain. One clear advantage of physical modalities is the lack of (systemic) side effects caused by pharmacologic or surgical interventions. Unfortunately, several authors concede that biofeedback, electrical stimulation, Hubbard tank, microwave, infrared, ultrasound therapy, cold treatments, and others have not been particularly effective in the treatment of central pain in SCI (42,43). However, there is good evidence for the effectiveness of transcutaneous electrical neurostimulation (TENS) in the treatment of pain of peripheral nerve and musculoskeletal origin (44,45,46).

Surgical Intervention

Multiple procedures are utilized to prevent or interrupt nociceptive input or serve to destroy abnormally functioning deafferented neurons. Examples of the former include operations such as rhizotomy, cordotomy, and cordectomy. Examples of the latter include lesions of the dorsal route entry zone (DREZ) and thalamotomy. A third category includes modulatory treatments such as chronic stimulation of peripheral nerves, the dorsal spinal cord, and other pathways. Numerous surgical procedures have been described for pain control. The efficacy of these procedures is variable, most likely because of the numerous neural factors involved in pain development. Neurosurgical lesions may sometimes produce new pains or aggravate existing pain, rather than diminish the pathologic pain for which they were intended. Any neurosurgical procedure for pain (neurectomy, rhizotomy, cordotomy) is essentially a deafferenting process and may actually provide the substrate for subsequent pain (16).

In 1947, Davis (10) first reported on twenty-three operations for pain on eighteen patients with SCI; only one patient received lasting relief from burning pain. His conclusion was that a cordotomy above the level of injury failed to give relief from pain, specifically burning pain. Botterell (12) first described bilateral tractotomy to treat the jabbing, shooting pains felt by patients with SCI. However, it was found that burning pain was uninfluenced. Subsequently, Porter (13) found that performing lateral spinothalamic tract lesions was very effective (61 percent of patients reported good to fair relief of pain) in relieving sharp lancinating pain, but was not effective in treating burning pain in lower extremities. Additionally, these lesions created complications of their own, including loss of motor power, development of spasms, and loss of sexual function. There are conflicting reports regarding dorsal root entry zone (DREZ) lesions in the treatment of pain following SCI. Nashold (47) reported that eleven of thirteen patients sustaining SCI describe good to excellent pain relief with DREZ procedure. Friedman et al. (48) reported that postoperative results in patients with diffuse SCI pain were disappointing, however patients with pain confined to dermatomes just below the level of spinal injury did well with DREZ lesions. In short, destructive neurosurgical procedures may be appropriate for specific pain syndromes, but their effectiveness cannot be generalized for all patients with pain.

Spinal cord stimulation has been useful in some deafferentation syndromes such as phantom limb pain. Cole et al. (49) found spinal cord stimulation not to be an effective technique for the relief of chronic deafferentation pain below the level of SCI. Richardson (45,46) also concluded that neurostimulation in the modulation of intractable paraplegic and traumatic neuroma pain resulted in no pain relief.

Finally, deep brain stimulation for intractable pain in selected patients may provide long-term pain control. In the United States, however, deep brain stimulation is no longer available for use and, in one study, patients with SCI did not do well with deep brain stimulation (50).

Frequently, patients suffering from gunshot wounds ask whether "taking the bullet out" will relieve the pain. Sued (51) divided SCI patients into two treatment groups, those who received surgical intervention and those who did not. He found that surgical intervention did not result in a decreased incidence of pain as a result of spinal stabilization. The effect of bullet removal on pain is very important, because it is known that gunshot-wound patients report more pain (4,5) postoperatively. Although it would be beneficial to know if removal of the bullet decreases the *perceptions* of pain, unfortunately, bullet removal does not appear to be associated with an actual reduction of pain. In fact, there is a trend in patients with the bullet removed to be more likely to develop deafferentation pain (5).

Pharmacologic Intervention

The use of oral medications for the treatment of pain in SCI is largely based on clinical experience. There is little scientific support for the use of specific medications and only recently has an emerging body of literature regarded the possibilities of drug classes that may be beneficial in treating specific pain patterns or syndromes. Several papers refer to the utilization of nonsteroidal antiinflammatory agents (NSAIDs) (52,53,54). Although these medications appear to offer little to no efficacy regarding the treatment of central pain and SCI, there is definitely a role for these medications in the treatment of musculoskeletal pain.

In their frustration at being unable to treat pain in their patients, many physicians resort to prescribing narcotic medication. Indeed, it is common for patients to be on significant doses of a narcotic with little or no relief of central pain. Alterations in their bowel programs, impaired alertness, as well as the potential for addiction and abuse may occur. Abuse and addiction is a particular problem, because many spinal cord–injured persons have premorbid substance abuse problems. There does not appear to be a role for opiates in the long-term treatment of central pain. Although there is significant literature evaluating psychotropic medication for neuropathic pain, the literature examining cord injury is rather limited (55). Maury (1977) recommended that "when the pain seems too difficult to bear, it is recommended to use antidepressive drugs." Additionally, he recommends the association of an antidepressive drug with a neuroleptic one. However, he includes no description of methodology, dosage, or description of pain syndrome. Tricyclic antidepressants such as amitriptyline are the most commonly studied medications (3,52–54,56). Davidoff's highly specific randomized double-blind placebo-controlled study examined the efficacy of antidepressant medication in the spinal cord injured population (27). Utilizing several pain instruments, Davidoff's group compared trazodone to a placebo for the treatment of central pain and found that there were no significant differences in the pain reported between the placebo and treatment group.

The utilization of tricyclic antidepressant medication combined with anticonvulsant medication appears to be more promising. Sanford et al. (52) noted that utilizing amitriptyline at doses of 25 mg, increasing to 200 mg per day, combined with carbamazepine in doses of 100 to 200 mg twice a day, had a substantial effect on decreasing central pain. Attempts to discontinue either drug immediately resulted in the return of the burning sensation below the level of injury. Amitriptyline and clonazepam were utilized in a step program to treat central pain (53). A program of nonsteroidal antiinflammatories and TENS, in conjunction with amitriptyline in doses of up to 75 mg per day with clonazepam in doses up to 1.5 mg a day, resulted in approximately 60 percent of patients finding some pain relief. Several other stepwise programs have been reported that utilize oral medications beginning with analgesics, then adding antidepressants and subsequently anticonvulsants (54); if there is no response, intravenous phentolamine and lignocaine are added. This group reported that 74 percent of patients required more than one pain management strategy, with analgesics used in 91 percent of cases

(63 percent of those utilized codeine), antidepressants used in 41 percent, and anticonvulsants in another 32 percent. Pain intensity increased across the board after discontinuation of medication. Response to carbamazepine was successful in some spinal cord–injured patients with segmental nerve pain (3,57). However, those with central pain or burning pain below the level of injury were found to respond much better to tricyclic antidepressants combined with epidural stimulation at high frequency (3).

Exploration of treatment with other anticonvulsant medications reveals that valproic acid—beginning at doses of 600 mg and increasing up to 2400 mg per day—demonstrated a trend towards improvement in pain in the valproate subgroups in a double blind cross-over study, but this did not reach statistical significance (56).

Although not specifically evaluated in the SCI literature, gabapentin is found more and more useful for the treatment of multiple painful neuropathies. Gabapentin monotherapy was found to be effective for the treatment of pain as well as the sleep interference associated with diabetic peripheral neuropathy (58) as well as for the treatment of postherpetic neuralgia (59). Gabapentin dosages began at 900 mg per day up to a total of 3600 mg per day by the fourth week of the study. Anecdotally, our center has had excellent results with the utilization of gabapentin for the treatment of central pain in SCI. Treatment is initiated at 900 mg per day, in three divided doses; we typically find that after approximately three weeks of treatment, we are able to taper and discontinue this medication in approximately two-thirds of our patients, particularly those with incomplete cervical spine injuries.

Other medications with theoretical usefulness in certain pain syndromes include dependent sodium channel blockers such as lidocaine and mexiletine. Intravenous lidocaine has been found to predict the efficacy of oral mexiletine (57). Doses as high as 750 mg per day or 10 mg per kilogram have been demonstrated to reduce neuropathic pain in peripheral nerve injury, including diabetic neuropathy (60,61). Chiou-Tan et al. (24) demonstrated no significant effect of mexiletine in doses of 450 mg per day versus a placebo in SCI dysesthetic pain scales. Mexiletine may not be appropriate for central pain in SCI. It appears to be more appropriate for radicular segmental pain after SCI rather than central pain (60).

Pain in cauda equina injury may be in part a segmental or radicular pain pattern rather than a true central pain; thus it requires a more customized approach than SCI pain, per se. Beric (62) discusses the possibility of preemptive analgesia via early spinal blocks in cauda equina injury to prevent the development of early and late neurogenic pains. Several other authors discuss the utilization of intrathecal medication in SCI as well as cauda equina injury. The utilization of intrathecal morphine was demonstrated to result in 66 percent of patients exhibiting improvement in cord deafferentation pain (53). However, pain classification, dosage, and long-term follow-up were not reported on. Spinal anesthesia delivered proximal to the injury should be effective if the pain-generating mechanisms are the result of deafferentation (63). However, this is a theoretical approach and no studies have been performed. The utilization of intrathecal (IT) morphine alone demonstrated no change in pain (64). However, the addition of clonidine to the pump reservoir resulted in good relief of pain. The use of intrathecal baclofen on chronic SCI pain has been evaluated in one small study with variable results. Intrathecal baclofen has been demonstrated to have no effect on chronic neurogenic SCI pain (65), but reduces chronic musculoskeletal pain associated with spasticity. In contrast, Herman et al. (25), in an even smaller study group, document that IT baclofen significantly depressed dysesthetic pain, but did not influence musculoskeletal pain. In an additional study, one patient with severe intractable anal spasm as well as pain who was initially treated with intrathecal baclofen did not exhibit improvements in symptoms. Intrathecal clonidine was added, with immediate improvement to both spasm and pain (66). The utilization of clonidine as an alpha-2 adrenal receptor modulator requires further study.

Alternative Medicine

Alternative medicine is receiving increased interest for numerous medical problems. Many believe it is no longer an option to ignore traditional or folk remedies, or to treat them as something outside the normal process of science and medicine (67). Although there are no specific studies of the many alternative or complementary options available, there is some suggestion that pain and phantom sensation in spinal paralysis may frequently be relieved by acupuncture (68). Anecdotally, in our center we have utilized acupuncture for a C4 complete tetraplegic with fair results in pain relief. Additionally, the utilization of biomagnets in magnetic pillows and mattress overlays has had reasonable success in one patient and good success in a nonspinal cord–injured trauma surgeon.

Wainapel et al. (69) reported that nearly one-third of rehabilitation patients were using alternative therapies. Almost all of those do so secondary to pain syndromes. Fifty-three percent of patients reported some degree of efficacy from the alternative therapies they had received. Above all, unless there is concern about the negative effect of an alternative or complementary procedure, patients should not be deterred from seeking such care. Indeed, alternative medical therapies may represent a vast potential in the practice of physical medicine and rehabilitation for integration with more traditional medical therapies.

Patients asking about the use of marijuana in pain relief can be referred to a marijuana policy project (MPP) Web page that describes the use of cannabis for pain, particularly for SCI (http://www.mpp.org/FDA.html or http://www.18c.org/mpp/patients.html). Currently there is no specific literature regarding central pain to support this, but studies may be underway to evaluate the effectiveness of Marinol for various syndromes associated with cancer and AIDS.

CONCLUSIONS

There is still much to be accomplished in conquering SCI pain, for there is still much to be delineated. As this chapter has outlined, today's accepted mechanisms, and thus the treatments, for SCI central pain are not based on double-blinded cross-over studies. The majority of the outlined studies have been small, retrospective, and poorly controlled. The application of new methods in studying SCI patients and new treatment techniques such as intrathecal agents and neuroactive drugs, will hopefully make the future of treating SCI pain promising.

REFERENCES

1. Rossier AB. Rehabilitation of the spinal cord injury patient. *Documenta Geigy Acta Clinica,* No. 3 North American Series, 1964; 80–82.
2. Roth EJ. Pain in spinal cord injury. In: Yarkony GM (ed.), *Spinal Cord Injury Medical Management and Rehabilitation.* Gaithersburg, Md.:Aspen Publishers Inc., 1994; pp 181–155.
3. Donovan WH, Dimitrijevic MR, Dahm L, Dimitrijevic M. Neurophysiological approaches to pain following spinal cord injury. *Paraplegia* 1982; 20:135–146.
4. Davidoff G, Roth E, Guarracini M, et al. Function-limiting dysesthetic pain syndrome among traumatic spinal cord injury patients: A cross-sectional study. *Pain* 1987; 29:39–48.
5. Richards JS, et al. Psychosocial aspects of chronic pain in spinal cord injury. *Pain* 1980; 8: 355–366.
6. Jensen LL, Halar E, Little JW, et al. Neurogenic heterotopic ossification. *Am J Phys Med* 1988; 66:351–363.
7. Biyani A, Masry WS. Posttraumatic syringomyelia: A review of the literature. *Paraplegia* 1994; 32:723–731.
8. Frost FS. Gastrointestinal dysfunction in spinal cord injury. In: Yarkony GM (ed.), *Spinal Cord Injury Medical Management and Rehabilitation.* Gaithersburg, Md.: Aspen Publishers Inc., 1994.
9. Holmes G. *Pain of Central Origin in Contributions to Medical and Biological Research.* New York: P.B. Hoeber, 1919, 1:235–246.
10. Davis L, Martin J. Studies upon SCI: The Nature And Treatment Of Pain. *J Neurosurg* 1947; 4:483–491.
11. Pollock LJ, Brown M, Bushes B, Finkelman I, Chor H, Arieff AJ, Finkle JR. Pain below the level of injury of the spinal cord. *Arch Neurol and Psychiatry* 1951; 65:319–322.
12. Botterell EH, Callaghan JC, Jousse AT. Pain in paraplegia: Clinical management and surgical treatment. *Proc Royal Soc Med* [Toronto]; September 1953; 47: 281–288.
13. Porter RW, Hohmann GW, Bors E, French JD. Cordotomy for pain following cauda equina injury. *Arch Surg* 1966; 92:765–770.
14. Loeser, JD. Definition, etiology, and neurological assessment of pain origination in the nervous system after deafferentation. *Pain* 1981; 81.
15. Druckman R, Lende R. Central pain of spinal cord origin: Pathogenesis and surgical relief in one patient. *Neurology* 1965; 15:518–522.
16. Melzack R, Loeser JD. Phantom body pain in paraplegics: Evidence for a central pattern generating mechanism for pain. *Pain* 1978; 4:195–210.
17. Melzack R, Wall PD. Pain mechanism: A new theory. *Science* 1965; 150:971–979.
18. Beric A, Dimitrijevic MR, Lindblom U. Central dysesthesia syndrome in spinal cord injury patients. *Pain* 1988; 34 (2): 109–116.
19. Tasker, RR. Pain resulting from central nervous system pathology. In: Bonica JJ (ed), *The Management of Pain,* Vol.1, 2nd ed. New York: Lea & Febiger, 1990; p.264–286.
20. Pagni, CA. Central pain due to spinal cord and brainstem damage. In: Wall PD and R Melzack (eds.), *Textbook of Pain,* 2nd ed. Edinburgh, Scotland: Churchill–Livingston, 1987; 637–655.
21. Segatore, M. Understanding chronic pain after spinal cord injury. *J Neuroscience Nursing* 1994; 26 (4):230–236.

22. Eide PK, Stubharg A, Stenehjen AE. Central dysesthesia pain after traumatic spinal cord injury is dependent on N-methyl-D-aspartate receptor activation. *Neurosurgery* 1995; 37 (6): 1080–1087.

23. Xu, XJ, Hau JX, Aldsuogius H, Seiger A, Wiesenfeld-Hallin Z. Chronic pain-related syndrome in rats after ischemic spinal cord lesion: A possible animal model for pain in patients with spinal cord injury. *Pain* 1992; 48:279–290.

24. Chiou-Tan FY, Tuel SM, Johnson JC, Priebe MM, Hirsch DD, Strayer JR. Effects of mexiletine on spinal cord dysesthetic pain. *Am J PM&R* 1996; 75(2):84–87.

25. Herman RM, D'Luzansky SC, Ippolito R. Intrathecal baclofen suppresses central pain in patients with spinal lesions: A pilot study. *Clin J Pain* 1992; 8:338– 345.

26. Xu, XJ, Hau JX, Seiger A, Arnes S, Lindblom U, Wiesenfeld-Hill, Z. Systemic mexiletine relieves chronic allodynialivie symptoms in rats with spinal cord injury. *Anesthesia Analgesic* 1992; 74:649–652.

27. Davidoff G. Trazodone hydrochloride in the treatment of dysesthetic pain in traumatic myelopathy: A randomized, double-blind, placebo-controlled study. *Pain* 1987; 29:151–161.

28. Waters, RL, Adkins RH. The musculoskeletal system. In: Whiteneck GG et al. (eds.), *Aging with Spinal Cord Injury*. New York: Demos Publications, 1993; pp. 53–71.

29. Ken S, Lewis MM, Main WK, Hermann G, Abdelwahab IF. Neuropathic arthropathy of the shoulder mimicking soft tissue sarcoma. *Orthopedics* 1993; 16:133–136.

30. Sie IH, Waters RL, Adkins RH, Gellman H. Upper extremity pain in the post–rehabilitation spinal cord injured patient. *Arch Phys Med Rehab* 1992; 73:44–48.

31. Nichols PJR, Norman PA, Ennis JR. Wheelchair user's shoulder? *Scand J Rehab Med* 1979; 11:29–32.

32. Scott JA, Donovan WH. The prevention of shoulder pain and contracture in the acute tetraplegic patient. *Paraplegia* 1981; 12:313–319.

33. Bayley JC, Cochran TP, Sledge CB. The weight-bearing shoulder:The impingement syndrome in paraplegics. *J Bone Joint Surg* 1987, 69A(5):676–678.

34. Davidoff, G, et al. Compressive mononueropathies of the upper extremity in chronic paraplegia. *Paraplegia* 1991, 29:17–24.

35. Gellman H, et al. Carpal tunnel syndrome in paraplegic patients. *J Bone Joint Surg* 1988, 70A:517–519.

36. Wylie EJ, Chakera TMH. Degenerative joint abnormalities in patients with paraplegia of duration greater than twenty years. *Paraplegia* 1988, 26:101–106.

37. Ragnarsson KT, Sell GH. Lower extremity fractures after spinal cord injury: A retrospective study. *Arch Phys Med Rehabil* 1981, 62:418–423.

38. Garland DE, Stewart CA, Adkins RH, et al. Osteoporosis following spinal cord injury. *J Orthop Res*. In press.

39. Rintala D, Loubser P, Castro J, Hart K, Fuhrer M. Chronic pain in a community- based sample of men with spinal cord injury: Prevalence, severity, and relationship with impairment, disability, medical, and subjective well-being. *Arch Phys Med Rehab* 1998; 79:604–614.

40. Elliott TR, Hawkins SW. Psychosocial concomitants of persistent pain among persons with spinal cord injuries. *Neurorehabilitation* 1991; 1:7–16.

41. Mariano AJ. Chronic pain and spinal cord. *Clin J Pain* 1997; 8:87–92.

42. Nepomuceno C, Fine PR, Richards S, Gowens H, Stover S, Rantanuabol U, Houston R. Pain in Patients with spinal cord injury. *Arch Phys Med Rehab* 1979; 60:605–609.

43. Kaplan LI, Grynbaum BB, Lloyd KE, Rusk HA. Pain and spasticity in patients with spinal cord dysfunction. *JAMA* 1962; 182:120–126.

44. Long DM. Stimulation of the peripheral nervous system for pain control. *Clin Neurosurg* 1983; 31:323–343.

45. Richardson RR, Meyer PR, Cerullo LJ. Neurostimulation in the modulation of intractable paraplegic and traumatic neuroma pains. *Pain* 1980; 8:75–84.

46. Richardson RR, Meyer PR, Cerullo LJ. Transcutaneous electrical neurostimulation in musculoskeletal pain of acute spinal cord injuries. *Spine* 1980: 5:42–45.
47. Nashold B, Bullit E. Dorsal root entry zone lesions to control central pain in paraplegics. *J Neurosurg* 1981; 55:414–419.
48. Friedman A, Nashold BS. Dorsal root entry zone lesions for relief of pain related to spinal cord injury. *J Neurosurg* 1986; 65:465–69.
49. Cole JD, Sedgewick EM. Intractable central pain in spinal cord injury is not relieved by spinal cord stimulation. *Paraplegia* 1991; 29:167–172.
50. Kumar K, Toth C, Nath RK. Deep brain stimulation for intractable pain: A fifteen-year experience. *Neurosurg* 1997; 40:736–474.
51. Sued P, Siddall PJ, McClelland J, Cousins MJ. Relationship between surgery and pain following SCI. *Spinal Cord* 1997; 35:526–530.
52. Sanford PR, Lindblom LB, Haddox JD. Amitriptyline and carbamazepine in the treatment of dysesthetic pain in spinal cord injury. *Arch Phys Med Rehab* 1992; 73:300–301.
53. Fenollosa P, Palares J, Cervera J, Pelegrin F, Ingio V, Giner M, Forner V. Chronic pain in the spinal cord injured: Statistical approach and pharmacological treatment. *Paraplegia* 1993; 31:722–29.
54. New PW, Lim, TC, Hill ST, Brown DJ. A survey of pain during rehabilitation after acute spinal cord injury. *Spinal Cord* 1997; 35:658–663.
55. Roth EJ. Practical pain management strategies. In:Yarkony GM (ed.), *SCI Medical Management and Rehabilitation*. Gaithersburg, Md.: Aspen Publishers Inc., 1994; pp. 159–166.
56. Drewes AM, Andreasen A, Poulsen LH. Valproate for treatment of chronic central pain after spinal cord injury: A double-blind cross-over study. *Paraplegia* 1994; 32:565–569.
57. Tanelian DT, Brose WG. Neuropathic pain can be relieved by drugs that are use- dependent sodium channel blockers: Lidocaine, carbamazepine, and mexiletine. *Anesthesiology* 1991; 74:949–951.
58. Backonja M, Beydovn A, Edwards K, Schwartz S et al. Gabapentin for the symptomatic treatment of painful neuropathy in patients with diabetes mellitus. *JAMA* 1998; 280:1831–1836.
59. Rowbotham M, Harden N, Stacey B, Bernstein P, Magnus-Miller L. Gabapentin for the treatment of postherpetic neuralgia. *JAMA* 1998; 280:1837–1842.
60. Chabal C, Jacobson L, Mariano A, Chaney E, Britell C. The use of oral mexiletine for the treatment of pain after peripheral nerve injury. *Anesthesiology* 1992; 76:513–517.
61. Oskarsson P, Ljunggren JG, Lins PE. Efficacy and safety of mexiletine in the treatment of painful diabetic neuropathy. *Diabetes Care* 1997; 20:1594–1597.
62. Beric A. Post–spinal cord injury pain states, editorial. *Pain* 1997; 72:295–298.
63. Yezierski, RP. Pain following spinal cord injury: The clinical problems and experimental studies. *Pain* 1996; 68:185–194.
64. Siddall PJ, Gray M, Rutkowski S, Dousins MJ. Intrathecal morphine and clonidine in the management of spinal cord injury pain: A case report. *Pain* 1994; 59:147–148.
65. Loubser PG, Akman NM. Effects of intrathecal baclofen on chronic spinal cord injury pain. *J Pain Symptom Management* 1996; 12:241–247.
66. Middleton JW, Siddall PJ, Walker S, Molloy AR, Rutkowski SB. Intrathecal clonidine and baclofen in the management of spasticity and neuropathic pain following SCI: A case study. *Arch Phys Med Rehab* 1996:77:824–826.
67. Jonas W.Research in alternative medicine will help identify what is safe and effective and will further the understanding of biology by exploring rather than marginalizing unorthodox medical claims and findings; editorial. *JAMA* 1998; 280:1616–18.
68. Burke DC, Woodward JM. Pain and phantom sensation in spinal paralysis. In: Vinkin PS, Bruyn GW (eds.), *Handbook of Clinical Neurology*. New York: John Wiley & Sons, pp. 489–498.
69. Wainapel SF, Thomas AD, Kahan BS. Use of alternative therapies by rehabilitation outpatients. *Arch Phys Med Rehab* 1998; 79:1003–1005.

5 Poststroke Pain

Trilok N. Monga, M.D.
Anthony J. Kerrigan, Ph.D.

Cerebrovascular accidents (CVA) are the third most common cause of death in North America. CVAs are one of the major causes of long-term disability. Although stroke is generally considered a neurologic disorder, it is associated with a variety of musculoskeletal complications and a multitude of pain problems. Pain following stroke is very common, especially in the upper extremities, and may be a major contributor to long-term disability. Pain can impact substantially on a patient's sense of well being. For many stroke patients, chronic pain is underestimated as a factor that significantly contributes to the overall quality of life and disability (1).

Pain in stroke patients may originate centrally (thalamic pain syndrome), but in most patients, the pain is caused by a peripheral mechanism. Pain is generally associated with spastic hemiplegia accompanied with contractures (2). Because stroke is common in the elderly, pain from concomitant chronic conditions such as arthritis and other musculoskeletal conditions must be considered as well. Furthermore, there are many associated medical conditions, such as venous thrombosis and peripheral neuropathies, that may contribute to poststroke pain. This chapter describes the common pain problems in stroke patients. The diagnosis, management, and impact of pain on rehabilitation outcomes will be described. Reference is also made to certain other diagnoses that are common causes of pain in elderly subjects.

HEADACHES

Within the first month poststroke onset, 18 to 34 percent of stroke patients may suffer from headaches (3–5). In a prospective study of headache in stroke patients, Jorgensen et al. (1994) reported that 28 percent of 867 patients had headache in relation to stroke onset (3). In patients whose headache was lateralized (46 percent), it was ipsilateral to the lesion in 68 percent of cases. There was no correlation between headache and initial stroke severity and lesion size. Headache was found to be more common in strokes confined to the vertebrobasilar than to the carotid artery territory. Stroke-related headache was associated with factors such as age and sex.

In another study by Ferro and associates (1995), 34 percent of 182 ischemic stroke patients complained of headache within 72 hours of stroke onset (4). Headache was more common in patients under 70 years of age, who had a past history of migraine.

Many aspects of stroke-related headache have been reported, such as its incidence, pathophysiology, risk factors, and relation to stroke severity and outcome. Exact pathogenesis and natural history of these headaches is not known. According to Kumral et al. (1995), headache in stroke patients may be explained in part by involvement of blood vessels (acute distension or distortion) and mechanical stimulation of intracranial nociceptive afferents (5). The influence of headaches on rehabilitation outcome is not known. Management is symptomatic.

TEMPORAL ARTERITIS

Giant cell arteritis is also known as temporal arteritis or cranial arteritis. It is sometimes associated with polymyalgia rheumatica. It is common in people over the age of 50 years. It is a disease of the medium- to large-sized arteries. Patients may present with severe temporal headache, jaw claudication, transient diplopia, and acute unilateral blindness. Physical examination may reveal a swollen and tender temporal artery. ESR is elevated, usually in the range of more than 100 mm/hr, and is a good indicator of disease activity. Biopsy of temporal artery is diagnostic and reveals inflammatory changes with the presence of macrophages, lymphocytes, and joint cells. The lumen of the artery is narrowed. Treatment of choice is high dose (60–80 mg/day) prednisone by mouth. The dose is reduced as improvement in clinical signs and ESR is evidenced. In some patients, maintenance therapy with low-dose prednisone may be required for a long time.

FACIAL PAIN

Cases of lateral medullary syndrome (Wallenberg's syndrome) most commonly demonstrate thrombosis of the vertebral artery at the origin of posterior inferior cerebellar artery. The syndrome is characterized by vertigo, nausea, vomiting, ipsilateral sensory loss, ataxia, nystagmus, hoarseness, dystonia, dysphasia, dysarthria, and ipsilateral Horner's syndrome. Additional physical findings include absent corneal reflex, vocal cord paralysis, and absent gag reflex. Diminished pin-prick sensation is found on the contralateral hemibody. Facial pain around the eye or the entire side of the face appears after the second week; the course tends to parallel the sensory loss. The pain is usually mild, but occasionally can be disabling and refractory to medications. Patients with a history of pain tend to have incomplete lesions. Some patients also have contralateral spontaneous trunk and extremity pain similar in intensity and duration to facial pain. The pain usually is burning or stinging in character. The symptoms in the lower extremities improve more readily than in the arms.

MacGowan et al. (1997) have described central poststroke pain (CPP) in patients with lateral medullary infarction (6). Sixteen of the sixty-three patients developed this syndrome within six months of the stroke. CPP was constant and severe with frequent allodynia. CPP affected the ipsilateral periorbital region most commonly either alone or in combination with contralateral limbs. CPP correlated significantly with the degree of clinical sensory loss but not with the size of infarction seen on MRI. This pain responded in all cases to amitriptyline and recurred promptly on attempted weaning.

SHOULDER AND UPPER EXTREMITY PAIN

Shoulder pain is a common problem following stroke (7–11). It usually starts early during the course of recovery, and the prevalence increases after discharge (11). The pain leads to immobilization of the shoulder followed by disuse muscle atrophy, contracture, and osteoporosis and varying degrees of disability. It appears that patients who require help in transfers are more likely to experience hemiplegic shoulder pain.

Good shoulder function is a prerequisite for successful transfers, maintaining balance, performing activities of daily living, and for effective hand function. Shoulder pain and associated restriction of range of motion of the shoulder interferes with achievement of optimal functional outcome and therefore increases the disability related to the neurologic deficit. In a recent study of seventy-six stroke patients, Roy and his associates concluded that hemiplegic shoulder pain was the most useful predictor of poor recovery of arm function and power and was a good predictor of inpatient stay, even after controlling for other stroke severity indicators (10).

The prevalence of hemiplegic shoulder pain has been reported to vary between 5 and 84 percent of the patients (7–15). The major limiting factor in determining a more reliable magnitude of the problem is the lack of an accepted set of diagnostic criteria. Furthermore, hemiplegic shoulder pain remains a nebulous clinical entity, defined differently by each investigator (16). Discrepancies between studies regarding the incidence of shoulder pain may arise partly from patient selection criteria. For example, Peszczynski et al. (1965), recorded tenderness rather than a complaint of pain in moderate to severe hemiplegic patients (7) whereas Tepperman included pain or tenderness (17). Timing of the study since onset of stroke may further contribute to the reported incidence in various studies.

Hemiplegic shoulder pain may develop at any time during the first year following stroke. Fifty-five to 72 percent of stroke patients develop shoulder pain in the affected limb within the first six to twelve months following stroke. In a study by Brocklehurst et al. (1978), 21 of 107 (20 percent) of stroke patients developed hemiplegic shoulder pain within 2 weeks of stroke onset and an additional 37 (35 percent) developed shoulder pain 1 year after the stroke, with an overall incidence of 55 percent (18). In a recent study by Wanklyn and associates, 63 of the 108 stroke patients (63.8 percent) developed hemiplegic shoulder pain at some time during the study period of 6 months duration (11). Thirty-nine of these patients had shoulder pain at the time of discharge from the hospital, fifty-nine at eight weeks and thirty-six at six months postdischarge. The authors concluded that

Table 5.1. Upper Extremity Pain

Shoulder pain
    Soft tissue lesions
        Bicipital tendinitis
        Supraspinatous tendinitis
        Subacromial bursitis
        Coracoiditis
    Rotator cuff tears
    Adhesive capsulitis
    Shoulder subluxation
    Shoulder-hand syndrome
    Brachial plexus injury
    Degenerative joint disease involving upper extremity
    Peripheral nerve compression

patients who required help with transfers were more likely to suffer with hemiplegic shoulder pain. Stroke patients and their care providers should be given advice about correct handling of the hemiplegic arm (11).

Despite the extensive interest in hemiplegic shoulder pain, there continues to be uncertainty about its etiology and appropriate treatment (15). It is often difficult to sort out the underlying cause of the shoulder pain, but the two factors that most frequently accompany shoulder pain are *glenohumeral subluxation* and *shoulder contractures*. Controversy exists regarding their causal relationship to shoulder pain. Patients with shoulder pain also manifest decreased motivation, depression, and poor motor recovery. These patients also have significantly more sleep disturbances and report less general well being than those stroke patients without shoulder pain (19).

When dealing with pain in a stroke patient, one must consider the common musculoskeletal problems seen in elderly patients. There are many conditions that may contribute to shoulder pain in a hemiplegic patient (see Table 5.1). Some are related to soft tissue lesions such as tendonitis, bursitis, rotator cuff or capsular tears, and heterotopic ossification. Other factors are related to the shoulder joint, such as disorders of the subacromial region, degenerative joint disease, humeral fracture, and restricted range of motion caused by glenohumeral subluxation, spasticity, and adhesive capsulitis. Neurogenic factors contributing to shoulder pain include brachial plexus injury, compressive mononeuropathy, reflex sympathetic dystrophy, and pain radiating from cervical radiculopathy. Shoulder pain may be part of diffuse thalamic pain (central pain).

Soft Tissue Lesions

Soft tissue lesions must be considered in a stroke patient with a painful shoulder. These include bicipital and supraspinatus tendinitis, subacromial bursitis, partial and complete rotator cuff tears, and acromioclavicular lesions. It is not clear whether soft tissue injuries are more common in stroke patients as compared with an age-matched control group without a history of stroke. The incidence of conditions such as arthritis involving acromioclavicular and glenohumeral joints, bicipital tendonitis, and subdeltoid bursitis in hemiplegic patients has been estimated to be 15 percent (9,11).

Bicipital Tendinitis

Bicipital tendinitis is a frequent cause of shoulder pain and is commonly overlooked. Pain is localized to the anteriolateral aspect of the shoulder. Pain becomes worse on range-of-motion movements of the shoulder, especially when moving the arm overhead and in an abducted externally rotated direction. There is localized tenderness over the bicipital groove. Pain may be reproduced by resisting forward flexion of the shoulder with the elbow extended and forearm supinated. Pain becomes worse when the patient is asked to supinate the forearm against resistance while the elbow is kept at 90 degrees of flexion with the shoulder in a neutral position. One may be able to feel or hear a click as the biceps tendon moves in and out of the groove.

Initial mild tenosynovitis of the long head of the biceps may be aggravated by aggressive range-of-motion exercises, and may progress to adhesive capsulitis. After a while, the adhesions may become firm and pain may subside, but range of motion also becomes very limited.

Supraspinatous Tendinitis/Calcific Tendinitis

Codman initially reported that the painful shoulder is caused by localized supraspinatous tendinitis followed by inflammation of the other components of the rotator cuff (20). Later, the subacromial bursa and the joint capsule are involved, eventually leading to a "frozen shoulder." There is localized tenderness over the supraspinatous insertion and pain is aggravated by abduction of the shoulder against resistance. The patient eventually may present as having a rotator cuff tear. Plain X-rays of the shoulder may show calcification near the greater tuberosity.

Subacromial Bursitis

Subacromial bursitis is a painful inflammation of the subacromial bursa. During abduction of the shoulder the patient complaints of pain through a 60- to 120-degree of range. Normally, full abduction is achieved by external rotation of the humerus, which helps to ease the subacromial bursa under the coracoacromial arch. In stroke patients the external rotation of the shoulder is usually restricted, causing impingement and inflammation of subacromial bursa. Abduction of the arm becomes painful and there is presence of localized tenderness in the subacromial region over the lateral aspect of the shoulder. Active abduction of the arm against resistance reproduces pain in the shoulder. A patient may experience more pain at night. At times it is difficult to differentiate subacromial bursitis from calcific tendinitis. Attempts should be made to prevent onset of this problem by a judicious range-of-motion exercise program.

Coracoiditis

Pain resulting from coracoiditis remains controversial; patients with either direct injury to the coracoid process or traction injury to the soft tissues attached to the coracoid process will present with pain localized at the coracoid process. Injury usually occurs when the arm is in an adducted and externally rotated position, which causes stretching of the corachobrachialis and short head of biceps. Pain is usually worse at night and aggravated by abducting, externally rotating, and elevating the shoulder against resistance. Tenderness is present over the coracoid process. In stroke patients the hemiplegic shoulder attains a position of adduction and internal rotation because of spasticity, thus resulting in restricted range of motion in abduction, elevation, and external rotation, and pain.

To manage soft tissue injuries in stroke patients, the same methods and techniques as in nonhemiplegic patients generally are used. These procedures, however, have not been fully evaluated in stroke patients. The treatment is directed to the underlying tissues that may be involved in causing pain. General measures include simple analgesics such as salicylates, acetaminophen, and nonsteroidal preparations like ibuprofen. Acetaminophen does not have any antiinflammatory action, whereas salicylates and NSAIDs reduce inflammatory response. Adequate control of pain during the acute stage is important so that the patient does not develop chronic pain syndrome. Pain can lead to muscle spasm that may produce more pain. Muscle relaxants are prescribed to relieve muscle spasm and interrupt the vicious cycle. It is recommended that analgesics be prescribed at regular intervals around the clock rather than on a PRN basis. Oral or intramuscular steroids are also valuable in controlling pain.

Various physiotherapy modalities such as local application of heat and cold helps to relieve pain and reduce muscle spasm. Heat also decreases joint stiffness by altering the physical properties of the fibrous tissues found in tendons, joints capsules, and scars (21). If one is dealing with tightness in these structures, optimum benefits are achieved by application of heat followed by stretch. Prolonged steady stretch is more effective than intermittent or short-term stretch. However, the effects of heat and stretching are transient, and application of therapeutic heat and cold is not a cure for the underlying disease process.

The various types of heating modalities are classified into those that heat the superficial tissues and those that heat the deeper structures. Ultrasound penetrates deeply and decreases articular pain. Local heat application is contraindicated over anesthetized areas or in comatose patients and should be used with caution in patients with inadequate blood supply.

Transcutaneous electrical nerve stimulation (TENS) may also be prescribed. It has been reported to relieve both acute and chronic pain (22–25). Electrode placement and stimulation parameters remain vague and controversial. Electrodes are usually placed at the painful sites. It is recommended to use acupuncture points for optimum effects. The decision regarding TENS equipment prescription should not be based upon a single therapy session. To establish whether or not TENS treatment is effective, one needs to provide a few therapy sessions using different stimulation parameters and electrode placements. Application of TENS has been classified into high frequency (60–100 Hz) and low frequency (0.5–10 Hz). High-frequency treatments are usually at low intensities whereas low-frequency treatments involve higher intensities in the order of three to five times the sensory threshold. Thus, high-frequency TENS can be tolerated for many hours and low-frequency stimulation is less comfortable. It is difficult to predict patient response with either of the two treatment options.

Short-term oral steroids (if not contraindicated) such as prednisone dosed at 30 to 60 mg/day for 3 to 4 days usually provides pain relief. This can be gradually tapered off over 7 to 10 days. Local steroid injections provide temporary relief. Precautions should be taken during steroid injections because inappropriate injections into tendons may cause collagen necrosis. The steroids should flow freely into the bursal space and tendon sheath and should never be forced.

Progressive resistive exercise programs should be avoided during the acute stages of coracoiditis to prevent exacerbation of symptoms. The first priority is to maintain joint mobility. When pain has become less severe, gentle range-of-motion exercises should be prescribed followed by an active stretching exercise program. Isometric exercises to maintain and restore strength should be taught to the patient.

Degenerative Joint Disease

Pain can occur from degenerative changes in the acromioclavicular joint. These changes may occur early in life, around third and fourth decade. Degenerative changes involve the acromioclavicular joint, glenoid labrum, and articular cartilage of the glenoid fossa. With increasing age, significant degenerative changes occur in the periarticular soft tissue, including thickening and shredding of the biceps tendon. The rotator cuff thins and calcific deposits may appear. These changes, along with the thickening of the adjacent bursae, result in reduced space under the coracoacromial arch and an increased likelihood of impingement and pain. The additional factors resulting from paralysis may activate or aggravate pain in a previously asymptomatic shoulder. For example, in the flaccid stage, the weight of the unsupported arm can lower the coracoacromial arch, causing an increased possibility of impingement during passive elevation of the arm. Pain is noted at the acromioclavicular joint. Tenderness may be elicited over the joint. Crepitation can be felt during range-of-motion movements. Pain is aggravated during elevation and depression of the shoulder. Injection of an anesthetic agent into the joint may relieve the pain and help in diagnosis.

Rotator Cuff Tears

Reported incidence of rotator cuff tears on arthrographic examination in stroke patients with shoulder pain range between 33 and 40 percent. Najenson et al. reported a 40 percent incidence of rotator cuff rupture on the hemiplegic side as compared with 16 percent incidence on the contralateral normal side (2). However, another study of thirty patients showed no evidence of rotator cuff tears on arthrographic examination (26). According to Hakuno et al. (1984), the incidence of rotator cuff tear in the hemiplegic shoulder may not be different than the incidence of tears in the contralateral shoulder (27). Furthermore, partial tears of the rotator cuff are common after 50 or 60 years of age. It appears probable that rotator cuff tears are no more common in poststroke patients than in the age-matched nonhemiplegic population. Forcible abduction of shoulder without lateral rotation can convert a partial tear to a complete rupture. A higher incidence of rotator cuff tear has been reported with the use of overhead pulleys.

Pain resulting from rotator cuff tear is severe, especially with passive abduction or flexion. Tenderness may be present at the rupture site. Muscle weakness and atrophy of lateral rotator and deltoid may be evident.

The prevention of rotator cuff tear is the key to management of the upper extremity in stroke patients. Forcible abduction of the shoulder without lateral rotation should be avoided. The use of overhead pulleys should be discouraged. Stroke patients and their caregivers need advice about correct handling of the hemiplegic arm to prevent shoulder injury and rotator cuff tear.

Local application of physical modalities such as heat, ice, and TENS should be tried. Weiss (1981) reported successful results in thirteen of fifteen patients treated with intra-articular injection of steroid during shoulder arthrography (28). Indications for and outcomes of surgical intervention for rotator cuff tear have not been studied in stroke patients, however, surgical procedures may be indicated to correct deformity, relieve pain, or improve function. If there has been a reasonable return of motor control but functional activity is limited because of pain, surgical intervention could be considered. The patient must be motivated and have good cognition before surgical intervention is attempted.

Adhesive Capsulitis

Patients with adhesive capsulitis present with pain and restricted range of motion. Although the pain may subside, restricted range of motion increases, followed by muscle atrophy. In hemiplegic patients, the precise cause of adhesive capsulitis remains obscure. Factors that have been implicated include paralysis leading to prolonged immobilization, impingement pain, subluxation, and spasticity. The cause of adhesive capsulitis even in nonhemiplegic patients is unknown. Bruckner and Ney (1981), showed that the frequency of adhesive capsulitis was associated with duration of unconsciousness and immobilization of a hemiplegic arm (29). It is common in patients between 40 and 60 years of age. It is believed that capsular adhesions are the consequence rather than the cause of restricted range of motion and pain. In a study by Neviaser (1983), only 22 percent of the patients were found to have the subsynovial fibrosis and focal degeneration of collagen that was indicative of capsulitis (30). The study was carried out by capsular biopsies through arthrotomies. The main finding was thickening and contracture of the capsule. The shoulder capsule volume decreases to 0.5 to 3.0 cc in patients with adhesive capsulitis when compared to normal values of about 35 cc.

Spasticity has been considered one of the main factors leading to restricted range of motion and pain. Spasticity in stroke patients is generally left untreated and contractures of the involved limbs are frequently seen in the neglected spastic hemiplegic patient (1). In the hemiplegic upper extremity, the shoulder joint acquires an adducted and internally rotated position and there is flexor deformities of the elbow, wrist, and fingers.

The frequency of adhesive changes on arthrography is reported to range between 55 and 77 percent. Rizk et al. (1984) carried out arthrographic studies of thirty patients with stiff and painful shoulders (26). In 77 percent of these patients the changes of adhesive capsulitis were noted. In their study, there was no evidence of rotator cuff rupture (26). In a study by Hakuno et al. (1984), adhesive changes were noted in both hemiplegic and nonhemiplegic shoulders (27). However, 55 percent of the hemiplegic shoulders had multiple adhesions compared with 4 percent in nonhemiplegic shoulders. According to these investigators, patients with adhesions in the glenohumeral joint and subscapular bursae had restricted range of motion; adhesions in the bicipital tendon sheath were associated with significant subluxation but no restriction in range of motion (27).

Attempts should be made to prevent this adhesive capsulitis through proper positioning, range-of-motion exercise, and active assisted exercises during the acute stages of recovery. Application of heat, cold, and TENS may be effective in relieving pain and encouraging movement. Antiinflammatory and analgesic medications, oral steroids, and muscle relaxants should be tried. Antispastic drugs such as dantroline sodium should be prescribed in patients with marked spasticity. For those patients who do not respond to antispastic drugs and physical agents, Van Ouwenaller (1986) has recommended the use of lidocaine injections, supplemented by alcohol injections for shoulder girdle muscles. According to Van Ouwenaller, the latter measure does not paralyze the treated muscles (14).

Subscapular nerve block in painful hemiplegic shoulder has been described (31,32). The subscapular muscle is a major internal rotator of the shoulder and therefore plays a significant role in the flexor synergy pattern commonly seen in spastic hemiplegia. Hecht treated thirteen patients with spastic hemiplegia, limited range of motion, and painful shoulders (32). Percutaneous phenol blocks to the nerves to the subscapularis muscle were carried out. Immediate improvements in range of motion were observed and relief of pain was noted where there was previously painful movement (32).

Ekelund and Rydell (1992) reported the results of a combination treatment for adhesive capsulitis of the shoulder in twenty-two patients (33). The adhesive capsulitis of the glenohumeral joint was verified arthrographically. A combination of treatments included distension-arthrography, local anesthetics and intra-articular steroids, and manipulation. A rapid improvement was seen after treatment; at four to six weeks, 91 percent of the patients had slight to no pain, and 83 percent of the patients had normal, or almost normal range of motion (33). The treatment was well tolerated with no complications. The authors concluded that a combination treatment for adhesive capsulitis of the shoulder is safe, yields immediate results, and is cost effective. A similar approach has been investigated by Laroche and colleagues, who treated forty cases of adhesive capsulitis with joint distension during arthrography followed by intra-articular corticosteroids injection and high intensity physical therapy (34). These authors also concluded that this approach is effective in improving range of motion and pain. However, this combination approach has not been studied in stroke patients.

Shoulder Subluxation

Subluxation of the hemiplegic shoulder is a very common problem. The incidence of subluxation in hemiplegic shoulders is reported to be as high as 92 percent (35–41). Incidence varies depending on whether the diagnosis was clinical or radiological. Subluxation may only be demonstrated if the patient is X-rayed erect, with the arm unsupported.

Shoulder subluxation has been associated with shoulder pain, although it is controversial whether it is a common cause of pain in the hemiplegic shoulder. A large number of stroke patients may have subluxation but no pain. The study by Bohannon and associates in 1986 failed to demonstrate a significant relationship between shoulder subluxation and shoulder pain (8).

Subluxation may be noted in the flaccid as well spastic stage of hemiplegia. Inferior subluxation appears to be more common in hemiplegic patients. It appears to develop during the first few weeks of stroke when flaccid weakness prevents normal muscle response to loading (37). In these stroke patients the usual stabilizing mechanism of the glenohumeral joint becomes ineffective, thus permitting inferior displacement of the humeral head in relation to the glenoid fossa (42). This becomes more evident in an upright position, when the gravitation force is unopposed, and results in inferior subluxation. Overstretching of the superior glenohumeral capsule occurs, and ligaments as well as the supraspinatus and deltoid muscles are affected. Improper positioning of the arm in the supine and upright position and also inappropriate pulling on the flaccid hemiplegic arm during transfer and other activities may also cause subluxation in some patients. A study by Smith et al. (1982), of stroke patients within 24 hours of their admission found that 60 percent of the patients with complete paralysis had glenohumeral joint malalignment (38). Serial electromyographic studies demonstrated that subluxation develops during the flaccid stage of hemiplegia (43–45). Subluxation does not occur after the supraspinatous muscle demonstrates electromyographic activity in response to loading (43,45).

The relationship of pain to subluxation in unclear. It appears that subluxation of the shoulder joint is common; however, there is doubt whether it is a causative factor in pain production. Several investigators have suggested that the presence of shoulder subluxation is an important factor in the development of shoulder pain (14,39,40). Najenson and colleagues (1965) reported that 88 of the 280 patients studied showed radiological evidence of malalignment of the gleno-humeral joint (46). They believed that malalignment produced moderate pain. In their study, the malalignment was associated with severe paralysis. However, Peszczynski and colleagues (1965), found no statistical difference in the amount of subluxation in patients with or without pain (7). Similarly, Kumar and associates did not find a difference in the development of pain with or without subluxation (12). A recent study by Joynt (1992) failed to show a statistical relationship between the presence of subluxation and either the severity of pain or the amount of pain on passive movement (15). Zorowitz et. al. (1996) concluded that limitation of shoulder external rotation played an important role in shoulder pain after stroke, whereas shoulder subluxation did not (47). Their findings suggest that treatment should focus on shoulder range of motion. Ikai and associates (1998) arrived at similar conclusions—no relationship was found between shoulder subluxation and pain (48). In their opinion, adhesive capsulitis was considered the main cause of shoulder pain (48). The authors recommended that correct positioning and shoulder range-of-motion exercises should be carried out.

The diagnosis of subluxation is a clinical one when a palpable gap is detected between the acromion and the humeral head on the affected side. The severity of subluxation can be assessed by radiological examination of the shoulder.

Management of subluxation in a painful hemiplegic shoulder is frequently less than satisfactory (49). Prevention of subluxation and maintaining range of motion is very important. During acute stages, proper positioning of the hemiplegic upper extremity is crucial. The shoulder should be kept in a slightly abducted and externally rotated position. The arm is positioned in a slight elbow flexion, forearm pronation, wrist and finger extension, and thumb abduction. While sitting in the wheelchair, the use of a trough is recommended. An arm trough helps to prevent adduction and internal rotation of the shoulder. It is imperative to prevent excessive downward pull on the humeral head by proper handling of the upper extremity during range-of-motion exercises and transfer activities. There is a need for meticulous attention to seating prescriptions and the positioning of the patient in a wheelchair. The emphasis is on maintaining anatomical alignment and on preventing injury to the insensate limb. A proper wheelchair armrest is required. If the trough is too low, functional scoliosis may develop. Humeral head impaction may occur if the armrest is too high. Similar guidelines apply if a lapboard is prescribed instead of the trough.

Range-of-motion exercises should be prescribed in the early stages of recovery and should be maintained for an indefinite period. It is recommended that these exercises should not be overly vigorous. Care should be taken in transfer activities.

Supporting and protecting the involved shoulder in the initial flaccid stage is important. Traditionally a sling has been used to prevent or treat subluxation. The use of slings remains controversial (38,50–52), and some believe that the use of a sling is contraindicated (53) because it may increase flexor synergy by maintaining the arm in a flexed position. Slings have been claimed to impair body image (2) and predispose the patient to reflex sympathetic dystrophy (54). A sling may be prescribed to support a flaccid arm, however, when the patient is ambulating. If used continuously without frequent range-of-motion exercises, it may play a role in developing contractures. In a study by Brooke et al. (1991), a Harris hemisling provided consistent correction of subluxation in the hemiplegic shoulder (55). According to these investigators, the Bobath sling did not correct the vertical subluxation and the arm trough tended to overcorrect. Other forms of supports also failed to correct subluxation (56,57). Brundy has reported good results with a much more complex device (58).

Functional electrical stimulation (FES) has been used to treat glenohumeral subluxation and pain (59,60). In a controlled study of 24 months duration, Chantraine et al. (1999) concluded that the FES program was significantly effective in reducing the severity of subluxation and pain and possibly may have facilitated recovery of shoulder function (60). Neuromuscular electrical stimulation of the shoulder-stabilizing muscles also has been reported to decrease shoulder subluxation and promote recovery of function (61). The discomfort of surface neuromuscular stimulation, however, significantly limits the clinical implementation of this modality for persons with hemiplegia (62). Chae and Hart (1998) compared surface and percutaneous intramuscular electrical stimulation and concluded that the percutaneous intramuscular stimulation was significantly better tolerated than surface stimulation and that the percutaneous technique may enhance patient compliance with neuromuscular stimulation treatments (62). Chae and Walker (2001) described the use of percutaneous, intramuscular neuromuscular electrical stimulation for the treatment of shoulder subluxation and pain in a patient with chronic hemiplegia (63). Myoelectric biofeedback from upper trapezius and middle and anterior deltoid muscles has been reported to decrease and often eliminate subluxation. Range of motion and spasticity may also be improved with biofeedback (64,65). A beneficial effect of electroacupuncture on shoulder subluxation and shoulder pain has been reported by Chen and colleagues (66).

Shoulder–Hand Syndrome (SHS): Reflex Sympathetic Dystrophy

The terms *reflex sympathetic dystrophy* and *causalgia* have been used in many different ways (67,68). The revised classification puts them under the umbrella of *complex regional pain syndrome* (CRPS) (69). Shoulder–hand syndrome (SHS) describes a clinical picture that is characterized by shoulder pain, distal limb pain, edema, changes of vasomotor instability, hyperalgesia, and dystrophic skin changes (70). The subject has been recently reviewed (71). The trophic changes include skin atrophy, hyperhidrosis, skin pigmentary abnormalities, and changes in the nails. The exact pathophysiology remains controversial. Peripheral and central nervous system etiologies have been proposed. The CVA may disturb central vasomotor regulation, thus resulting in arteriolar vasodilation of the upper extremity. The sympathetic nervous system has frequently been implicated because of vasomotor instability in the hand, and SHS has been widely considered as a sympathetic mediated pain often seen in the hemiplegic upper extremity following stroke. Pain, however, may or may not be dependent on the sympathetic nervous system. Campbell et al. (1992) have described sympathetically maintained pain on the basis of whether the pain is eliminated by sympathetic blockade (72).

The exact incidence and prevalence of shoulder–hand syndrome in hemiplegic patients is unclear (73). Van Ouwenaller and colleagues (1986) cite incidence rates from 12 to 70 percent (14); in their own study the incidence rate was 23 percent (14). The disparity regarding incidence may result from different definitions and reports of so-called partial forms. Most stroke patients who develop SHS do so between two and four months following stroke. It has been reported more commonly in patients with sensory loss, marked weakness, presence of spasticity, and confusion. SHS is usually unilateral. In 20 to 35 percent of patients, it is bilateral. In the hemiplegic patient the syndrome may occur along with flaccidity as well as spasticity.

The primary signs and symptoms of SHS include distal pain, swelling, and discoloration of the skin. These must be present to make a presumptive diagnosis. The clinical picture of shoulder–hand syndrome may be described in three phases (74). During Phase One there is severe burning pain and limited range of motion. Passive and active range of motion is most restricted in shoulder extension and abduction, wrist dorsiflexion, and flexion of the metacarpophalangeal and proximal interphalangeal joints. This is associated with swelling, stiffness, and increased skin temperature. Swelling is usually confined to the dorsum of the hand, wrist, and finger joints. The swelling is firm and the skin becomes shiny and moist. The skin temperature over the hand varies and is usually high in the early stages of the syndrome. There is increased sweating and vasomotor instability. Tenderness may be elicited over the dorsum of the hand.

During Phase Two, the shoulder pain may subside. The range of motion improves with residual restriction. The hand swelling subsides and becomes brawny in nature. The joint stiffness becomes progressively worse in the fingers and is difficult to treat. The hand becomes cold. There may be evidence of hair loss and atrophy of the nail. The skin shows atropic changes and becomes pale and shiny. X-rays may show patchy osteoporosis.

During Phase Three, there is progressive atrophy of the bones. There is also significant atrophy of the skin and decreased sweating. Intrinsic muscle wasting is evident. When the pain subsides, there is a marked restriction in range of motion. At this point the functional loss is essentially irreversible.

Early recognition, based on by proper interpretation of symptoms and clinical signs, is the key to prevention and successful treatment. No one sign or symptom, however, can establish the diagnosis. Awareness on the part of the physician regarding signs and symptoms is the first essential step in diagnosis of this syndrome. Technetium diphosphonate bone scan demonstrates periarticular uptake in the wrist and metacarpalphalangeal joints of the involved limb. Bone scan abnormalities appear at the same time as the onset of clinical signs and symptoms. According to Tepperman et al. (1984), 25 percent of hemiplegic patients demonstrated evidence of SHS in the involved upper extremity on bone scan although only two-thirds went on to develop the clinical syndrome (17).

Symptoms and signs of SHS may resolve spontaneously, but an early management of the condition carries a better prognosis. Most treatments are directed at reducing pain so that function can be maintained and restored. A comprehensive approach towards relieving pain, maintaining range of motion and maximizing function should be implemented. Treatment of SHS includes range of motion exercises, mobilization of the involved limb, and optimal positioning of the joints. Joint mobilization is essential and must be performed with great care. Control of swelling is accomplished with elevation, wrapping, and intermittent compression. Use of local heat may help in mobilization. Active exercises are encouraged and should be performed within the limits of pain tolerance. Transcutaneous electrical nerve stimulation can be helpful to relieve pain (52). Nonsteroidal drugs are prescribed to control pain. A short course of high oral dose of steroids is prescribed (52,73,75). The usual dose varies from 60 to 100 mg of steroids daily for 7 to 10 days, gradually tapering over 3 to 4 weeks. Response to oral steroids has been reported to be better in those patients who have positive bone scan (70). Precautions should be taken in prescribing steroids for patients who have a history of diabetes mellitus and peptic ulcer.

Alternatively, sympathetic blockade may be performed either by a regional sympathetic block or intravenous injection of agents to produce a chemical sympathectomy. Two drugs that have been reported to relieve the pain are guanethidine and reserpine. Double-blind studies have shown guanethidine significantly reduces pain in comparison to saline controls. Because of associated cardiac problems in stroke patients, some investigators caution the use of alpha adrenergic blockers such as guanethidine and phentolamine in these patients (76–78). Sympathetic blockade can also be attained by surgical stellate sympathectomy in selected cases. The stellate ganglion block requires a thorough anatomic knowledge and experience in performing the procedure. Many patients require more than one block. Other options that have been reported include local corticosteroid injection and surgical sympathectomy. Hamamci et al. (1996) reported beneficial effects of calcitonin in patients with reflex sympathetic dystrophy (79). Salmon calcitonin, 1 × 100 IU/day intramuscularly for 4 weeks, was administered to 25 stroke patients and the results were compared with intramuscular injection of physiological saline in 16 patients. In the calcitonin group a significant decrease in pain and tenderness resulted in improvement of range of motion and motor function. Patients who are not treated or those who respond incompletely to treatment are left with varying degrees of pain and contractures of the upper extremity (79). Acupuncture in the treatment of chronic pain has been described (80).

SHS is often accompanied by mood disturbance and, according to Savage (1982), depression more frequently accompanies this diagnosis than other categories of shoulder pain (81). Clinical depression often requires appropriate treatment that may also relieve pain. SHS persisting longer than 6 months has a poor prognosis.

Brachial Plexus Injury

Nerve injury to the brachial plexus and suprascapular nerve has been implicated as a possible cause for shoulder pain (82,83). Brachial plexus injury may be caused either by lack of support of the paralyzed flaccid limb, subluxation, or caused by inadvertent traction during the flaccid phase of hemiplegia. Patients who are unconscious are more prone to have traction injury. The exact pathophysiology of pain in traction injury is not known. Jaeger et al. reported that traction injury could cause both physiologic and anatomic dysfunction (77). There may be myelin sheath disruption and loss of continuity of the endoneurial tubes. According to these authors, when the myelin sheath loses continuity and the endoneural tube remains intact, a "spindle neuroma" is produced. In more severe traction injuries, the endoneural tubes can be damaged. The cellular response yields a firm, irregular nodule referred to as a *neuroma in continuity*. This type of lesion may be quite painful and resistant to surgical excision (77).

Chino (1981) reported that 75 percent of his hemiplegic patients with subluxation demonstrated neuropathic responses in the deltoid and supraspinatus muscles (44). Kaplan and associates found EMG abnormalities that were consistent with injury to the upper trunk of the brachial plexus in hemiplegic patients with flaccid paralysis (82). Some investigators have found no electrophysiologic evidence of brachial plexus injuries in hemiplegic patients (50,84).

Clinically, brachial plexus injury may not be recognized in the presence of marked weakness and decreased tone resulting from hemiplegia. Brachial plexus injury should be suspected in the presence of an abnormal pattern of recovery. Usually, proximal recovery is followed by distal recovery. In patients with brachial plexus injury, however, this sequence is reversed. Brachial plexus injury leads to atrophy of proximal shoulder muscles, with fair to good recovery of hand and fingers. In these patients, the usual adduction and internal rotation of the shoulder is not present. Electromyographic examination may help to diagnose brachial plexus injury. Involvement of the lower motor neuron in the presence of an upper motor neurone lesion increases the likelihood for the development of painful contractures (83).

Injury to the brachial plexus may influence functional outcome and result in a prolonged rehabilitation. Thus it is very important to maintain range of motion by passive or active assistive exercise program. Pain should be controlled by prescribing appropriate analgesics and modalities. The shoulder should be splinted in 45 degrees of abduction.

HAND AND WRIST PAIN

Hand and wrist pain may result from trauma, infection, and inflammation of the joints. Pressure neuropathy of ulnar and median nerve may cause pain not only in the hand and forearm, but around the shoulder joint as well. Usually there is associated paresthesia in the effected hand. Flexion contractures of the hand and wrist are common and may cause pain. Pain may increase spasticity. Pain, spasticity, and contractures limit return of functional activity in the hemiplegic hand.

Contractures should be prevented through range-of-motion exercise and optimal positioning of the wrist and fingers. The wrist is maintained in 20 to 30 degrees of extension. If splinting is prescribed, care should be taken that the splint fits properly and does not cause pain.

Table 5.2. Lower Extremity Pain

Heterotopic ossification
Degenerative joint disease
Genu recurvatum
Polymyalgia rheumatica
Spinal stenosis
Fractures
Deep venous thrombosis
Foot deformities

LOWER EXTREMITY PAIN

Lower extremity pain is common in spinal cord injury patients and may take several forms. The most common causes of lower extremity pain are described in this section (see Table 5.2).

Heterotopic Ossification (HO)

Although heterotopic ossification is common in patients with spinal cord injury, traumatic brain injury, burns, or direct trauma, it is rare following cerebrovascular accidents. It may affect the elbow, shoulder, and hip (85–88). Some believe that HO is associated in patients with decubiti and is more common in debilitated patients. During the acute stage, the clinical picture includes local pain, tenderness, swelling, and increased skin temperature. Later, a hard mass may be palpable. Range of motion is painful and restricted. Blood work shows an elevated sedimentation rate and alkaline phosphatase. HO at the elbow should be suspected when there is an elbow extension contracture rather than the more typical flexion contracture. Infection should be ruled out. Diagnosis and maturity of HO is confirmed by bone scan. Treatment includes maintaining range of motion to prevent contractures. Delay in diagnosis and treatment results in a poor functional outcome. Surgical removal is indicated in patients with mature ossified tissue and if removal of the ossified tissue is expected to enhance function. Immature resected HO usually reoccurs. The maturity is best determined by decreased activity on bone scan. When a bone scan is not available, maturity may be verified by serial estimation to show that alkaline phosphatase has become stable. Although etidronate sodium has been reported to be effective in preventing HO in spinal cord injury and traumatic brain injury, its role in preventing HO in stroke patients is less clearly defined.

Degenerative Joint Disease

Stroke is common in elderly people and as such other common causes of pain in this population must be considered in differential diagnosis. Degenerative joints are common in the elderly. Osteoarthritis of the hip and knee joints on the affected side is usually aggravated with the onset of hemiplegia and spasticity (89). Because of increased mechanical demands on the unaffected side, there is exacerbation of pre-existing osteoarthritis and aggravation of pain in the hip and knee joints.

Symptoms are localized to the involved joints. Pain is usually the presenting symptom. Pain is relieved by rest and increases with activity. During the course of the disease the patient may experience more pain at night. One or more joints may be involved. Examination of the joint may reveal swelling, restricted range of motion, and palpable crepitus. In advanced cases there may be muscle wasting and deformity with evidence of contractures. The patient usually complains of limited mobility and difficulty in performing activities of daily living. Radiologic examination shows an irregular and narrow joint space, subchondral sclerosis, osteophytes, and cyst formation. Radiologic changes of degenerative arthritis are present in 85 percent of those between the ages 75 to 79 years. Radiologic changes, however, do not always correlate with the clinical picture (90). Degenerative joint disease involving hip and knee joints is a common source of limited functional activities because of pain that is aggravated by walking.

Lower extremity pain in a stroke patient may interfere in gait training. Irrespective of whether the pain is on the hemiplegic or normal side, the patient may have difficulty with weight bearing and may develop balance problems while protecting the painful extremity. Severe pain may increase spasticity.

In addition to an appropriate assisstive device for walking, local heat should be prescribed. TENS may help control the pain. Analgesics and NSAIDs should be prescribed with special care because of a higher incidence of gastrointestinal bleeding and renal failure in the elderly. Intra-articular injection of steroids may help to reduce pain and swelling. Replacement arthroplasty of knee and hip joint should be considered.

Genu Recurvatum

Genu recurvatum is a posterior bowing of the knee and is caused by impaired tone and lack of knee control. An increased extensor tone about the knee, plantar flexion of the ankle caused by a tight gastrocnemius muscle, decreased proprioception about the knee, and weak quadriceps mechanism contribute to hyperextension of the knee. To prevent knee collapse while weight bearing during the stance phase of the gait, patients may often hyperextend the knee. Hyperextension may lead to progressive stretching of the posterior capsule and ligaments of the knee. If allowed to continue for some time, this often leads to a painful knee. Another contributing factor for knee pain is degenerative changes within the knee joint (as described above) caused by the change in weight-bearing surfaces within the knee joint.

Management involves gait training, strengthening of the quadriceps muscle, and ensuring adequate ankle dorsiflexion. An ankle–foot orthosis may be prescribed with 5 degrees of dorsiflexion. Care should be taken to prevent excessive knee flexion, which might lead to collapsing of the knee during stance phase. This can be achieved by quadriceps strengthening or adding an anterior stop to a double-action ankle–foot orthosis.

Polymyalgia Rheumatica

Because stroke is common in the elderly, it is important to understand some of the other causes of common pain that may be coincidental but significant in limiting rehabilitation outcomes. Polymyalgia rheumatica is one of these syndromes. The peak incidence occurs at 70 to 79 years of age. It is more common in females. Presenting history includes sudden onset of pain in the neck, back, and proximal parts of the upper and lower extremities. The pain may be associated with morning stiffness. Some patients may also complain of anorexia, weight loss, lethargy, and depression. The physical examination is usually noncontributory. The ESR is elevated, often greater than 100 mm/hr. Other laboratory work is normal including normal muscle enzymes, electromyography, and muscle biopsy.

Response to oral steroids is excellent. If pain is not relieved within 7 to 10 days, another diagnosis should be considered. Appropriate range-of-motion exercise should be prescribed to prevent contractures. Disuse muscle weakness should be prevented by strengthening exercises.

Spinal Stenosis

Spinal stenosis is another comorbid condition in the elderly stroke patient that must be kept in mind during rehabilitation. The patient presents with history of pain, numbness, and weakness in the gluteal region and thigh. The symptoms are usually bilateral. Symptoms are worse when walking or standing and are relieved with rest and flexion of the lumbosacral spine. There is a slow progression of the symptoms. Physical examination may reproduce pain on extension of the spine. In the presence of hemiplegia, the neurologic findings resulting from spinal stenosis may be difficult to interpret. CT scan and MRI are helpful in diagnosis and may show narrowing of the spinal canal. Needle electromyography may help to confirm the diagnosis.

Management includes prescription of range-of-motion exercise, local physical modalities, and nonsteroidal antiinflammatory drugs. Surgical decompression may be required in patients with severe spinal stenosis and intractable pain.

Fractures

Fracture involving femur, humerus, and distal radius are common in the elderly. Fractures occur more often on the hemiplegic side. The significant bone-mass reduction that occurs on the hemiplegic side of stroke patients, caused by disuse, may explain the increased poststroke incidence of fractures. It appears that skeletal remodeling is accelerated in patients with hemiplegia (91). This may be the result of vitamin D deficiency and insufficient compensatory hyperparathyroidism stimulating skeletal turnover in immobilized stroke patients (92). There is often osteoporosis present, caused by decreased weight bearing, throughout the affected side.

Perceptual deficits may not play a major role, because the incidence of hip fractures is thought to occur equally in both right- and left-hemiplegic patients. A fracture in the lower extremity may cause some increase in spasticity and may result in a decline in functional activities. After a history of fall, fracture should be considered as a source of pain in the stroke patient. Most of these fractures occur as a result of a minor fall. Hip fractures are associated with high morbidity and mortality. Prevention of falls and fractures is crucial to a successful rehabilitation outcome. High-risk patients must be identified and closely monitored during their rehabilitation program. Proper management of deteriorating vision and hearing will help to prevent falls and subsequent fractures. Improving muscle strength and balance may also reduce the incidence of falls. Sato and associates (1997) evaluated the efficacy of 1 alpha-hydroxyvitamin D3 and supplemental elemental calcium in maintaining bone mass and decreasing the incidence of hip fractures (93). The authors conclude that treatment can reduce the risk of hip fractures and can prevent further decrease in bone mineral density on the hemiplegic side of patients with a long-standing stroke. Poplingher and Pillar (1985) found no difference in incidence of concurrent disease, hospitalization time, mortality, and functional recovery between hip fracture patients with or without a history of stroke (94). An interval of less than a week between stroke and fracture, however, was associated with poor functional recovery (94).

Surgical intervention appears to be the choice of treatment. Hooper (1979) found that internal fixation was technically satisfactory in trochanteric fractures, but failed in cervical fractures (95).

Leg Pain

Stroke patients are at high risk of developing deep venous thrombosis (DVT) in the paralyzed lower extremity. Deep venous thrombosis is a common consequence of immobility and as such, may cause significant morbidity after stroke. The reported incidence of DVT following stroke varies depending on the type of patient population studied. The patient may present with leg pain and swelling. Prevention with an appropriate anticoagulation regimen is the key to success. For a detailed description of screening, prevention, and treatment refer to the recent reviews by Brandstater et al. (1992) and Clagett et al. (1992) (96,97).

Many patients go on to develop some form of postphlebitic sequelae following a DVT. The initial symptoms of postphlebitic syndrome are swelling and an aching pain in the leg. Pain is more marked when the leg is left in a dependent position. In severe cases, venous claudication may occur in the calf during exercise. Patients with postphlebitic syndrome are best treated with pressure gradient stockings and leg elevation.

Foot Pain

Equinovarus deformity is quite common in patients with cerebrovascular accidents secondary to the common extensor reflex pattern of the lower extremity. Equinus is caused by overactivity of the gastrocnemius and soleus. This contributes to genu recurvatum caused by the extensor moment placed on the knee by the plantar flexion deformity. Ankle varus may be caused by spasticity of the tibialis anterior, flexor hallucis longus, flexor digitorum longus, soleus, and—less commonly—tibialis posterior muscles. Ankle varus also causes the patient to walk on the anterolateral aspect of the foot. Consequently, stress fractures and pain may result. Pressure sores may develop on the lateral aspect of the foot. Local foot pain may result even without the stress fracture. Foot pain may be a major limiting factor in gait training.

During the early stages, treatment options include correction of equinus by a locked ankle–foot orthosis. There are many commercial and custom orthoses available, and these include conventional dual-channel double-upright adjustable ankle AFO, single-adjustable ankle joint with dorsiflexion assist, and molded plastic posterior AFO. In less severe cases, providing lateral flares and lateral wedging to the patient's footwear helps to improve gait and relieve pain.

In severe and selected cases of equinus deformity surgical correction is performed by lengthening of the Achilles tendon (98). At the time of the Achilles tendon lengthening, release of the toe flexors should be performed to prevent toe curling from the tenodesis effect of ankle dorsiflexion. Preoperative EMG studies are helpful to determine the specific muscles responsible for the varus deformity, usually the tibialis anterior. For varus deformity, a split anterior tibial transfer for spastic equinovarus foot deformity improves the ability to ambulate independently and decreases the need to wear orthopedic shoes and orthosis. This procedure has been reported to be safe and yields good results with minimal complications (99).

Toe flexion deformity is a common problem. Usually both extrinsic and intrinsic toe flexors are responsible. Excessive toe flexor may cause pain and is difficult to treat. Prescription of a deep, wide shoe may help to relieve the pain. If the pain is disabling and a contracture and associated pain cannot be corrected with physiotherapy, an ankle–foot orthosis or surgical intervention should be considered. Toe flexor release is performed through a medial midfoot incision. Occasionally, an intrinsic plus deformity is present that may required intrinsic release through plantar incision at the base of the toes.

CENTRAL PAIN (THALAMIC PAIN)

Central pain following a cerebrovascular accident is often mistakenly referred to as thalamic pain, despite the fact that in many patients with central poststroke pain the thalamus is not affected (100). Central pain has been described following lower brainstem, thalamic, and suprathalamic cerebrovascular accidents. When the thalamus is involved, generally the lesion is in the posterolateral or posterior thalamus. Involvement of this area, however, does not necessarily lead to central pain (101).

Dejerine and Roussy described a clinical syndrome caused by a thalamic lesion (102). Pain is the cardinal symptom. Pain is described as spontaneous, severe, paroxysmal, and burning. Central pain is also described as ripping, pressing, aching, and lacerating. Spontaneous dysesthesias occur in the majority of patients with central pain problem. Patients also complain of overreaction to noxious tactile stimuli (hyperalgesia) as well as painful sensation to non-noxious stimuli. Features of thalamic involvement, such as hemiparesis, hemiataxia, hemichoreoathetosis, and hemihypoesthesia on the affected side are present. Pain may involve the face, tongue, and thorax and the affected limbs. Pain is exacerbated by emotional states and tactile, visual, auditory, or thermal stimuli. Vasomotor changes may be present. The patient may give a history of cyclic skin changes such as coolness, pallor, and hyperhidrosis, alternating with warmth, rubor, and edema (103).

Pathophysiology of Central Pain

The pathophysiology of central pain remains unknown. The most widely accepted explanation is loss of inhibitory influences on somatosensory pathways. Presence of hyperesthesias and allodynia suggest that many of these patients may have components of sympathetic mediated pain.

In a study by Nasreddine, thalamic pain was more common with right-sided thalamic lesion; this laterality was more evident in men when compared with women (104). The frequency of components of the syndrome such as sensory impairment, hemiparesis, ataxia, and choreoathetosis, did not significantly differ between right and left stroke. Pain onset was within the first week poststroke in 36 percent of the patients. All patients had vascular lesions, 71 percent had ischemic infarction, and 29 percent parenchymal hemorrhage. Lesions were confined to the thalamus in about 52 percent of the patients and an additional 21 percent had extension to the internal capsule.

For prognostic and treatment purposes various investigators have attempted to classify the syndrome in different nosologic entities. For example, Mauguiere and Desmedt (1988) examined thirty patients with thalamic vascular lesions and, based on the clinical sensory disturbance and examination of somatosensory evoked potentials (SEPs), identified four nosological clinical thalamic syndromes (101). Group One had complete hemianesthesia and loss of SEPs, but no central pain. In Group Two there was severe hypoesthesia and loss of SEPs with a history of central pain. Group Three had central pain and hypoesthesia with intact, although delayed, SEPs on the affected side. The fourth group had central pain with preserved touch and joint sensations and normal SEPs. The authors conclude that the proposed nosologic differentiation provides a reference frame for treatment and pathophysiologic studies of central pain (101). According to these investigators, larger thalamic lesions usually did not result in central pain, and patients with smaller lesions in the same area seemed to be at higher risk of developing central pain. Patients with identical lesions, however, often do not go on to develop central pain.

Similarly, Wessel et al. (1994) correlated the clinical symptoms, somatosensory evoked potentials, and computed tomography (CT) findings (105). They divided the syndrome into three groups (a) those with somatosensory deficits, central pain, and abnormal SEPs (classic thalamic pain syndrome); (b) those with somatosensory deficits, no central pain, and abnormal SEPs (analgetic thalamic syndrome); and (*c*) those with almost normal sense perception, central pain, and normal SEPs (pure algetic thalamic syndrome). Patients with CT evidence of a paramedian or anterolateral thalamic lesion manifested with central pain. Holmgren and colleagues (1990) studied somatosensory evoked potentials in twenty-seven stroke patients and nineteen healthy controls and concluded that lesions of the spinothalamic pathways are crucial for the development of central poststroke pain (106).

The exact incidence and prevalence of central pain is unknown. According to Gonzales (1995) roughly 90 percent of all cases of central pain are caused by strokes (107). It is estimated to occur in 2 to 16 percent of cases. The frequency of thalamic pain is relatively more common in lesions involving geniculothalamic artery. Examination may reveal marked proprioceptive loss and body neglect on the hemiplegic side.

Treatment of Central Pain

Management of central or thalamic pain has been a particularly difficult problem. At times the goal of treatment should be pain reduction rather than complete pain relief. Analgesics, opioids, and psychotropic drugs have yielded variable but generally inconsistent and ineffective results. Pharmacological treatment may take the form of stepwise addition of various agents: the sequence of prescription usually starts with antidepressants, followed by phenothiazines, and anticonvulsants. Tricyclic antidepressant medications have been shown to have a beneficial effect on central pain. According to Andersen et al. (1985), the most effective treatment is with adrenergically active antidepressants, such as amitriptyline and nortriptyline (108). Dosage is gradually increased from 10 or 25 mg/day to 50 or 75 mg/day (109). Patients not responding to antidepressants may benefit by adding mexiletine. Phenothiazines (chlorpromazine) and anticonvulsants (phenytoin) may also help in relieving pain. Vick and Lamer (2001) reported a case of 68-year-old female patient with refractory central poststroke pain who responded to a ketamine trial (110). Apomorphine also has been reported effective, but it is associated with significant adverse effects and has a tendency to lose its beneficial effects over time.

Other available options that may provide some temporary relieve include transcutaneous electrical nerve stimulation (TENS) and sympathetic blockade. Sympathetic blockade with stellate ganglion and lumbar sympathetic blocks or local venous guanethidine blocks may temporarily relieve pain. Electroconvulsive therapy was found to be ineffective in relieving pain in three subjects with intractable poststroke thalamic pain (111). Taira et al. (1994) described their experience with spinal intrathecal injections of baclofen in five stroke patients with central pain (112). Four of the five subjects reported pain reduction.

Several operative procedures have been described in selected patients. These procedures include brain stimulation, electrical stimulation of precentral cortical area (113), stereotaxic thalamotomy (114), and stereotaxic chemical hypophysectomy. Overall, neurosurgical procedures have demonstrated a 25 percent success rate in permanently relieving central pain. These procedures are associated with a significant risk of brain injury.

Motoi et al. (1997) have described a case of posthemiplegic painful dystonia following thalamic infarction with good response to botulinus toxin (115).

Treatment of psychological problems resulting from CP is necessary because depression and the risk of suicide is significant in these patients.

PAINFUL TONIC SPASMS

Tonic spasms typical of those seen in multiple sclerosis have been reported in patients with lacunar infarcts involving putamen and pons (116–118). Paroxysmal painful spasms may involve upper and lower extremities and are associated with dull occipital headache and nausea. These spasms usually are brief, frequent, and intensely painful. Spasms may be precipitated by attempts to move. Increased weakness and tone may follow a spasm. Carbamazepine may relieve the spasm and, during a prolonged episode, rapid relief may be obtained with intravenous administration of diazepam.

CONCLUSIONS

Pain following stroke is very common, especially in the upper extremities, and may be a major contributor to long-term disability. Pain can impact substantially on a patient's sense of well being. For many stroke patients, chronic pain is underestimated as a factor that significantly contributes to the loss of overall quality of life and disability. Attempts should be made to prevent certain problems that may lead to acute and chronic pain. Early recognition of underlying causes and application of appropriate interventions is crucial to prevent morbidity.

REFERENCES

1. Teasel RW. Pain following stroke. *Crit Rev Phys Med Rehab* 1992; 3:205–217.
2. Najenson T, Yacubovich E, Pikielni SS. Rotator cuff injury in shoulder joints of hemiplegic patients. *Scand J Rehab Med* 1971; 3:131–137.
3. Jorgensen HS, Jespersen HF, Nakayama H, Raaschou HO, Olsen TS. Headache in stroke: The Copenhagen Stroke Study. Neurology 1994; 44:1793–1797.
4. Ferro JM, Melo TP, Oliveira V, Salgado AV, Crespo M, Canhao P, Pinto AN. A multivariate study of headache associated with ischemic stroke. *Headache* 1995; 35:315–319.
5. Kumral E, Bogousslavsky J, Van Melle G, et al. Headache at stroke onset: the Lausanne Stroke Registry. *J Neurol Neurosurg Psychiatry* 1995; 58:490–492.
6. MacGowan DJL, Janal MN, Clark WC, Wharton RN, et al. Central poststroke pain and Wallenberg's lateral medullary infarction: Frequency, character, and determinants in 63 patients. Neurology 1997; 49: 120–125.
7. Peszczynski M, Rardin TE, Jr. The incidence of painful shoulder in hemiplegia. *Polish Medical Science and History* 1965; 29:21–23.
8. Bohannon RW, Larkin PA, Smith MB, Horton MG. Shoulder pain in hemiplegia: Statistical relationship with five variables. *Arch Phys Med Rehab* 1986; 67:514–516.

9. Roy CW. Shoulder pain in hemiplegia: A literature review. *Clin Rehab* 1988; 2: 35–44.

10. Roy CW, Sands MR, Hill LD, Harrison A et al. The effect of shoulder pain on outcome of acute hemiplegia. *Clin Rehab* 1995; 9: 21–27.

11. Wanklyn P, Forster A, Young J. Hemiplegic shoulder pain: Natural history and investigation of associated features. *Disability and Rehabilitation* 1996; 18:497–501.

12. Kumar R, Metter EJ, Mehta AJ, Chew T. Shoulder pain in hemiplegia: The role of exercise. *Am J Phys Med Rehab* 1990: 69:205–208.

13. Braun RM, West F, Mooney V, et al. Surgical treatment of painful shoulder contracture in stroke patients. *J Bone Joint Surg* [Am] 1971; 53:1307–1312.

14. Van Ouwenaller C, Laplace PM, Chantraine A. Painful shoulder in hemiplegia. *Arch Phys Med Rehab* 1986; 67: 23–26.

15. Joynt RL. The source of shoulder pain in hemiplegia. *Arch Phys Med Rehab* 1992; 73:409–413.

16. Griffin JW. Hemiplegic shoulder pain. *Phys Ther* 1984; 66:1884–1893.

17. Tepperman PS, Greysen D, Hilbert L, Jimenez J, Williams JI. Reflex sympathetic dystrophy in hemiplegia. *Arch Phys Med Rehab* 1984; 65: 442–447.

18. Brocklehurst JG, Andrews K, Richards B, et al. How much physical therapy for patients with stroke? *Br Med J* 1978; 1307–1310.

19. Kuecuekdeveci AA, Tennant A, Hardo P, Chamberlain MA. Sleep problems in stroke patients: Relationship with shoulder pain. *Clin Rehab* 1996; 10: 166–172.

20. Codman EA. *The Shoulder.* Boston:Todd, 1934.

21. Gersten JW. Effect of ultrasound on tendon extensibility. *Am J Phys Med* 1955; 34:362–369.

22. Davis R, Lentini R. Transcutaneous nerve stimulation for treatment of pain in patients with spinal cord injury. *Surg Neurol* 1975; 4:100–101.

23. Lewis D. Lewis B, Sturrock RD. Transcutaneous electrical nerve stimulation in osteoarthrosis: A therapeutic alternative: *Ann Rheum Dis* 1984; 43:47–49.

24. Hansson P, Ekblom A, Thomson M, Fjellner B. Influence of naloxone on relief of acute oro-facial pain by transcutaneous electrical nerve stimulation (TENS) or vibration. 1986; 323–329.

25. Carabelli RA, Kellerman WC. Phantom limb pain: Relief by application of TENS to contralateral extremity. *Arch Phys Med Rehab* 1985; 66:466–467.

26. Rizk TE, Christopher RP, Pinals RS, Salazar JE, Higgins C. Arthrographic studies in painful hemiplegic shoulders. *Arch Phys Med Rehab* 1984; 65: 254–256.

27. Hakuno A, Hironobu S, Ohkawa T, Itoh R. Arthrographic findings in hemiplegic shoulders. *Arch Phys Med Rehab* 1984; 65: 706–711.

28. Weiss JJ. Intra-articular steroids in the treatment of rotator cuff tear: Reappraisal by arthrograph. *Arch Phys Med Rehab* 1981; 62:555–557.

29. Bruckner FE, Nye CJS. A prospective study of adhesive capsulitis of the shoulder (frozen shoulder) in a high-risk population. *QJ Medicine* 1981; 74: 191–204.

30. Neviaser RJ. Painful conditions affecting the shoulder. *Clin Orthop* 1983; 173:63–69.

31. Chironna RL, Hecht JS. Subscapularis motor point block for the painful hemiplegic shoulder. *Arch Phys Med Rehab* 1990; 71:428–429.

32. Hecht JS. Subscapular nerve block in the painful hemiplegic shoulder. *Arch Phys Med Rehab* 1992; 73:1036–1039.

33. Ekelund AL, Rydell N. Combination treatment for adhesive capsulitis of the shoulder. *Clin Orthop Sep* 1992; (282): 105–109.

34. Laroche M, Ighilahriz O, Moulinier L, Constantin A, Cantagrel A, Mazieres B. Adhesive capsulitis of the shoulder: An open study of 40 cases treated by joint distension during arthrography followed by an intra-articular corticosteroids injection and immediate physical therapy. *Rev Rhum Engl Ed* 1998; 65:313–319.

35. Carpenter GI, Millard PH. Shoulder subluxation in elderly inpatients. *J Am Geriatr Soc* 1982; 30:441–446.

36. Miglietta O, Lewitan A, Rogoff GB. Subluxation of the shoulder in hemiplegic patients. *NJ State J Med* 1959; 59:457–460.

37. Chaco J, Wolf E. Subluxation of the glenohumeral joint in hemiplegia. *Am J Phys Med* 1971; 50:139–143.

38. Smith RG, Cruikshank JG, Dunbar S, et al. Malalignment of the shoulder after stroke. *Br Med J* 1982; 284:1224–1226.

39. Shai G, Ring H, Costeff H, Solzi P. Glenohumeral malalignment in the hemiplegic shoulder. *Scan J Rehab Med* 1984; 16:133–136.

40. De Courval LP, Barsauskas A, Berenbaum B, et al. Painful shoulder in the hemiplegic and unilateral neglect. *Arch Phys Med Rehab* 1990; 71:673–676.

41. Chaco J, Wolf E. Subluxation of the glenohumeral joint in hemiplegia. *Am J Phys Med* 1971; 50:139–143.

42. Moskowitz E. Complications in rehabilitation of hemiplegic patients. *Med Clin North Am* 1969: 53:541–559.

43. Basmajian JV, Bazant FJ. Factors preventing downward disclocation of the adducted shoulder joint. *J Bone Joint Surg* [Am] 1959; 41:1182–1186.

44. Chino N. Electrophysiological investigations on the shoulder subluxation in hemiplelgics. *Scan J Rehab Med* 1981; 13:17–21.

45. Ring H, Leillen B, Server S, et al. Temporal changes in electrophysiological, clinical and radiological parameters in the hemiplegic's shoulder. *Scan J Rehab Med* 1985; 12(suppl):124–127.

46. Najenson T, Pikielni SS. Malalignment of the glenohumeral joint following hemiplegia: Review of 500 cases. *Ann Phys Med* 1965; 8:96–99.

47. Zorowitz RD, Hughes MB, Idank D, Ikai T, Johnston MV. Shoulder pain and subluxation after stroke: Correlation or coincidence? *Am J Occup Ther* 1996; 50:194–201.

48. Ikai T, Tei K, Yoshida K, Miyano S, Yonemoto K. Evaluation and treatment of shoulder subluxation in hemiplegia: Relationship between subluxation and pain. *Am J Phys Med Rehab* 1998; 77:421–426.

49. Rizk TE, Pinals RS. Frozen shoulder. *Semin Arthritis Rheum* 1982; 11:440–452.

50. Hurd MM, Farrell KH, Waylonis GW. Shoulder sling for hemiplegia: Friend or foe? *Arch Phys Med Rehab* 1974; 55:519–522.

51. Voss DE. Should patients with hemiplegia wear a sling? *Phys Ther* 1969; 49:1030.

52. Varghese G. Evaluation and management of shoulder complications in hemiplegia. *Karela Med Soc* 1981; 82:451–453.

53. Johnstone M. *Restoration of Motor Function in Stroke Patients*. Edinburgh: Churchill Livingstone, 1983.

54. Flatt A. Shoulder–hand syndrome in hemiplegia. *Lancet* 1974; 1:1107–1108.

55. Brooke MM, deLateur BJ, Diane-Rigby GC, Questad KA. Shoulder subluxation in hemiplegia: Effects of three different supports. *Arch Phys Med Rehab* 1991; 72:582–586.

56. Sodring KM. Upper extremity orthoses for stroke patients. *Int J Rehab Res* 1980; 3:33–38.

57. Rajaram V, Holta M. Shoulder forearm support for the subluxed shoulder. *Arch Phys Med Rehab* 1985; 66:191–192.

58. Brudny J. New orthosis for treatment of hemiplegic shoulder subluxation. *Orthotics and Prosthetics* 1985; 39: 14–20.

59. Benton LA, Baker LL, Bowman BR, Waters RL. *Functional Electrical Stimulation: A Practical Clinical Guide*, second edition. Rancho Los Amigu Engineering Center, Calif.: Downey, 1981.

60. Chantraine A, Baribeault A, Uebelhart D, Gremion G, Shoulder pain and dysfunction in hemiplegia: Effects of functional electrical stimulation. *Arch Phys Med Rehab* 1999; 80:328–331.

61. Baker LL, Parker K. Neuromuscular electrical stimulation of the muscles surrounding the shoulder. *Physical Therapy* 1986; 66: 1930–1937.

62. Chae J, Hart R. Comparison of discomfort associated with surface and percutaneous intramuscular electrical stimulation for persons with chronic hemiplegia. *Am J Phys Med Rehab* 1998; 77:516–522.

63. Chae J, Yu D, Walker M. Percutaneous, intramuscular neuromuscular electrical stimulation for the treatment of shoulder subluxation and pain in chronic hemiplegia: A case report. *Am J Phys Med Rehab* 2001; 80:296–301.

64. Inglis J, Donald MW, Monga TN, Sproule M, Young MJ. Electromyographic feedback and physical therapy of the hemiplegic upper limb. *Arch Phys Med Rehab* 1984; 65: 755–759.

65. Williams JM. Use of electromyographic biofeedback for pain reduction in the spastic hemiplegic shoulder: A pilot study. *Physiotherapy Canada* 1982;34:327–333.

66. Chen CH, Chen TW, Weng MC, Wang WT, Wang YL, Huang MH. *Kaohsiung J Med Sci* 2000; 16:525–532.

67. Wesselmann U, Raja SN, Campbell JN. Sympathetically maintained pain. In: Teasell RW (ed.), *The Autonomic Nervous System, State of the Art Reviews*. Philadelphia: Hanley & Belfus, 1996, 10:1, pp 137–151.

68. Monga TN, Zimmermann KP. Autonomic nervous system function in stroke and traumatic head injury patients. In: Teasell RW (ed.), *The Autonomic Nervous System, State of the Art Reviews*. Philadelphia: Hanley & Belfus, 1996, 10:1, pp 81–110.

69. Merskey H, Bogduk N. *Classification of Chronic Pain: Description of Chronic Pain Syndromes and Definition of Pain Terms*, 2nd ed. Seattle: IASP Press, 1994, pp 40–43.

70. Kozin F, Ryan LM, Carrera GF, Soin JS, Wortmann RL. The reflex sympathetic dystrophy syndrome (RSDS) III. Scientigraphic studies, further evidence for the efficiency of systemic corticosteroids and proposed diagnostic criteria. *Am J Med* 1981; 70: 23–30.

71. Philip PA, Philip M, Monga TN. The reflex sympathetic dystrophy in central cord syndrome. *Paraplegia* 1990; 28:48–54.

72. Campbell JN, Meyer RA, Raja SN. Is nociceptor activation by alpha-1 adrenoceptors the culprit in sympathetically maintained pain? *Am Pain Soc J* 1992; 1:3–11.

73. Davis SW, Pestrillo CR, Eischberg RD, Chu DS. Shoulder–hand syndrome in a hemiplegic population: A 5–year retrospective study. *Arch Phys Med Rehab* 1977; 58:353–355.

74. Kozin F, McCarty DJ, Sims JE, Genant HK. The reflex sympathetic dystrophy syndrome: I. Clinical and predictable response to corticosteroids. *Am J Med* 1976; 60:321–331.

75. Steinbrocker O. The shoulder–hand syndrome: Present perspective. *Arch Phys Med Rehab* 1968;49:388–395.

76. Hannington-Kiff JG. Relief of Sudeck's atrophy by regional intravenous guanethidine. *Lancet* 1977; 1132–1133.

77. Jaeger SH, Singer DI, Whitenack SH. Nerve injury complications: Management of neurogenic pain syndrome. *Hand Clin* 1986; 2:217–236.

78. Arner S. Intravenous phentolamine test: Diagnostic and prognostic use in reflex sympathetic dystrophy. *Pain* 1991; 46:17–22.

79. Hammasi N, Dursun E, Ural C, Cakci A. Calcitonin treatment in reflex sympathetic dystrophy: A preliminary study. *Br J Clin Pract* 1996; 50:373–375.

80. Monga TN, Jaksic T. Acupuncture in phantom limb pain. *Arch Phys Med Rehab* 1981; 62:229–231.

81. Savage R, Robertson L. The relationship between adult hemiplegic shoulder pain and depression. *Physiotherapy Canada* 1982; 34: 86–90.

82. Kaplan PE, Meridith J, Taft G, et al. Stroke and brachial pexus injury: A difficult problem. *Arch Phys Med Rehab* 1977; 58:415–418.

83. Moskowitz E, Poter JI. Peripheral nerve lesions in the upper extremity in hemiplegic patients. *N Eng J Med* 1963; 269: 776–778.

84. Alpert S, Idarraga S, Orbegozo J, et al. Absence of eletromyographic evidence of lower motor neuron involvement in hemiplegic patients. *Arch Phys Med Rehab* 1971; 52:179–181.

85. Hajek VE: Heterotopic ossification in hemiplegia following stroke. *Arch Phys Med Rehab* 1987; 68:313–314.

86. Botte MJ, Waters RL, Keenan M, et al. Orthopedic management of the stroke patient. Part II: Treating deformities of the upper and lower extremities. *Orthop Rev* 1988; 17:891–910.

87. Nakajo et. al. Heterotopic ossification with hemiplegia caused by cerebral apoplexy *Seikei Geka* 1969; 20:1193–1201.

88. Berrol S. Heterotropic ossification. *Arch Phys Med Rehab* 1987; 68:746.

89. Rana NA. Orthopedic surgical management of stroke. In: Kaplan PE, Cerullo LI (eds.), *Stroke Rehabilitation.* Stoneham, Mass.: Butterworth, 1986; 373.

90. Monga TN. Geriatric disorders: Musculoskeletal diseases of the elderly. In: Mehta AJ (ed.), *Common Musculoskeletal Problems.* Philadelphia: Hanley & Belfus, Inc. 1996; 103–106.

91. Sato Y, Kuno H, Ohshima Y, Asoh T, Oizumi K. Increased bone resorption during the first year after stroke. *Stroke* 1998; 29:1373– 1377.

92. Fujimatsu Y. Role of the parathyriod gland on bone mass and metabolism in immobilized stroke patients. *Kurume Medical Journal* 1998; 45:265–270.

93. Sato Y, Maruoka H, Oizumi K. Amelioration of hemiplegic associated osteopenia more than 4 years after stroke by 1 alpha-hydroxyvitamin D3 and calcium supplementation. *Stroke* 1997; 28:736–739.

94. Poplingher AR, Pillar T. Hip fracture in stroke patients: Epidemiology and rehabilitation. *Acta Orthoped Scand* 1985; 56:226–227.

95. Hooper G. Internal fixation of fractures of the neck of the femur in hemiplegic patients. *Injury* 1979; 10:281–284.

96. Brandstater ME, Roth EJ, Siebens HC. Venous thromboembolism in stroke: Literature review and implications for clinical practice. *Arch Phys Med Rehab* 73 (Suppl): 1992; 379–389.

97. Clagett GP, Anderson FA, Levine MN, Salzman EW, Wheeler HB. Prevention of venous thromboembolism. *Chest* 102 (Suppl): 1992; 391S-407S.

98. Waters RL, Penny J, Garland DE. Surgical correction of gait following stroke. *Clin Orthop* 1978; 131:54–63.

99. Vogt JC. Split anterior transfer for spastic equinovarus foot deformity: Retrospective study of 73 operated feet. *J Foot Ankle Surg* 1998; 37:2–7.

100. Teasell RW. Long-term consequences of stroke. In: *State of the Art Reviews: Physical Medicine and Rehabilitation.* Philadelphia: Hanley & Belfus, 1993, 140.

101. Mauguiere F, Desmedt JE. Thalamic pain syndrome of Dejerine-Roussy: Differentiation of four subtypes assisted by somatosensory evoked potential data. *Arch Neurol* 1988; 45: 1312–1320.

102. Dejerine J, Rousay G. Le syndrome thalamique. *Review Neurology* 1906; 12: 521–532.

103. Griffin JW, Reddein G. Shoulder pain in patients hemiplegia: A literature review. *Physical Therapy* 1981; 61:1041–1045.

104. Nasreddine ZS, Saver JL. Pain after thalamic stroke: Right diencephalic predominance and clinical features in 180 patients. *Neurology* 1997; 48: 1196–1199.

105. Wessel K, Vieregge P, Kessler C, Kompf D. Thalamic stroke: Correlation of clinical symptoms, somatosensory evoked potentials, and CT findings. *Acta Neurol Scand* 1994; 90:167–173.

106. Holmgren H, Leijon G, Boivie J, Johansson I, et al. Central poststroke pain: Somatosensory evoked potentials in relation to location of the lesion and sensory signs. *Pain* 1990; 40:43–52.

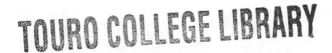

107. Gonzales GR. Central pain: Diagnosis and treatment strategies. *Neurology* 1996; 45: S11–S16.

108. Andersen LT: Shoulder pain in hemiplegia. *Am J Occup Ther* 1985; 39:11–19.

109. Bowsher et al. Central poststroke pain. *CNS Drugs* 1997; 5:160–165.

110. Vick PG, Lamer TJ. Treatment of central poststroke pain with oral ketamine. *Pain* 2001; 92:311–313.

111. McCance S, Hawton K, Brighous D, Glynn C. Does electroconvulsive therapy have any role in the management of intractable thalamic pain? *Pain* 1997; 68: 129–131.

112. Taira T, Tanikawa T, Kawamura H, Iseki H et al. Spinal intrathecal baclofen suppresses central pain after stroke. *J Neurology, Neurosurgery, and Psychiatry* 1994; 57: 381–382.

113. Peyron R, Garcia L, Deiber MP, Cinotti L, et al. Electrical stimulation of precentral cortical area in the treatment of central pain: Electrophysiological and PET study. *Pain* 1996; 62: 275–286.

114. Levin AB, Ramirez LF, Katz J. The use of stereotaxic chemical hypophysectomy in treatment of thalamic pain syndrome. *J Neurosurg* 1983; 59:1002.

115. Motoi Y, Hattori Y, Miwa H, Shina K, Mizuno Y. A case of post-hemiplegic painful dystonia following thalamic infarction with good response to botulinus toxin. *Rinsho Shinkeigaku* 1997; 37:881–886.

116. Merchutt MP, Brumlik J. Painful tonic spasms caused by putaminal infarction. *Stroke* 1986; 17: 1319–1321.

117. Kaufman DK, Brown RD, Karnes WE. Involuntary tonic spasms of a limb due to a brainstem lacunar infarction. *Stroke* 1994; 25:217–219.

118. Kellett MW, Young GR, Fletcher NA. Painful tonic spasms and pure motor hemiparesis due to Lacunar Pontine Infarct. *Movement Disorders* 1997;12:1094–1096.

Pain Management in Traumatic Brain Injury

Cindy B. Ivanhoe, M.D.
Zoraya M. Parrilla, M.D.

The evaluation and treatment of pain in the traumatic brain injured (TBI) patient poses an interesting challenge for those physicians not familiar with this population. The array of cognitive and communicative deficits that can be encountered after TBI may limit the patient's ability to accurately characterize his or her complaints, and the physician's ability to ascertain the source of pain. Often the presence of pain is manifested solely as agitation. Pain may have different causes, further complicating the diagnosis and treatment plan. Another issue that arises in the treatment of pain syndromes is the effect of many medications on cognition and arousal following a brain injury. This is a major consideration for the rehabilitation specialist selecting among the various treatment alternatives.

POSTTRAUMATIC HEADACHES (PTHA)

Headaches are quite common after TBI. They may result from injury to diverse intracranial and extracranial structures. Both the diagnosis and treatment of PTHA can be challenging. PTHA should also be considered as a cause of pain in severely injured patients who cannot communicate or identify their needs. Often different structures can contribute to the development of PTHA, and a comprehensive approach must be undertaken to successfully treat this condition.

Epidemiology

It is difficult to obtain a true estimate of the incidence of PTHA, although it is more frequently reported after mild brain injury (MBI) (1–3), with an incidence between 30 and 90 percent (4–5). The incidence and prevalence of PTHA is probably underestimated, because many patients are not hospitalized after a MBI or do not seek medical attention. To further complicate the picture, the occurrence of headaches is common in the general population, thus making the distinction between PTHA and primary headache difficult.

Pathophysiology

Any trauma to the head or neck may injure the surrounding soft tissues, leading to traction, displacement, inflammation, or ischemia of pain-sensitive structures. These sequelae may lead to pain referred to the head. This occurs through a complex process mediated by several vasoactive substances and neuropeptides responsible for the transmission of nociceptive stimuli to the central nervous system and cerebral vasomotor regulation. This is the basis of the neurovascular theory that has been proposed to explain the pathogenesis of vascular-type headaches and PTHA.

Classification and Headaches Types

The most commonly used classification system of headaches is that proposed by the International Headache Society (IHS) (6–7). One of the goals of this system is to allow the clinician to categorize the headache based on symptoms and clinical presentation, thus facilitating an appropriate treatment plan. The term *posttraumatic headache* is assigned to the type of headache that develops shortly after head trauma. However, the IHS classification system does not provide further descriptions of the different types of headache presentations that develop after trauma, including the mixed types of headache seen frequently with the postconcussive syndrome. The reader is referred to the work of Barcellos and Rizzo (7) for a more detailed classification system.

History. As is true in the management of any other medical condition, the history and physical examination are the most important steps in determining the diagnosis and appropriate treatment plan for PTHA. The initial assessment is aimed at identifying ominous causes of headache, such as intracranial hemorrhages and vascular pathologies, because the correction of such conditions may not only be lifesaving, but can eliminate or significantly alleviate the source of pain.

During the interview (see Table 6.1), the clinician should obtain a description of the original trauma, which may suggest the possible mechanisms of injury that can contribute to the development of pain. For example, contact (impact) injuries may result in face and skull fractures, joint dislocation, lacerations, and local damage to the various soft-tissue structures of the head and neck. Acceleration–deceleration injuries tend to produce distraction of these structures, with more diffuse involvement and less obvious trauma. Most injuries are mixed and thus can produce a mixed clinical picture of PTHA (1).

The characterization of the pain is key to assigning the headache to a particular category. The use of the acronym COLDER is useful to get a description of the pain: it stands for Character, Onset, Location, Duration, Exacerbating, and Relieving factors (see Table 6.1). In addition to this description, the physician should note any associated symptoms that can be included within a particular syndrome, such as nausea or vomiting. Factors that can modify the presentation, treatment, and perception of pain should also be sought, such as premorbid

Table 6.1. Key Elements in the Headache Interview

Mechanisms of trauma
Description of the pain
- Character (quality, intensity)
- Onset (temporal relation to the trauma as well as evolution)
- Location (including any pattern of referred pain)
- Duration (including frequency)
- Exacerbating factors (including medications)
- Relieving factors (including over-the-counter medications)

Associated signs and symptoms
Modifying factors
- Medical conditions (including psychiatric conditions and medications)
- Psychosocial stressors (including family and society support net)
- Patient's response to trauma and losses and future expectations

Complete medical history

medical conditions, medications, psychosocial factors, and the patient's current level of functioning and expectations. It is also important to recognize changes in the characteristics of the pain in patients who suffered from headaches prior to the occurrence of trauma.

Tables 6.2 and 6.3 depict the key points that help in differentiating among the different headache types most commonly encountered after trauma to the head and neck. However, the physician involved in this process needs a high degree of suspicion to identify the etiology of pain, because often the most common indication of ongoing pathology in these patients is the evidence of declining cognitive and overall functional status.

Physical Examination. The physical examination starts with a general assessment of the patient's current status as compared to baseline evaluations. Evaluations of the patient's sensorium, mood, and reaction to pain are important to note during the examination process. General body habitus, deformities, asymmetries, and obvious signs of trauma should be noted as well.

The examination of the musculoskeletal structures of the head and neck, including the temporomandibular joint, is of utmost importance because cervicogenic headache is a very common etiology of PTHA. It is always important to look for signs of myofascial pain syndrome (MPS), because this is one of the most common causes of cervicogenic headache after trauma. The muscles most commonly associated with MPS after trauma are the splenius cervicis and capitis, semispinalis capitis, suboccipital muscles, trapezius, sternocleidomastoid, temporalis, masseters, occipitofrontalis, and the pterigoids (8). Although the clinician might concentrate on these structures, the contribution of distal structural abnormalities to the development and perpetuation of pain should not be overlooked.

Table 6.2. PTH: Key Points in Patient History

Type of Headache	C	O	L	D	E	R	Associated Symptoms	Comments
Vascular Migraine-like	Throbbing, severe (may prohibit activity)	Early morning Develops slowly	Usually unilateral and temporal	All day	Valsalva, coughing, bending, local heat, exertion	Local cold application	Nausea +/- vomits, photo/phono-phobia, mood changes, anorexia, Transient, neurological symptoms/ mental status deterioration (aura)	More common in women and children after MBI Should rule out more ominous causes of headaches
Tension-type	Usually dull, variable intensity (may inhibit, but not prohibit activity)	Very rapid	Bilateral	Frequency >1/wk (recurrent type)	Psychosocial stressors		Depression and/or anxiety	Strong relationship with myofascial pain
Cluster	Severe, gnawing	Unilateral (supraorbital, orbital, or temporal)	Chronic or episodic; Relatively brief with a frequency of 1 every other day to 8/day			Autonomic symptoms		The episodic variant often responds well to conventional treatment

Cervicogenic	Mild to severe; steady sensation of pressure	Neck and occipital regions; possible projection to the forehead, orbital region, vertex, or temple	Intermittent or relatively constant; may last several days with exacerbations	Neck movements, sustained neck position, and palpation of neck structures	Physical modalities, analgesics, or local injections		Among other sources, myofascial pain and somatic dysfunction of C_{1-3} are very common
Temporo-mandibular joint (TMJ) syndrome	Mild to severe; steady sensation of pressure	Localized to the affected TMJ	Related to mouth movements	Movements of the mouth		Bruxism, mouth malocclusion, TMJ noise on movement, pain on jaw function	Myofascial pain of mastication muscles can coexist
Neuritic Occipital neuritis/neuralgia	Continuous, aching, throbbing or stabbing	Hemicranial, periocular, or suboccipital	Intermittent	Palpation around the nerve	Local anesthetic nerve blocks		Can coexist with myofascial pain of the cervical extensors
Neuroma	Sharp, shooting or "electrical" pain	Circumscribed to scar's area		Scalp/scar palpation	Local anesthetic	Pain when brushing hair	Lesser occipital nerve distribution overlaps that of the greater occipital nerve but is lower on the skull and produces less retro-ocular complaints
C_1-C_2 root Impingement		Dermatomal distribution C_1: orbitofrontal C_2: back and base of head		Movements of neck	Nerve block (invasive)		

Table 6.3. Intracranial Etiologies of PTHA and Their Evaluation

Etiology	History	Physical Examination	Comments
Increased intracranial Pressure (ICP)	• Chronic, progressive and constant HA; variable location • Vomiting > nausea • Declining cognition/function; (acute mental changes less common) • Classic triad for HCP (dementia, ataxia, incontinence; may not be apparent)	• Declined mental status as compared to baseline evaluations • Worsened spasticity • Papilledema • Focal neurologic deficits	• Key to diagnosis is comparison to baseline evaluations • Causes: intracranial hematomas, extension of a contusion and associated edema, hydrocephalus, pneumocephalus, shunt malfunction, meningitis/cerebritis, abscess formation
Low ICP	• Periauricular or frontal location • Exacerbated with positional changes to the upright position • Decreased hearing/tinnitus • Salty taste in mouth	• Rhinorrhea/raccoon's eyes (anterior fossa fracture) • Otorrhea/Battle's sign (petrous bone fracture) • Hemotympanium, decreased hearing and vestibular dysfunction • Halo sign • Cerebrospinal fluid (CSF) leak with valsalva	• Causes: shunt malfunction (excessive drainage), CSF leaks • CSF fistulas
Vascular Carotid Dissection	• Focal, unilateral HA (orbital or periorbital) • Amaurosis fugax • Cervical pain	• Horner's syndrome • Neck bruising • Carotid bruit • Mandibular dysfunction • Cervical carotid bruit	• Mechanism: hyperextension injuries, local neck trauma • Consider it in patients sustaining basilar skull, mandibular, and facial fractures, and penetrating injuries to the neck
Carotid Cavernous Fistula	• Frontal or periorbital HA • Diplopia, proptosis, visual dysfunction, chemosis	• Ocular bruit	• Results from blunt trauma • Most common traumatic injury to the carotid artery

Vertebral Artery Dissection	• Severe, unilateral pain; cervical or occipital in location • Acute or delayed onset • Vertebral basilar ischemic symptoms	• Lateral Medullary Syndrome (most commonly found)	• Mechanism: acute head rotation and stretching at the atlanto-occipital and atlanto-axial joints
Traumatic Aneurysm	• Severe HA; lateral • Nausea • Neck stiffness/discomfort • Delayed deterioration after trauma	• Focal neurologic deficits • Meningismus • Signs of increased ICP (see above)	• Relatively rare compared to nontraumatic counterparts
Vasospasm	• Diffuse HA of relatively acute nature • Lateral location • New neurologic deficits	• Focal neurologic deficits	• Associated to subarachnid hemorrhages (SAH); usually 4-14 days after injury.
Dural Sinus Thrombosis	• Severe HA; located at vertex or back of head • Seizures associated with HA • New neurologic deficits	• Focal neurologic deficits	• Common after penetrating head injury
Infectious	• Focal HA; pounding (in abscesses) • Varying time course • Fever, malaise (may not be apparent in osteomyelitis) • Vomiting and progressive lethargy (space-occupying lesions)	• Low grade fever • Wound drainage • Meningismus • Signs of increased ICP • Focal neurologic deficits (in abscesses)	• Particular concern in patients with penetrating head trauma and neurosurgical instrumentation

A full neurologic examination completes the assessment and should include palpation of the scalp and any incision to look for neuroma formation. Palpation of the greater and lesser occipital nerves, as well as the supraorbital nerve can lead to a diagnosis of neuralgia or neuritis. In addition, abnormalities of the eyes, ears, nose, and throat must be appropriately assessed and treated.

Further Assessment. After physical examination, several diagnostic tests may help to confirm the etiology of the pain. Serologies search for infectious or inflammatory disease of the central nervous system. Plain radiographs of the cervical spine may add to the diagnosis, although findings on X-rays should be carefully correlated with the symptoms and timing of the injury.

Computed tomography (CT) of the cervical spine, brain, and at times, skull, may be useful. Magnetic resonance imaging (MRI) is helpful in detecting herniated disks and disruption of the soft tissues of the neck. MRI is more sensitive than CT in detecting brain contusions, diffuse axonal injury, small or transversely oriented fluid collections, and subacute or chronic injury (9). It is also more sensitive in the detection and localization of intracranial infections and abscesses (8). Used in conjunction with magnetic resonance angiography, MRI is useful in the detection of vascular lesions and malformations, including those of the venous sinuses, and to evaluate the extent of cerebral ischemic lesions. Angiogram is reserved for the diagnosis and evaluation of vascular lesions. Indium scan is useful for the diagnosis of osteomyelitis, if standard bone scan and imaging procedures are nondiagnostic and the diagnosis is strongly suspected.

Treatment. Several points must be stressed before treatment of PTHA is undertaken. The treatment of PTHA follows the concepts of regular headache management, because there is little research done in this area (10). Modifications to this basic scheme are based on empirical experience. The presentation of information to the patient may need to be provided in a manner adjusted for the patient's cognitive level of functioning. Factors that can modify the perception of pain or its treatment (depression, level of stress, exercise and leisure activities, diet, caffeine use, sleep patterns) should be discussed with an individualized plan of care. Drug interactions and side effects, which may be magnified in this patient population, must be considered.

Treatment into acute and prophylactic phases. The goal of the acute phase of treatment should be towards prompt and appropriate pain alleviation to avoid risk for habituation and perpetuation of pain and the eventual development of rebound headaches. This is crucial particularly when treating migraine headaches. Use of scheduled medications can minimize the negative effects of headache on a patient's functioning in both the rehabilitation setting and the normal setting of his life. Regular reevaluation of medications, as well as the use of single-subject experimental trials, helps determine efficacy and adjustments in the treatment regimen. The decision to treat prophylactically is based on the frequency, severity, and chronicity of headaches, nature of associated symptoms, and inherent limitations in the use of some of the medications used for acute treatment, especially migraine-specific medications.

Vascular-type Headache. Details about the most commonly used medications for acute and prophylactic treatment in vascular headaches are presented elsewhere (7,10). Acetaminophen and nonsteroidal antiinflammatory drugs (NSAIDs) can be used as first-line agents in uncomplicated or early cases of migraine, although the most successful medications for the treatment of these types of pain are the agonists and antagonists of serotonin (5-HT) receptors. The most common limiting factor in the use of these agents is that they tend to induce headaches if used too frequently, whereas others may cause rebound headaches or dependence. In general the 5-HT_1 receptor agonists are useful in the acute treatment, whereas the 5-HT_2 receptor antagonists are useful for prophylaxis. Ergotamine is a potent vasoconstrictor with $5\text{-HT}_{1,2}$, alpha-adrenergic, and dopaminergic activity (11). It stabilizes the release of serotonin from the dorsal raphe nucleus and blocks the neurogenic inflammation of the dura mater (7). It is often used in combination with caffeine to increase its bioavailability. Dihydroergotamine (DHE) is the parenteral form and also comes in a suppository preparation for those patients who cannot tolerate the oral medication. It is better tolerated and absorbed when compared to ergotamine, because it has less 5-HT_2, adrenergic, and dopaminergic activity. These agents have potent vasoconstrictive effects and this, along with nausea and vomiting, are the major side effects. The use of antiemetics is recommended to lessen the nausea and vomiting, although their cognitive side effects are well known. Sumatriptan is another 5HT_1 agonist available in injectable form; it is better tolerated than other oral agents. Among the serotonin antagonists, methysergide and cyproheptadine are treatment options, although their side-effect profile is unappealing, not only in brain injured patients, but also in the general population.

Tension-type Headaches. The use of NSAIDs is discouraged in tension-type headaches in view of the chronic nature of the headache, but NSAIDs are useful during the period of drug withdrawal for treatment of rebound headache (7). For tension-type headaches, prophylactic treatment is preferred. The use of tizanidine has recently been found effective in the treatment of this particular type of pain and may be considered as an alternative if side effects are tolerated (12). For acute cluster headaches, sumatriptan, oxygen, and intranasal lidocaine are recommended. By definition, the headaches in chronic paroxysmal hemicrania are completely responsive to indomethacin.

Choices for prophylaxis include the beta-adrenergic blockers (BB), which moderate the discharge of serotonin neurons, and the tricyclic antidepressants (TCAs), which are direct antagonists of the 5-HT_2 receptor. The cognitive side effects of these groups of drugs are well established. The use of calcium channel blockers may be more reasonable in patients with contraindications to the use of BB or TCA. Anticonvulsants and selective serotonin reuptake inhibitors (SSRIs) are more appropriate in the TBI population, because they have a safer side effect profile, and they can treat other conditions that may coexist in this population, such as agitation, seizures, mood and movement disorders, and neuropathic pain.

Fluoxetine has been suggested to have some benefit in chronic PTHA although corticosteroids, calcium-channel blockers, methysergide, and lithium are more commonly used for prophylaxis.

Neuralgias, Neuritis, and Cervicogenic Headache. These conditions can coexist, and the treatment aimed towards one condition may in fact treat the others. Local injections of anesthetics with or without steroids are helpful for the treatment of occipital neuralgia and neuromas. This can be combined with the use of oral medications. Physical modalities, including stretching, strengthening, and flexibility exercises, and manual medicine (massage) techniques can help bring the muscle to its normal length and biomechanical position.

In cases of cervical dysfunction, manipulative techniques can be undertaken to restore the normal anatomical alignment of the affected segments. In cases of cervicogenic headache, the use of NSAIDs and acetaminophen is preferred; these provide analgesic and antiinflammatory effects. Different classes of NSAIDs should be tried and used for at least a few weeks before a decision is made concerning efficacy. The use of opiates is indicated in cases where pain is severe, but the sedative effects of opiates may be accentuated in this patient population. The use of muscle relaxants in TBI is discouraged because they may cause excessive sedation in these patients; muscle relaxants should be considered as an adjuvant treatment only for a short period of time.

As in the treatment of neuralgia and neuritis, the use of oral agents and injections coupled with the use of therapeutic exercises and physical modalities is effective. When pain is a major factor contributing to behavioral problems, treatment of the pain can outweigh the need to enhance cognition for a time.

Myofascial Pain. Focus in the treatment of myofascial pain is aimed at the elimination of trigger points. This can be addressed with the use of modalities including acupuncture, ischemic pressure, massage, ultrasound, transcutaneous electrical nerve stimulation (TENS), diathermy, and heat or ice applications, either alone or in combination (13). In particular, the use of manipulative techniques, such as spray-and-stretch, strain–counterstrain, soft tissue mobilization, and myofascial releasing techniques have proved effective (14). Trigger point injections may be performed using dry needling, anesthetics, and botulinum toxin-A, which has been reported to be effective, particularly for the cervical paraspinal and shoulder girdle muscles (15–16). Sleep habits, emotional and psychologic status, and physical and biomechanical factors should be addressed, although symptoms of depression, such as slowness of thought processing, poor sleep, and memory deficits can result from brain injury alone. Goals of the individualized pain treatment program should include patient education and independence.

Psychologic Considerations in PTHA

The natural course of most PTHA situations is one of improvement during the first year (17). Some cases can become permanent, secondary to the complex relationship between organic pathology and the individual's psychosocial circumstances. The patient suffering from PTHA may display cognitive deficits similar to those found after MBI (1,18). Thus, neuropsychologic interventions should be part of the management of PTHA and should be aimed at improving the individual's coping skills and minimizing the detrimental effects of cognitive deficits. Those factors that modify or aggravate the pain experience (e.g., depression, anxiety, stress, nutrition, sleep, etc.) must be addressed. It is imperative that the patient is educated about the process that has led to her symptoms, thus giving her validation and hope while avoiding enablization. Many brain-injured patients with PTHA may appreciate an explanation of their symptoms, and support and reassurance as much as pain relief (19). Expected goals and outcomes can be reassuring.

SPASTICITY

Spasticity is more common after severe and moderate traumatic brain injury. It can cause pain and deformity, and may increase medical complications and limit function. Spasticity can present with flexor and extensor patterns. Although it is usually considered an issue in the limbs, the muscles of the face and trunk can also be affected. Pain can present with stretch, weight-bearing, positioning, and other rehabilitation interventions. Pain can also result from abnormal postures that are allowed to progress. For example, pain at the elbow may be related to internal rotation of the shoulder. Patients may develop ongoing difficulties with neck positioning secondary to the combinations of visual deficits and cervical spasticity.

Treatment

Treatments for spasticity caused by brain injury are best delivered via an interdisciplinary approach. Whereas a pyramidal approach of services was previously advocated, techniques for spasticity management are most effective when delivered as part of an organized plan. Oral medications generally recommended for spasticity treatment are not well tolerated in the brain-injured population, particularly at the doses necessary to gain a beneficial result. These medications, such as dantrium, diazepam, baclofen, and tizanidine, are associated with cognitive side effects and weakness. The specific side effect profiles and characteristics are available elsewhere.

Casting. Serial and inhibitory castings are a mainstay of spasticity management. These techniques combined with chemodenervating injections with botulinum toxin and chemoneurolysis with phenol or alcohol (motor or nerve blocks) can produce maximal effects (20–21).

Botulinum Toxin-A. Botulinum toxin-A was approved for the treatment of ocular disorders but its indications have been expanded to include dystonia, spasticity, anismus, spasmodic dysphonia, and other ailments associated with excessive muscle tone. Botulinum toxin acts by irreversibly binding to prevent presynaptic release of acetylcholine. To avoid development of antibodies, injections should not be repeated more often than every 3 months and doses should be kept as low as possible to obtain the desired effect (22–23). Side effects of botulinum toxin include weakness, bleeding, and flu-like symptoms. However, these injections are generally very well tolerated and there are no specific postprocedure restrictions.

Motor Point and Nerve Blocks. Motor point and nerve blocks are invasive techniques that have been available for much longer. They are usually performed with alcohol or phenol with stimulation to locate the best injection site. The art of performing these injections is dying out, and they require a degree of skill more difficult to achieve than that necessary for the performance of botulinum toxin injections. Side effects associated with these neurolytic procedures include bleeding, dysesthesias, pain and tenderness, swelling, and deep venous thrombosis. Patients usually rest the injected limb for 24 to 48 hours after injections.

Whether patients are undergoing botulinum toxin injections, motor point blocks or both, it is common to follow the procedures with weight-bearing, stretching, and other activities to work on improved motor control.

Intrathecal Baclofen (ITB). Baclofen administered via an implanted pump is the most effective way to manage spasticity across multiple joints and the trunk. Initial studies originally recommended that cerebral-origin spasticity patients be at least one year from the date of onset before an ITB trial and implant were performed. If a patient is medically stable and there do not appear to be significant factors contributing to their spasticity, such as hydrocephalus or infections, an implant trial can be performed sooner. The benefits of ITB therapy are most apparent in the lower extremities partially because the concentration of medication in the lumbar region of the spinal cord is approximately four times greater than in the cisterns (24). The incidence of complications is low with ITB therapy (25).

Orthopedic Procedures. Orthopedic procedures to relieve spasticity include tendon transfers and lengthenings. These procedures also have a place in the management of pain associated with brain injury, because malalignment of joints can be a significant contributor to pain. The most common area where this is an issue is the ankle, where equinovarus can lead to tendon strains and positions that interfere with wheelchair positioning and transfers. If a corrective surgical procedure is contemplated, it is vital that the spasticity be managed simultaneously or the deformity will recur. Any orthotic management should be arranged prior to surgery.

HETEROTOPIC OSSIFICATION

Heterotopic ossification (HO) is a common source of pain in the TBI population. Its incidence is reported to be between 11 and 76 percent (26), although it seems to be clinically significant in about 11 to 35 percent of patients (26–28). HO is believed to originate from metaplasia of the pericapsular soft tissues into true osseous tissue by fibroblasts that convert from osteoblasts (29). The actual stimulus for this transformation is not known. It has been suggested that in the TBI population, a mechanical influence from spastic muscles create a tension–stress effect that induces fibroblasts to initiate the formation of HO (30–32). Risk factors for the development of HO include prolonged coma, spasticity, immobilization, and associated limb fractures. The hips are usually most affected after TBI, followed by elbows, knees, and shoulders (33–34). The average length of time between injury and the diagnosis of HO is 50 to 120 days, with 90 percent of cases diagnosed by 7 months (35).

Clinical Presentation

HO manifests as an inflammatory process with the appearance of edema, warmth, and erythema in the involved limb, with or without low-grade fever. The differential diagnoses include thrombophlebitis, deep venous thrombosis, and cellulitis. Induration of the area along with decreased and painful range of motion is also characteristic. Not only is HO a painful process it can also predispose the patient to the development of pressure ulcers and the compression of adjacent nerves and vessels. This adds other sources of pain for consideration.

Methods of Detection

The diagnosis is typically made by clinical presentation and confirmed by radiographic studies. Measurement of serum alkaline phosphatase may be useful in early detection of HO. Serum levels may be elevated as early as 7 weeks prior to clinical presentation (33). However, this enzyme is increased whenever osteogenic activity is increased and is therefore a nonspecific indicator of HO, particularly after trauma. Decreased levels correlate with decreased metabolic bone activity, and although still nonspecific, decreased levels can serve as a gauge of HO activity.

Triple-phase bone scan is the most sensitive method of HO detection. This method detects early HO formation 4 to 6 weeks before ossification is detected on plain film (36). It may be performed serially to demonstrate evolution of HO. When HO has reached maturity the intensity of uptake diminishes, demonstrating stabilization of the ectopic bone. Two-dimensional CT scanning has been used to localize exact sites of HO in relation to muscle planes and specific muscles. This technique is useful in determining the proximity of HO to surrounding neurovascular structures.

Management

Management of HO usually involves a combination of pharmacologic treatment and physical modalities, including range-of-motion (ROM) exercises, positioning, and splinting. It has been evidenced that ROM exercises and manipulation under anesthesia decreases the risk of joint ankylosis without promoting further development of HO (37–38). Among the pharmacologic agents used to treat HO, indomethacin and salicylates provide both analgesic and preventive effects, especially after orthopedic surgery in pediatric TBI patients (39–40). Etidronate disodium is also used to inhibit the formation of HO, by blocking the aggregation, growth, and mineralization of hydroxyapatite crystals (33). Etidronate disodium is effective in delaying the process after spinal cord injury as well as TBI (41–42). Biopsy studies from patients with HO suggest that diphosphonates may be beneficial when given early in the course of HO, whereas NSAIDs should be given during the intermediate stage (30). Suggested dosing is 20 mg/kg per day for 3 months, followed by 10 mg/kg per day for a total of 6 to 9 months. Prophylaxis is not routine in the United States.

Surgery for removal of ectopic bone is the standard of treatment of HO (41). It should be undertaken only for clear functional goals, usually not earlier than 18 months after injury to allow for the maturation of the ectopic bone and lessen the risk of recurrence. The process appears to stabilize after 5 to 14 months following onset of neurologic injury (42). Those patients who remained severely cognitively and physically impaired have a high rate of recurrence after surgical resection of HO (43).

NEUROPATHIC PAIN

As with all issues related to brain injury, the physician often must rely on reports from the rehabilitation team to monitor the patient for subtle physical findings and functional issues that may suggest the etiology of the pain and response to interventions.

Neuropathic pain can be perceived as true pain or as painful dysesthesias. These sensations are usually described as "burning," "shocklike," or "pins-and-needles." The pain itself may be provoked by nonpainful or minor stimuli, in the form of allodynia or hyperalgesia. When faced with the possibility of neuropathic pain it is important that the physician recognize the most frequent etiologies, because there are certain key differences in the treatment approach depending on the entity being addressed.

Central Pain Syndrome (CPS)

Also known as thalamic or deafferentiation pain, this type of pain was originally described in patients after thalamic infarcts, but can occur after any lesion of the central nervous system (CNS) (44), especially of the ascending somatosensory pathways, thalamus, thalamocortical connections, and cortex. Its incidence is low; no more than 8 percent in the stroke population (45).

The diagnosis of CPS is based on clinical presentation. The onset of pain is usually delayed after the central nervous system (CNS) injury, as long as 1 to 2 months (46–47). The pain is usually localized within a residual area of sensory deficit and is not influenced by peripheral or spinal blocks or deafferentiation procedures (47). Findings of allodynia and hyperalgesia are helpful in the diagnosis, as is the findingof sensory loss, although the latter is not required for purposes of diagnosis. There are no laboratory tests useful for the diagnosis of CPS, but electrodiagnostic tests can exclude peripheral nerve injury. MRI is useful in detecting CNS lesions alongside the spinothalamic tract pathways, but some lesions may go undetected.

Complex Regional Pain Syndrome (CRPS)

CRPS I, formerly known as *reflex sympathetic dystrophy* (RSD), usually occurs after minor injuries of the limbs or areas distant from the limbs, including the brain. CRPS II develops after an injury to a peripheral nerve. The most prominent feature of CRPS is pain out of proportion to the degree of injury. There is severe hyperalgesia, allodynia, and hyperpathia, poorly localized and frequently progressing to a diffuse distribution. In CRPS II, the pain is usually limited to the territory of the involved nerve. The overall incidence of CRPS after TBI is 12 percent, and the mean time from the injury to its diagnosis is approximately 4 months (48).

The diagnosis of CRPS is primarily clinical. Patients usually present with pain that is described as burning, throbbing, pressing, shooting, or aching. Movements and pressure at one or more joints such as the fingers, hands, toes, or foot typically elicit the pain, even if these were not affected directly by the preceding lesion. Spontaneous paroxysms of pain are also frequent. Autonomic signs and symptoms include swelling, hyperhydrosis, abnormalities of skin coloration and temperature, osseous demineralization, sensitivity to cold, muscle weakness, and atrophy. Trophic changes of the skin include abnormal nail and hair growth, hyperkeratosis, and thin shiny skin.

The signs and symptoms of CRPS may be subtle, especially at an early stage. For this reason it should be suspected in any patient with hyperalgesia as described above. Relief of pain and modification of signs after sympathetic nerve blockade is virtually diagnostic. Three-phase bone scan is the preferred method for diagnosis, especially in atypical or early cases, and should reveal increased uptake of radioactive material during the delayed phase.

Peripheral Neuropathy

Peripheral neuropathy usually results from systemic conditions such as diabetes, nutritional deficiencies, or from the use of alcohol and medications toxic to the neural tissue. Localized injuries (which may initially go undetected), HO, and other iatrogenic causes abound after trauma. Suspicions may be peaked based on the patient's history and complaints: there may be evidence of foot or wrist drop after prolonged periods of immobilization, which raises the possibility of nerve compression; poor motor return of the proximal upper extremity despite good function distally, which brings the suspicion of brachial plexopathy; and the like. A good neurologic exam should be the primary diagnostic tool, but electrodiagnostic testing is particularly useful to differentiate this condition from other sources of neuropathic pain and for purposes of prognostication.

Pharmacologic Treatment. The treatment of neuropathic pain follows the same approach as that for PTHA. Early detection and treatment is crucial to avoid the evolution toward chronicity and the development of maladaptive coping skills. A multidisciplinary approach is often necessary to achieve this goal. Therapeutic interventions usually start with conservative measures, including the use of pharmacologic agents and physical modalities, followed by more invasive approaches, such as intrathecal analgesic drug delivery, spinal cord, or deep brain stimulation, and finally surgical ablative procedures.

The pharmacologic treatment of neuropathic pain is essentially the same regardless of the etiology, although there may be some key differences in determining the first line of treatment. For example, the pain in CPS is neither influenced by peripheral or spinal blocks, nor by deafferentiation procedures (47) as opposed to that of CRPS. On the other hand, CPS does not respond well to steroids, whereas improvements are expected with the use of low dose antidepressants (47); the opposite is true for CRPS. The following is a summary of the most common treatment alternatives for neuropathic pain and its applicability in the brain-injured population. Table 6.4 highlights some general principles in the pharmacologic management of neuropathic pain.

Tricyclic Antidepressants (TCAs). Tricyclic antidepressants are the most widely used of all the medications available for the treatment of painful neuropathies. Their efficacy is proven, mostly in diabetic neuropathies. Amitriptyline is the most effective in this group, but also demonstrates the most anticholinergic side effects. A very low starting dose (10 mg at bedtime) with gradual increments is suggested to minimize its secondary effects. Despite their theoretic benefit, especially in the treatment of CPS, many patients obtain suboptimal pain relief and intolerable side effects. For this reason, TCAs are not often of benefit for patients with brain injury.

Table 6.4. General Principles of Pharmacotherapy in Neuropathic Pain

- Use scheduled medications
- Start with low doses
- Increase dosages slowly (every 3-7 days)
- Optimize dosage until reaching:
  - Maximal pain relief
  - Appearance of side effects/toxicity
- If no therapeutic effect, try other medication from the same family before considering switching to another drug group
- Simplify program; avoid polypharmacy
- In cases of partial pain relief with one drug, adjuvant therapy or a second analgesic is considered for synergistic effects
- Continue treatment for 3 to 6 months if the patient has demonstrated functional improvement secondary to pain relief
- Try tapering medication after 3 to 6 months of successful treatment; if pain recurs, reinstitute treatment indefinitely

Selective Serotonin Reuptake Inhibitors (SSRIs). The usefulness of SSRIs seems to derive from the treatment of coexistent depression, especially when pain becomes chronic. An exception to this statement is the use of venlafaxine, which is not only a serotonin uptake inhibitor, but also a norepinephrine-uptake inhibitor. It may produce pain relief similar to that of TCAs without the anti-cholinergic or histaminergic side effects (49). The use of venlafaxine in the treatment of painful neuropathies is relatively novel and controlled studies in this area are underway.

Anticonvulsants. Although the clinical experience of classic agents in this group is suboptimal in the general population, anticonvulsants may actually be the first choice—along with corticosteroids—in patients with brain injury. In comparison with TCAs, anticonvulsants have a relatively acceptable side-effect profile in addition to treating concomitant comorbid conditions associated to TBI, such as movement disorders, PTHA, agitation, and seizures. Phenytoin, carbamazepine, and valproic acid have been tried, although the cognitive side effects associated with phenytoin make its use less desirable.

Newer agents such as lamotrigine and especially gabapentin, have also been tried empirically and found to be beneficial. The use of gabapentin deserves special attention, because this drug appears to be a major breakthrough in the treatment of the various types of neuropathic pain. Its efficacy has surpassed the empirical experience and several studies demonstrate its usefulness (50–52). The drug is not metabolized in the liver, decreasing the risk of drug–drug interactions and toxicity in patients who often have elevated liver enzymes following trauma and anticonvulsant administration. An additional benefit includes the elimination of laboratory monitoring, which makes this drug a convenient therapeutic option. The recommended starting dose is 100 to 200 mg three times a day, tritrated by 300 mg every 3 to 7 days until therapeutic effects are noticed. There is virtually no ceiling dose; the maximum recommended dose is 6000 mg and patients usually respond to lower dosages. In our experience, brain-injured patients obtain relief within a range of 900 to 1500 mg per day, which is a lower range when compared to other populations; this may support the fact that brain-injured patients are more sensitive to the effect of centrally acting medications.

Corticosteroids. Corticosteroids are widely used in the treatment of CRPS. The use of tapering doses (e.g., Medrol® pack) is very popular, but there is still variability as to the duration of the tapering schedule.

Opioids. Opioids can be considered in conjunction with NSAIDs as adjuvant treatment, especially during peaks of pain (47), such as during physical therapy in patients with polytrauma. Long-acting, pure opioids such as extended-release oxycodone and extended-release morphine can be prescribed. Tolerance and addiction does not seem to develop if used in a time-contingent manner and if there is no history of substance abuse or addiction. It is best if these medications are used for a limited time such as during the acute phase of rehabilitation.

GABA-agonist Agents. GABA-agonist agents such as valium have been used to control pain, but their cognitive side effects are unacceptable in people with preexisting cognitive impairment. Intrathecal baclofen (ITB) has an analgesic effect in SCI patients, but the contribution of spasticity to the perception of pain and success of treatment should be considered a confounding factor.

Surgical Treatment. When considering CRPS, the most effective treatment is a sympathetic nerve block. For pain in upper limbs or areas above the thorax, a stellate ganglion block or a cervical sympathetic block at the C6 level may be used. For pain in the abdominal area, a celiac plexus block is indicated and a lumbar paravertebral block is indicated for the lower extremities. For refractory cases, neurolytic and ablative procedures are considered. Nerve blocks are not only therapeutic but also diagnostic. Local anesthetics or combined use of anesthetics and steroids are used depending on the physician's experience. In cases of neuroma formation, scar massage and mobilization to provide prolonged or sustained relief of symptoms follows these injections.

Rehabilitation Interventions. Despite the indications for physical therapy, it is often difficult if not impossible to carry out rehabilitative efforts in the acute stages of pain of neuropathic origin. At this point, more passive interventions can be undertaken, including resting of the involved limb with efforts aimed at pain relief, positioning, and edema control. When pain is under better control, it is reasonable to start gentle activity.

There are various physical modalities available for the treatment of pain with variable degree of usefulness. TENS is commonly used, although not adequately researched (53–54). Other modalities that result in pain control while allowing the performance of ROM exercises are fluidotherapy and paraffin or contrast baths. Desensitization techniques can be an important therapeutic intervention, but may not be well tolerated. Techniques aimed at preventing or relieving pressure on compressed nerves are helpful as part of the entire therapeutic program. Although bracing may be appropriate early in the course of pain, it causes atrophy in supported muscles when used long-term. Special garments, orthotics, and retrograde massage are useful for edema control, which, if left untreated, can produce stiffness of the affected limb. Because active muscle strength of all muscles of the involved extremity is often decreased, the performance of ROM exercises is recommended to avoid the development of contractures and impaired function of the affected extremity.

VENOUS THROMBOEMBOLISM

Venous thromboembolism (VTE), which includes deep venous thrombosis (DVT) and pulmonary embolism (PE), is a well-known cause of pain, morbidity, and mortality among hospitalized patients, including those with traumatic brain injury (TBI). The incidence of DVT after major head injury is 53.8 percent (55); in patients admitted to the brain-injury rehabilitation unit, incidence is between 7.8 and 20 percent (56–57). Studies assessing the incidence of PE in the trauma population found it to be between 4 and 22 percent (58–60). Despite these numbers, there is a low incidence of symptomatic and clinically significant VTE among TBI patients (55,61).

In addition to the commonly known risk factors for the development of VTE, there are factors inherent to the TBI population that makes them prone to the development of thromboembolic events. These factors include trauma, prolonged surgery, protracted immobility and coma, paralysis, fractures, gram-negative sepsis, shock, and transfusions (62). It is believed that spasticity is protective against VTE. Despite the fact that its incidence is low in upper extremities and spastic limbs (63–64), it can still develop secondary to trauma caused by venous catheterization, dissection, and in the presence of flexion contractures that limit the venous return of the affected limb.

Screening and Diagnostic Methods

Because the clinical diagnosis of VTE is unreliable and many cases are asymptomatic, screening is necessary to avoid potential complications, particularly from untreated DVT prior to mobilization of the patient. Routine screening for DVT is safe and cost-effective (56–57). After considering the sensitivity, specificity, cost-effectiveness, and safety of the various tests used for screening and diagnosis of DVT, impedance plethysmography and duplex ultrasound are the preferred methods. For details in relation to the diagnosis of DVT and PE, the reader is referred to the work by Brandstater et al. and Ginsberg (65–66).

Prophylaxis and Treatment

Debate still exists as to the best way to prevent and treat VTE in TBI patients in view of the high risk of intracranial hemorrhage in this population. In addition to the risks inherent to the original trauma and surgery, other conditions such as agitation, impulsiveness, decreased safety awareness, poor judgment, and gait disturbances further increase the risks of intracranial hemorrhage and other injuries. The same is true regarding the duration of prophylactic treatment; individual evaluation of the ongoing risks for DVT after the acute trauma phase is the gauge that determines the need for continued prophylaxis. Some investigators have found that anticoagulation can be safely started early after injury, usually within a few days to about 2 weeks after injury, provided that the initial coagulation parameters are normal and hemorrhagic lesions have stabilized (67–70). For the treatment of VTE, intravenous heparin followed by warfarin is the standard of care. When anticoagulation is contraindicated, inferior vena cava filter placement is recommended. This can be implanted with minimal loss of time from therapy. The prophylactic use of filters in patients with polytrauma is also debatable. Considerations about this practice must be individualized and research is needed in this area.

The use of mechanical compression devices in combination with anticoagulation therapy is the most common method of prophylaxis for VTE.

POSTPHLEBITIC SYNDROME

Although this is an uncommon condition, it is still another source of pain after DVT, especially in low-level patients with limited mobility. The pain usually occurs when the extremity is placed in a dependent position or upon weight-bearing activities. Edema and skin pigment changes are common associated findings; without treatment, postphlebitic syndrome can progress to skin ulceration.

The treatment of postphlebitic syndrome is aimed at the control of edema and pain relief. Several physical modalities are available to decrease edema such as use of external compression devices or garments and retrograde massage. In addition, the patient may need bed rest coupled with leg elevation. For pain control, the use of NSAIDs may serve the purposes of providing analgesia, diminishing inflammation, and as a method of delivering mild anticoagulation. Becuase this condition tends to occur late in the course of injury (when the risk of intracranial bleeding has decreased), anticoagulation with warfarin may be safely started. Use of other anticoagulation agents can be considered as well, to decrease the risk of recurrent thrombosis.

FRACTURES AND OTHER MUSCULOSKELETAL CONDITIONS

The occurrence of fractures and other musculoskeletal injuries goes hand in hand with traumatic brain injury. Approximately 71 to 80 percent of the TBI population suffer from additional injuries, fractures being one of the most common (71–72). Some of these injuries are missed during the acute hospitalization period, because the focus at this time is on medical stabilization and life-saving procedures. At the same time, patients tend to be immobile and unable to relate complaints of pain because of their cognitive–linguistic impairments, the use of sedatives, and their altered level of arousal and consciousness. It is not surprising then to diagnose previously unrecognized fractures in the rehabilitation setting, once the patient is more mobile and communicative. The incidence of such findings has been found to be about 11 percent (73).

Diagnosis

Again, a high degree of suspicion is necessary to diagnose fractures and other soft tissue injuries. Agitation and other physical reactions is commonly seen when the affected body part is being manipulated or upon weight-bearing activities, and careful examination may reveal areas of edema or deformities. A similar clinical picture can be found in heterotopic ossification and—as noted before—fractures are one of the risk factors for HO development. Recommendations on the best way to screen for unrecognized fractures vary. Some authors suggest screening radiographs including cervical and thoracic spine, pelvis, hips, and knees (71–74). Others advocate for the use of bone scans, 7 to 10 days after injury (75). This latter approach helps with the detection of both missed fractures and early HO. However, patients often demonstrate nonspecific findings secondary to the diffuse trauma they have sustained. There is therefore no substitute for a thorough clinical examination. When suspicion of ligamental and meniscal tears or joint dislocation arises, magnetic resonance imaging or computed tomography is preferred.

Treatment

Appropriate orthopedic consultation is required after a fracture is detected because fracture stabilization (usually by open reduction and internal fixation) is desirable for early mobilization and decreased risk for development of comorbid conditions associated with immobilization (75). If casts are required, they should be applied with the limb in a functional position (76). If spasticity interferes with adequate positioning in the cast, botulinum toxin injections and motor point blocks should be considered.

NSAIDs, acetaminophen, and opioid analgesics are the mainstay of pharmacologic treatment of pain of musculoskeletal origin. In general, brain-injured patients are often more susceptible to the effects of opioid agents, so low doses should be initiated, usually in conjunction with acetaminophen on a scheduled basis. There are times however, when pain relief and sedation can be less impairing cognitively and functionally than inadequately treated pain. In these cases long-acting opioids are recommended. Higher breakthrough doses, usually prior to therapy, may allow for greater participation and more appropriate movement patterns. Dosage varies depending on the patient's age, body habitus, and extent of injuries and BI.

Two entities that can commonly be encountered either as a direct result of trauma or secondary to neuromuscular deficits are shoulder subluxation and rotator cuff tendinitis or tear. These can occur in isolation but often occur concomitantly. Their diagnosis is usually clinical, but can be confirmed by radiographic studies and (in the case of rotator cuff tears) MRI. In terms of management, a conservative approach is indicated first, including symptomatic treatment with analgesics and physical modalities to reduce pain. In cases of shoulder subluxation, joint support is of utmost importance to alleviate pain as well as to promote good biomechanical alignment and avoid complications such as frozen shoulder. In cases of rotator cuff tear, surgery may be indicated, but is usually delayed until the intracranial insult is stable. It is then important to concentrate in preserving the arc of motion and conditioning of shoulder structures by means of therapeutic exercises.

MISCELLANEOUS SOURCES OF PAIN

Problems with constipation and urinary retention are the most common and most preventable causes of pain in patients with any neurologic condition including brain injury. The principles of bowel and bladder training are beyond the scope of this chapter, but it is important to stress that the use of indwelling catheters should be discouraged and, especially with regard to the gastrointestinal tract, patients should be treated pharmacologically to induce regular bowel movements and avoid fecal impaction. Patients admitted to the rehabilitation unit are started on a bowel and bladder routine suitable to their level of activity and current cognitive deficits, and this routine is tailored according to the patient's progression to achieve either modified or complete continence.

CONCLUSIONS

The diagnosis and management of pain in the brain-injured patient can be challenging in view of the limitations imposed by the cognitive, behavioral, and linguistic deficits found in this population. A high degree of suspicion is also needed to rule out sources of pain that are not obvious to the examiner. Patients who are unable to express their needs or even understand their situation may manifest pain as hypertension, tachycardia, or agitation. Disruption of the blood–brain barrier can contribute to the potential for an exaggerated incidence of side effects from medication.

The principles of pain management in the general population also apply to patients with brain injury. However, the therapeutic effects of any treatment proposed must be weighed against possible detrimental effects on cognitive recovery. Behavioral deficits such as poor judgment, decreased awareness, and perseveration may be mistaken for "pain behaviors" but do not lessen the value of seeking the cause and treating appropriately.

REFERENCES

1. Packard RC. Epidemiology and pathogenesis of posttraumatic headache. *J Head Trauma Rehabil* 1999; 14(1):9–21.
2. Zasler ND. Posttraumatic headache: Caveats and controversies. *J Head Trauma Rehabil* 1999; 14(1): 1–8.
3. Horn LJ. Postconcussive headache. *Phys Med Rehabil State* 1992; 6(1):69–78.
4. Evans RW. The postconcussion syndrome and the sequelae of mild head injury. *Neurol Clin* 1992; 10:815–847.
5. Packard RC, Ham LP. Posttraumatic headache. *J Neuropsychiatry Clin Neurosci* 1994; 6(3):229–236.
6. Headache Classification Committee of the International Headache Society. Classification and diagnostic criteria for headache disorders, cranial neuralgias, and facial pain. *Cephalagia* 1988; 8 (suppl. 7):1–96.
7. Barcellos S, Rizzo M. Posttraumatic headaches. In: Rizzo M, Tranel M (eds.), *Head Injury and Post–Concussive Syndrome*. New York: Churchill Livingstone, 1996.
8. Zafonte RD, Horn LJ. Clinical assessment of posttraumatic headaches. *J Head Trauma Rehabil* 1999; 14(1):22–33.
9. Landy SH, Donovan TB, Laster RE. Repeat CT or MRI in posttraumatic headache. *Headache* 1996; 36(1):44–47.
10. Bell KR, Kraus EE, Zasler ND. Medical management of posttraumatic headches: Pharmacological and physical treatment. *J Head Trauma Rehabil* 1999; 14(1):34–48.
11. Tfelt-hansen P, Johnson ES. Antiemetics and prokinetic drugs. In: Olesen J, Tfelt-Hansen P, Welch KMA (eds.), *The Headaches*. New York: Raven Press, 1993.
12. Fogelholm R, Murros K. Tizanidine in chronic tension-type headache: A placebo controlled double blind cross-over study. *Headache* 1992; 32 (10):509–513.
13. Covey MC. Posttraumatic myofascial pain syndrome. *Phys Med Rehabil State* 1998; 12(1):73–84.

14. Travell JG, Simons DG. *Myofascial Pain and Dysfunction: The Triggger Point Manual.* Baltimore: Williams & Wilkins, 1983.
15. Acquandro MA, Borodic GE. Treatment of myofascial pain with botulinum A toxin. *Anesthesiology* 1994; 80:706–707.
16. Cheshire WP, Abashjan SW, Mann JD. Botulinum toxin in the treatment of myofascial pain syndrome. *J Pain* 1994.
17. Packard RC. Posttraumatic headache: Permanency and relationship to legal settlement. *Headache* 1992; 32:496–500.
18. Martelli MF, Grayson RL, Zasler ND. Posttraumatic headache: Neuropsychological and psychological effects and treatment implications. *J Head Trauma Rehabil* 1999; 14(1):49–69.
19. Packard RC. What does the headache patient want? *Headache* 1979; 19:370–374.
20. Booth BJ, Doyal M, Montgomery J. Serial casting for the management of spasticity in the head-injured adult. *Phys Ther* 1983; 63(12):1960–67.
21. Lehmkuhl LD, Thoi LL, Baize C, et al. Multimodality treatment of joint contractures in patients with severe brain injury: Cost, effectiveness and integration of therapies in the application of serial/inhibitive cast. *J Head Trauma Rehabil* 1990; 5(4):23–42.
22. Pierson SH, Katz DI, Tarsy D. Botulinum toxin A in the treatment of spasticity: Functional implications and patient selection. *Arch Phys Med Rehabil* 1996; 77(7):717–721.
23. Koman LA, Mooney JF, Smith BP, et al. Management of spasticity in cerebral palsy with botulinum toxin: Report of a preliminary randomized double blind trial. *J Pediatr Orthop* 1994; 14(3):299–303.
24. Meythaler JM, DeVivo MJ, Hadley M. Prospective study on the use of bolus intrathecal baclofen for spastic hypertonia due to acquired brain injury. *Arch Phys Med Rehabil* 1996; 77(5):461–466.
25. Becker R, Alberti O, Bauer BL. Continuous intrathecal baclofen infusion in severe spasticity after traumatic brain injury. *J Neurol* 1997; 244(3):160–166.
26. Rogers RC. Heterotopic ossification in severe head injury: A preventive programme. *Brain Inj* 1988; 2:169–173.
27. Garland DE. Periarticular heterotopic ossification in head-injured adults: Incidence and location. *J Bone Joint Surg (Am)* 1980; 62(7):1143–1146.
28. Gennarelli TA. Heterotopic ossification: A subject review. *Brain Inj* 1988; 2:175–178.
29. Bagley S.L. Funny bones: A review of the problem of heterotopic bone formation. *Orthop Rev* 1979; 8:113–120.
30. Keenan MAE, Haider T. The formation of heterotopic ossification after traumatic brain injury: A biopsy study with ultrastructural analysis. *J Head Trauma Rehabil* 1996; 11(4):8–22.
31. Ilizarov GI. The tension–stress effect on the genesis and growth of tissues: Part I. The influence of stability of fixation and soft-tissue preservation. *Clin Orthop* 1989; 238:249–281.
32. Ilizarov GI. The tension–stress effect on the genesis and growth of tissues: Part II. The influence of the rate and frequency of distraction. *Clin Orthop* 1989; 239: 263–285.
33. Citta-Pietrolungo TJ, Alexander MA, Steg NL. Early detection of heterotopic ossification in young patients with traumatic brain injury. *Arch Phys Med Rehabil* 1992; 73:258–262.
34. Garland DE. Clinical observations on fractures and heterotopic ossification in the spinal cord and traumatic brain injured populations. *Clin Orthop* 1988; 233:86–101.
35. Mendelson L, Grosswasser Z, Najenson T, et al. Periarticular new bone formation in patients suffering from severe head injuries. *Scand J Rehabil Med* 1975; 7(4):141–145.
36. Freed JH, Hahn H, Menter R, et al. The use of three-phase bone scan in the early diagnosis of heterotopic ossification (HO) and in the evaluation of didronel therapy. *Paraplegia* 1982; 20(4):208–216.

37. Stover SL. Heterotopic ossification in spinal cord-injured patients. *Arch Phys Med Rehabil* 1975; 56:199–204 .

38. Garland DE. Forceful joint manipulation in head-injured adults with heterotopic ossification. *Clin Orthop* 1982; 169:133.

39. Ritter MA. Prophylactic indomethacin for the prevention of HO formation following total hip arthroplasty. *Clin Orthop* 1985:196:217–225.

40. Mital MA, Garber JE, Stinson JT. Ectopic bone formation in children and adolescents with head injuries: Its management. *J Pediatr Orthop* 1987; 7:83–90.

41. Stover SL. Disodium etidronate in the prevention of HO following SCI (preliminary report). *Paraplegia* 1976; 14:146–56.

42. Spielman G. Disodium etidronate: Its role in preventing HO in severe head injury. *Arch Phys Med Rehabil* 1983; 64:539–542.

43. Garland DE, Hanscom DA, Keenan MA, et al. Resection of heterotopic ossification in adults with head trauma. *J Bone Joint Surg [Am]* 1985; 67 :1261–1269.

44. Merskey H, Bogduk N (eds). *Classification of Chronic Pain: Descriptions of Chronic Pain Syndromes and Definitions of Pain Terms,* 2nd edition. Seattle: IASP Press 1994, pp 207–213.

45. Andersen G, Vestergaard K, Ingeman-Nielsen M, et al. Incidence of central poststroke pain. *Pain* 1995; 61(2):187–193.

46. Bowsher D. Central pain: Clinical and physiological characteristics. *J Neurol Neurosurg Psychiatry* 1996; 61(1):62–69.

47. Beric, A. Central pain and dysesthesia syndrome. *Neurol Clin* 1998; 16(4):899–918.

48. Gellman H, Keenan MA, Botte MJ. Recognition and management of upper extremity pain syndromes in the patient with brain injury. *J Head Trauma Rehabil* 1996; 11(4):23–30.

49. Galer BS. Painful polyneuropathy. *Neurol Clin* 1998; 16(4):791–811.

50. Merren MD. Gabapentin for treatment of pain and tremor: A large case series. *South Med J* 1998; 91(8):739–744.

51. Samakoff LM, Daras M, Tuchman AJ, et al. Amelioration of refractory dysesthetic limb pain in multiple sclerosis with gabapentin. *Neurology* 1997: 49:304–305.

52. Mellick GA, Mellick LB. Reflex sympathetic dystrophy treated with gabapentin. *Arch Phys Med Rehabil* 1997; 78:98–105.

53. Sjolund BH, Eriksson M, Loeser JD. Transcutaneous and implanted electrical stimulation of peripheral nerves. In: Bonica JJ (ed.), *The Management of Pain,* 2nd edition Vol 2. Philadelphia: Lea & Febiger, 1990, pp 1852–1861.

54. Woolf CJ, Thompson JW. Stimulation-induced analgesia: Transcutaneous electrical nerve stimulation (TENS) and vibration. In: Wall PD, Melzack R (eds.), *Textbook of Pain,* 3rd edition. New York: Churchill Livingstone, 1994, pp 1191–1208.

55. Geerts WH, Code KI, Jay RM, et al. A prospective study of venous thromboembolism after major trauma. *N Eng J Med* 1994; 331(24):1601–1606.

56. Cifu DX, Kaelin DL, Wall BE. Deep venous thrombosis: Incidence on admission to a brain injury rehabilitation program. *Arch Phys Med Rehabil* 1996 Nov; 77:1182–1185.

57. Meythaler JM, DeVivo MJ, Hayne JB. Cost-effectiveness of routine screening for proximal deep venous thrombosis in acquired brain injury patients admitted to rehabilitation. *Arch Phys Med Rehabil* 1996; 77:1–5.

58. Schakford SR, Moser KM. Deep venous thrombosis and pulmonary embolism in trauma patients. *J Intensive Care Med* 1988; 3:87–98.

59. Kaufman HH, Satterwhite T, McConnel BJ, et al. Deep vein thrombosis and pulmonary embolism in head injured patients. *Angiology* 1983; 34:627–638.

60. Sobus KM. Pulmonary embolism in the TBI adolescent: Report of two cases. *Arch Phys Med Rehabil* 1994; 75:362–364.

61. Lai JM, Yablon SA, Ivanhoe CB. Incidence and sequelae of symptomatic venous thromboembolic disease among patients with traumatic brain injury. *Brain Inj* 1997; 11(5):331–334.

62. Hammond FM, Meighen MJ. Venous thromboembolism in the patient with acute traumatic brain injury: Screening, diagnosis, prophylaxis and treatment issues. *J Head Trauma Rehabil* 1998; 13(1):36–50.

63. Beck ER, Bell KR. Deep venous thrombosis in the spastic upper limb. *Brain Inj* 1995; 9(4):413–416.

64. Stone LR, Keenan MA. Deep venous thrombosis of the upper extremity after traumatic brain injury. *Arch Phys Med Rehabil* 1992 May; 73:486–489.

65. Brandstater ME, Roth EJ, Siebens HC. Venous thromboembolism in stroke: Literature review and implications for clinical practice. *Arch Phys Med Rehabil* 1992 May; 73:379S–391S.

66. Ginsberg JS. Management of venous thromboembolism: Review article. *N Eng J Med* 1996 Dec; 335(24):1816–1828.

67. Steinberg DP, Green D. Prophylactic anticoagulation in patients with intracranial hemorrhage: A retrospective review of bleeding risk. *Arch Phys Med Rehabil* 1993; 64:1243.

68. Narayan R, Wilberger J, Povlishock J. *Neurotrauma*. New York: McGraw-Hill 1996 pp. 94.

69. Marion D. Complications of head injury and their therapy. *Neurosurg Clin North Am* 1991:2(2):411–424.

70. Hamilton MG, Hull RD, Pineo GF. Venous thromboembolism in neurosurgery and neurology patients: A review. *Neurosurgery* 1994; 34:280–296.

71. Bontke CF, Lehmkhul DL Englander JS, et al. Medical complications and associated injuries of persons treated in Traumatic Brain Injury Model Systems Programs. *J Head Trauma Rehabil* 1993; 8:34.

72. Rimel RW, Jane JA. Characteristics of the head injured patient. In: Rosenthal M, Griffith ER, Bond MR, Miller JD (eds.), *Rehabilitation of the Head Injured Adult*. Philadelphia: FA Davis, 1983, pp 9–21.

73. Garland DE, Baley S. Undetected injuries in head-injured adults. *Clin Orthop* 1981; 155:162–165.

74. Garland D, Rhoades M. Orthopedic management of brain-injured adults: Part II. *Clin Orthop* 1978; 131:111.

75. Hanscom DA. Acute management of the multiply injured head trauma patient. *J Head Trauma Rehabil* 1987; 2:1.

76. Garland DE. Clinical observations on fractures and heterotopic ossification in the spinal cord and traumatic brain injured populations. *Clin Orthop* 1988; 233:86–101.

7 Pain in Multiple Sclerosis

Michael F. Saffir, M.D.
David S. Rosenblum, M.D.

Multiple sclerosis (MS) is an inflammatory demyelinating disease of the central nervous system (CNS) that creates focal lesions at multiple sites. It is estimated to affect over 250,000 people in the United States, and causes a wide range of disabilities and impairments. It is more common in women and generally affects young individuals: the average age is 30 at the time of diagnosis. There is a small increased risk of MS to family members of affected individuals, and the twin of an affected individual has a significantly higher risk of developing MS. Chromosomal locations of susceptibility loci have been identified that may be responsible for susceptibility to MS. Non-gene factors include the environment: geographic distribution studies indicate that those in a northern latitude have a higher risk of MS. Migration before adolescence results in acquiring the risk for the new location. It is not clear what the trigger is that causes the immune response to destroy myelin. The diagnosis of MS is based on the history, physical examination findings, and ancillary tests, which may for example include magnetic resonance imaging (MRI), LP, BSAER, and SSEP.

The pathophysiology of MS is characterized by episodes of inflammation in the CNS. Myelin is destroyed by an immune process, and plaques are formed. The plaques have inflammatory cells, and proinflammatory cytokines are released. Gliosis is formed in multiple areas, hence the term multiple sclerosis. The plaques are seen commonly around the ventricles, optic tracts, and cerebellum, but other sites may include the basal ganglia, gray matter, and any part of the white matter of the cerebrum. The plaques and central demyelination causes a slowing of conduction velocity—at times conduction block—and thus the symptoms of MS.

The treatment of multiple sclerosis has improved significantly over the past few years. Steroids are used to shorten the duration of acute exacerbations, but do not alter the course of the disease. Immune modulating agents, such as cyclophophamide and methotrexate, are used to suppress the immune system and impact on the autoimmune factors. Beta interferon 1a (Avonex®) and 1b (Betaseron®), Copolymer 1 (Copaxone®), and mitroxantone (Novantrone®) have been approved to treat MS. All have been shown to alter the course of the disease.

127

The clinical course of MS is quite variable. In its benign form, there are infrequent mild exacerbations with extensive remission and little disability. In the relapsing-remitting form, there are exacerbations with variable remissions, with increasing impairment. The relapsing–progressive type demonstrates ongoing relapses and residual impairment. The chronic–progressive type develops steadily without relapses. Many patients have different types of clinical courses at different times. Signs, symptoms, function, and pain clearly fluctuate because of the natural history of the disease.

Multiple sclerosis affects many systems, such as the pyramidal, cerebellar, brain stem, sensory pathways, visual system, and cerebral portions of the CNS. Therefore, the difficulties that people with MS face relate to white matter disease and are multiple. They may include, for example, weakness, numbness, fatigue, balance difficulty, bladder and bowel dysfunction, spasticity, ataxia, heat intolerance, diplopia, optic neuritis, sexual dysfunction, cognitive dysfunction, paresthesias, and pain. Independence in self-care and mobility may be threatened because of pain.

CLASSIFICATION OF PAIN IN MULTIPLE SCLEROSIS

Pain was identified in MS in the late 1800s in patients studied by the eminent neurologist Charcot and again 30 years later by Gowers in treatises on diseases of the nervous system. Pain has always been a highly subjective experience, and Gowers noted that pain transcends the vocabulary (1). To understand pain, it is essential to have a consistent set of definitions and basic concepts. This can best be done using three compatible approaches to pain.

The first is a multidimensional approach that looks at how pain manifests itself at four different levels. This approach is the four-level *Biopsychosocial* or *Seattle model* of pain, developed by Dr. John Loeser at the University of Washington (2). (See Figure 7.1.) The first and most basic level of pain originates as signal responses at the level of the peripheral nerve receptors—often termed *nociception*. The second level is the actual perception of pain above a particular threshold and discrimination of the nature of the painful signal within the CNS. The third level is the affective response of the individual to the pain signal. The fourth and last level relates to the sociobehavioral context of the individual's response to pain, with its external manifestations and modifiers. Overall, this model provides a framework for understanding the complete pain experience. The model can also be correlated with the underlying neuroanatomic substrate starting with the first order neurons coming into the dorsal horn and subsequent modulation of signal transmission. The second order neurons then travel up the spinothalamic tracts anteriorly and laterally to the brain stem reticular systems and thalamus. The anteromedial pathway projects more diffusely up to the thalamus and cortical regions, particularly the frontal lobe and associative cortex, and is related more with the affective and emotional response to pain. The lateral pathway projects more specifically to the somatosensory cortex and is related to discrimination of specific sensory modalities and localization. These signals are modulated by both

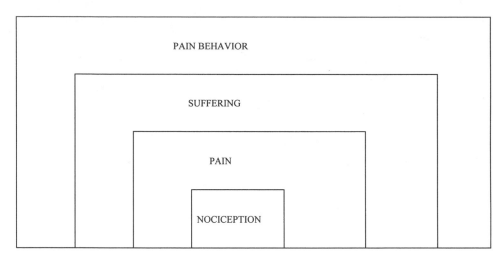

Figure 7.1. Components of pain.

ascending signals along the dorsal columns and descending signals along the dorsolateral funiculus (3). In patients with MS, lesions in the CNS may alter these pathways, change modulation, and result in pain syndromes.

Pain is also classified by its etiology at the most basic level of nociception: an intrinsic or primary disorder involving the nervous system can cause neurogenic pain; an extrinsic or secondary disorder may involve the musculoskeletal system or the visceral organs causing somatic or visceral pain. A third or tertiary category includes higher-level dysfunction with a psychogenic basis for a pain experience.

Finally, pain is typically broken down into acute and chronic categories. Acute pain is usually less than 3 to 6 months in duration and is usually associated with a specific triggering event. Chronic pain is ongoing beyond 6 months and may or may not be associated with ongoing triggers. Acute pain can be related to the Seattle model primarily at the lower two levels of nocioception and pain perception. Chronic pain is more related to levels 2 through 4, the affective response and social context, and may or may not have an active nociceptive trigger.

These classifications are critical to understanding the various types of pain related to MS. In reviewing the research on pain in MS, several categories of pain have been considered. These include studies by Moulin (4,5), Clifford (6), and Vermote (7). Typically, the types of pain are divided into acute and chronic categories. The former includes acute and often paroxysmal neuralgias, trigeminal neuralgia, optic neuritis, L'Hermitte's phenomenon, radiculitis, and tonic seizures and tetany. All of these are primarily neurogenic disorders. Nonneurogenic acute pain can occur with associated somatic disorders or injuries but have typically not been included in past studies. Chronic pain study categories include secondary somatic disorders, particularly those associated with postural problems including low back pain, joint pain, and myalgias, whereas primary neurogenic chronic pain includes persistent dysesthesias and spasms. In addition to studying pain in the context of these primary classifications, some of the studies also examine the affective component of pain and its social impact on quality of life. Thus, pain is a complex multidimensional phenomenon, which must be considered in a consistent and detailed manner.

PAIN EVALUATION/ASSESSMENT

Given the wide ranging, pleomorphic findings in MS, a comprehensive review of systems is essential in any treatment plan, and must include an assessment for pain. Many areas reviewed may include pain findings. Sensory disturbances such as dysesthesias can be caused by increased sensitivity and reduced thresholds that result in hyperpathia with increased pain perception. This can extend to allodynia with pain attributed to typically nonpainful stimuli. Delineation of the pain may help clarify its etiology such as focal low back pain vs. radiculitis or sciatica. Muscle and motor systems disorders can include spasms and other imbalances with weakness and postural disturbances resulting in pain. Myofascial pain syndromes and contractures may also be contributing problems. The head and neck is another region that is often associated with pain. Primary neurogenic pain may be seen with trigeminal neuralgia and retrobulbar neuritis in distinction to secondary musculoskeletal cervicalgia and temporomandibular disorders (TMD). Headache pain should be assessed for components related to cervicalgia, fatigue, and stress, or prodromal symptoms that may suggest migraine or possible vascular disorders, syncope, and dysautonomia. Visceral disorders can involve the gastrointestinal (GI) and genitourinary (GU) systems and may be a source of pain caused by distention and spasms (4). The psychologic domain is one of the most important systems to review, to assess individual coping skills, moods, stressors, family issues, support systems, and potential problem areas such as substance abuse. Detailed psychologic follow up may be indicated, including specialized assessment tools such as the Minnesota Multiphasic Personality Index (MMPI-2), the Symptom Check List (SCL-90R), or the Multidimensional Pain Index (MPI) (8).

Evaluation for pain focuses on two areas: the characterization of the pain and its impact on function. Pain may be characterized in terms of the perceived sensory disturbance, using an instrument such as with the McGill Pain Questionnaire (9), and its localization, for which a pain diagram may be used. The temporal course may be outlined graphically for both daily, diurnal variations and the overall course of the pain problem since its initial onset. Aggravating factors associated with worse pain and alleviating factors with reduced pain may be identified. These can include environmental influences, activities, foods, and specific interventions such as medication or other modalities. Assessment of daily activities should include sleep patterns and identify any relationships to pain problems. Functional limitations should be clarified at home and on the job. The patient may be asked to provide a pain rating with regard to specific problem areas. The pain history should also include any previous problems that included pain symptoms and identify the pain levels in those situations. This should include any interventions used previously and the outcome. Family history and dynamics often play a role and should be assessed. Identification of incentives and motivation surrounding a specific activity and associated responsibilities may help clarify problems. Finally, it is essential to ascertain with the patient how he perceives the problem and what his goals are in addressing the problem by seeking treatment.

Symptomatic management addresses such factors as spasticity, bowel and bladder dysfunction, decreased mobility and self-care, fatigue, and others. Rehabilitation approaches use comprehensive interdisciplinary interventions to address the multitude of issues that impact physical, psychosocial, vocational, avocational, and functional issues. Pain is an important "silent symptom" of MS that is often overlooked, inadequately addressed, and therefore poorly treated. It greatly impacts all aspects of function and care in the patient with MS.

Overall, a number of different types of interventions are utilized for the treatment of pain because of the complexity of pain syndromes and neuropathic disorders. Careful clinical delineation of the problem and an educated trial of treatment often produces the best results.

NEUROPATHIC PAIN OR CENTRAL-PERIPHERAL PAIN

Neuropathic or neurogenic pain is a primary pain source. It is distinct from the pain signals that are produced secondary to problems in other body systems and their subsequent transduction and transmission up through the nervous system that results in the perception of pain. Neurogenic pain can occur in either the peripheral or central nervous system. Central pain can result from tissue destruction and deafferentation with reorganization of receptors, altered signal transmission, loss of inhibition, amplification, and denervation hypersensitivity(4,10,11). Partial demyelination may produce axonal hypersensitivity and possibly ectopic impulse generation (12,13). Deafferentation caused by demyelination along the dorsal columns may affect gabinergic transmission along interneurons with the resulting disinhibition of afferent glutamatergic nociceptive fibers producing dysesthesias (14). In neuropathic disorders, Loeser indicates that the resulting pain is often caused by similar nervous system changes no matter what the underlying disease (15). Trigeminal neuralgia (TN) and sympathetically mediated pain such as complex region pain syndrome (CRPS) are distinct examples where pain signals may be generated spontaneously or so amplified from even a nonpainful stimuli to cause allodynia (16).

Central pain is most frequently seen in association with strokes or cerebral vascular accident (CVA), three-quarters of which are above the level of the brainstem (17). Central pain is fairly common in MS, possibly occurring in as many as 43 percent of patients and, in contrast to CVA, is usually the result of lesions and plaques along the spinal cord (14,18,19). Central pain is described as constant in 85 percent, burning in nature in 60 percent, a deep aching in 30 percent, a sharper shooting or lancinating pain in 25 percent, superficial in 30 percent, deep in 30 percent, or a combination of descriptors in 40 percent of MS patients (20,21).

The transition from the central nervous system to peripheral nervous system can be exemplified by TN, which may originate in the CNS along the trigeminal tract and dorsal root entry zone or more outward to the PNS in the trigeminal (or gasserian or semilunar) ganglion. Possible compression or entrapment may exist along these three branches as they exit the superior orbital fissure, foramen rotundum, and foramen ovale respectively. Peripheral disorders are often related to localized compression, which causes radiation of pain, but may also be caused by hypersensitivity at the dorsal root ganglion or distally from trauma resulting in a neuroma. In both cases there can be ectopic discharges possibly related to ephaptic transmission (22,23).

Peripherally radiating pain is exemplified by *radiculopathy*, which is a problem in the dorsal root zone. Radicular symptoms were identified in more than 10 percent of MS cases by Clifford et al (6). It was also found to be the presenting finding in 4 percent of newly diagnosed cases, with symptoms of segmental weakness and parasthesia occurring equally. Radiculopathy initially was associated with some type of traumatic injury with no skeletal abnormality or extraaxial lesion identified (24). *Myofascial disorders* often mimic neuropathic processes, producing radiating symptoms and referred pain related to segmental convergence and projection; they may also arise secondarily in association with neuropathic pain disorders (22,25).

PAIN MANAGEMENT AND TREATMENT OPTIONS

The treatment of neuropathic conditions is a significant challenge of pain management and centers on a variety of different kinds of medications. Pharmaceutical intervention is directed at the neurons that transmit and modulate pain signals and may involve as many as five or more different neurotransmitters including primary, secondary, and third order neurons (20).

The classic example of medications used for neuropathic pain are antidepressants such as tricyclic antidepressants (TCAs) amitriptyline and imipramine or their secondary amines nortriptyline and desipramine. Other antidepressants utilized include trazodone; the selective serotonin reuptake inhibitors (SSRIs) fluoxetine, sertraline, and paroxetine; and other newer reuptake inhibitors venlafaxine and nefazodone (22,26). These medications act to inhibit the reuptake of noradrenergic and serotonergic transmitters, which is believed to increase the inhibitor effects on the transmission of pain signals via descending and ascending pathways. The descending pathways may potentiate morphine-type analgesia (27). There can be independent effects for analgesic and antidepressant actions with these medications. Analgesia often occurs at lower doses and sooner after the initiation of treatment than do the antidepressant effects, which may result from stimulation of ascending pathways to the forebrain (27–30). Typically, the TCAs are most effective with the dull neuropathic pain and burning dysesthesias often seen in deafferentation. Occasionally they have been used with sharper, lancinating pain such as with trigeminal neuralgia (TN); here clomipramine is also found to be effective (31). Medication doses of TCAs generally start at 10 to 50 mg daily to produce pain relief. Doses can be gradually titrated up to usual antidepressant levels ranging from 80 to 200 mg daily per specific prescribing guideline and with close monitoring for side effects. In TCAs, side effects typically include anticholinergic effects, sedation, orthostasis, and cardiac conduction effects particularly at the higher doses. Slow titration may minimize side effects (22). Screening the medical history and consideration of an ECG evaluation, as appropriate, is necessary before initiating therapy. Contraindications to TCAs include closed-angle glaucoma, prostatic hypertrophy, and risk factors for cardiac conduction disturbances such as myocardial infarction (MI). Medication interactions should be considered. For example, individuals with MS may be on other medications with anticholinergic effects, such as oxybutinin for bladder control.

The SSRIs have a different side-effect profile, causing primarily GI disturbances, headache, and nervous system stimulation more than sedation. They are contraindicated with current or recent use of monoamine oxidase inhibitor (MAO-I) drugs. There is currently some debate over the efficacy of SSRIs, which focuses on the different receptor effects, with some experimental support of paroxetine use for neuropathic pain in diabetic neuropathy (32,33).

Anticonvulsant drugs (ACDs) are the other major class of medications that has been utilized for neuropathic pain. They tend to work best with paroxysmal, lancinating pain, which can be both acute and chronic-recurrent; the classic example is TN (12). Another paroxysmal condition seen in people with MS is *tonic seizures* or *dystonic spasms*. The first line of treatment for this condition is an ACD such as carbamazepine (CBZ, Tegretol®), which is similar to the TCA imipramine (27). Carbamazepine has been found effective in as many as 80 percent of cases with general TN, compared to 20 percent treated with dilantin (DPH), which had been tried prior to CBZ (12,13,34). Postulated mechanisms of action for ACD medication such as DPH include effects on neuronal signal transmission via altered calcium and sodium conduction and membrane stabilization effects, which can reduce ectopic signal generation, ephaptic transmission, and suppress high-frequency discharges (27). CBZ may also suppress posttetanic potentiation at central synapses such as the caudal trigeminal nucleus and the thalamic nuclei (27). Typical doses are 100 to 200 mg bid and can be increased to 1 gm daily to produce desired blood levels of 4 to 12 μg/ml of CBZ. A therapeutic response is often achieved at 6 to 8 μg/ml (35). Gradual titration while testing for blood levels, blood urea nitrogen (BUN), liver function, urinalysis, and complete blood cell count (CBC) is often necessary to monitor for potential side effects such as bone marrow depression. Other adverse effects most often include dizziness, nausea and vomiting, and drowsiness. Espir noted that while double-blind administration was difficult with CBZ because of its side effects, the therapeutic benefits usually preceded their onset by several days (13). Mexiletene is another medication with similar mechanisms of action via sodium channel blocking effects (36,37). It is an analog of lidocaine having anesthetic, antiarrhythmic, and anticonvulsant properties. It was found helpful in thalamic pain secondary to MS and causes limited side effects of nausea and dizziness (38,39). Doses can be titrated to reduce potential cardiac effects (38). Doses up to 900 mg/day have been used for antiarrhythmic purposes, but reduction in pain symptoms are seen at half that level and increasing side effects above 10 mg/kg have been noted (40).

Valproic acid (another traditional ACD), benzodiazepenes such as clon-azepam, and gabapentin (a new ACD) act via a distinct mode of action by potentiating the inhibitory effects of gamma-amino butyric acid (GABA). Benzodiazepenes may also facilitate serotonin production and potentiate central opiate effects. Gabapentin is effective in managing several types of pain, including pain in MS. This includes both acute neuralgias and chronic dysesthetic pain. The best responses with gabapentin were seen in 75 percent of patients with throbbing–cramping pains and, pins-and-needles type pain; those with burning and sharp or shooting pains showed slightly lower response rates of 60 percent; and 33 percent of patients showed no relief of neuropathic pain (41). Doses for gabapentin usually range from 300 to 2700 mg per day in three divided doses. Increases from 300 mg should be done gradually over several weeks because an increase from 300 to 900 over several days has been shown to produce increased side effects such as nausea, dizziness, and mental status changes. Side effects were seen in half of the patients taking gabapentin, and half of these discontinued treatment (41).

Benzodiazepenes have been used for chronic problems such as pain-producing spasms, and clonazepam has been found useful in acute neuralgias and peripheral nerve injuries (27), although some concern for developing tolerance has been noted (12). Baclofen is another medication typically used for spasms but which can also alleviate neuropathic pain. It can be taken systemically by mouth and or administered more directly to the central nervous system through intrathecal dosing. The latter route minimizes systemic side effects and has been found to be more effective in treating central disorders such as spasticity and pain. Baclofen is a GABA analog and has agonist action at postsynaptic receptors. A study of intrathecal baclofen for the treatment of dysesthetic pain and painful spasms has shown relief through possibly two different mechanisms of action, based on the differing time course for response and the recurrence of symptoms relative to changes in treatment (42). Baclofen has also been found useful with acute neuralgia and TN, but surprisingly not helpful with paroxysmal dystonic spasms, which do not appear to be related to classic spasticity (35,43). Two atypical medications that have been reported to help paroxysmal pain are bromocryptine and miso-prostol (a prostaglandin analog) (44). Another class of medication that has given some relief for both pain and spasm are the alpha-2 agonists clonidine and tizanidine (45–47). These provide inhibitory feedback to the adrenergic activity that plays a central role in pain induction and transmission. Sympathetically mediated pain can be treated directly with adrenergic alpha blockers such as phentolamine, prazosin, and hytrin. Amantadine has reportedly provided relief in chronic pain and fatigue by causing elevated serum levels of beta endorphins (48,49).

Although medications can mediate central neuropathic pain disorders, electrical stimulation has also been used to treat painful conditions in a variety of circumstances. It can be used peripherally, as with transcutaneous electrical nerve stimulation (TENS), percutaneously, or more centrally in the nervous system through dorsal column stimulation (DCS). DCS has been successfully used to relieve dysesthetic pain in MS, resulting in complete relief initially and relief of over 75 percent of pain beyond the first couple of years (50). There has been some limitation in the use of DCS because of tolerance, which can develop in the first 2 to 4 years (50). Electrical stimulation is usually tried first with TENS in a particular distribution. If TENS is reasonably successful, then DCS is more likely to provide relief (50,51). The beneficial effects of TENS have been postulated to involve two different mechanisms. Conventional TENS uses higher stimulation frequencies (50–100Hz), causing intensities sufficient to generate parasthesia sensations. This mechanism is postulated to reduce pain based on Melzack and Wall's gate theory, whereby stimulation of large myelinated A-alpha and beta afferents produce presynaptic effects at the dorsal horn and thus produce inhibition of ascending pain pathways. The other mechanism is characterized as acupuncture-type TENS, which uses a lower frequency stimulation and higher intensity, thus causing the release of endogenous endorphins and enkephalins and resulting in a longer lasting relief of pain (which is reversible by nalozone) (52). The latter is felt to be more useful in chronic pain conditions.

Acupuncture itself has also been used for pain relief in a number of conditions (53).

Finally, an invasive neuroablative procedure has been utilized for neuropathic pain. In MS this has been attempted primarily with trigeminal neuralgia.

SPECIFIC EXAMPLES OF PAIN IN MULTIPLE SCLEROSIS

Trigeminal Neuralgia

A patient with MS who reports intense pain in the face and jaw should be evaluated for trigeminal neuralgia (TN). Its incidence in the United States is 5 of 100,000 MS patients (20), and it is 400 times more common in people with MS than in the general population (54). TN is most common in women, and in middle and later life, although it may be found in younger patients with MS. It usually occurs after the diagnosis of MS, but may be a presenting symptom of MS (54). TN in MS is frequently bilateral (55). MS should be considered in a person with bilateral TN, especially if they are younger than 50. TN is associated with MS in 1 to 8 percent of cases of MS (55, 56). The course of TN is often exacerbating and remitting, just as MS often is, over many years. Spontaneous remissions do occur, and can last for years.

The pain of TN is often described as "electrical," paroxysmal, stabbing, lancinating, and intense. Other associated symptoms may include pruritis and hypersensitivity. Most commonly, the maxillary and mandibular divisions of the fifth cranial nerve are affected. In fact, involvement of the ophthalmic division is rare. The pain usually lasts for a few seconds, but can recur repetitively and last for many minutes. The frequency of painful attacks can vary, but can be many times a day. TN can be initiated by gentle sensory stimulus to the face, teeth, or mucosa—such as brushing the teeth—or by movements such as chewing, drinking, or even talking. In its most severe forms, patients may avoid brushing, shaving, washing, and even eating and drinking in their efforts to immobilize the mandible and prevent pain (57).

The pathophysiology of TN in MS is not clear. MS plaques containing macrophages and cytokines in the sensory pathways that cause interruption of central projecting fibers of the trigeminal system and plaques in the fifth nerve root entry zone are some possible etiologies (58,59). However, the etiology of TN in general is multifactorial. Most cases are considered idiopathic and may result from compression of the trigeminal nerve root as it passes over the petrous portion of the temporal bone, or from compression by an aberrant vessel (58). Other possible etiologies may include compression from vascular loops and local lesions such as schwannomas, meningiomas, and cerebellopontine angle tumors. It is therefore important to consider that TN in MS should not be assumed to be secondary to demyelination or plaques without considering other potential causes such as vascular etiologies or tumor (60).

The diagnosis of TN is based largely on the pain history. The pain should be confined to the fifth cranial nerve, usually the second and third divisions, should be paroxysmal with remission between attacks, and should be provokable by sensory stimulation (57). Observation may reveal facial guarding, or an area of the face which is unshaven or dirty from lack of hygiene in more severe cases. The neurologic examination will not reveal sensory loss of the trigeminal nerve in idiopathic TN, but decreased sensation may be seen with MS. Diagnostic imaging is important in the evaluation of both MS and TN. Computed tomography (CT), MRI, and X-ray may be useful in evaluating structural lesions. MRI is useful in the assessment of patients with TN to evaluate for lesions along the course of the trigeminal nerve and to evaluate the progress of MS (61).

The treatment of TN includes a change in lifestyle. The avoidance of exacerbating factors can occasionally give great relief and decrease the need for medical or surgical interventions (62). A dental examination may reveal exacerbating factors as well. Most individuals, however, require additional pharmacologic intervention.

Carbamazepine can be very effective in treating TN in patients with MS, with complete or partial relief in 60 to 80 percent of cases (54,57). Tachyphylaxis may occur with prolonged use. Most individuals report improvement within a few days. Side effects include ataxia, drowsiness, and vertigo, which may also be seen in MS. Although patients with MS often experience side effects, few have to stop taking carbamazepine as a result (54). Clinical monitoring should include blood work before instituting treatment, and should be repeated at regular intervals.

Other medications have been shown to be effective in the treatment of TN. Diphenylhydantoin has been used for over 50 years for TN. It may cause confusion, nystagmus, and ataxia, which can also be seen in MS. Additional side effects can include gastrointestinal disturbances and hematological abnormalities. Blood work and medication levels must be monitored periodically. Clonazepam and valproic acid have also been used to suppress TN attacks. Baclofen has been used alone or in combination with the above medications. Early experience with gabapentin suggests that it may be effective in TN (19) and other pain syndromes. Recent studies have shown it is also effective in the treatment of spasticity in MS. Carbamazepine, phenytoin, valproate, baclofen, and perhaps gabapentin reduce neuronal excitability and block ephaptic nerve conduction (59). Misoprostol, a long-acting prostaglandin E analog, has been shown to be effective in six out of seven patients with MS and TN who were refractory to conventional treatments (59). It may work by suppressing inflammation in MS plaques at or near the fifth cranial nerve. Side effects are minimal. Analgesics, such as opiates and nonsteroidal antiinflammatory medications (NSAIDs), are not as effective for prolonged treatment of TN.

Surgical treatments should be considered in patients who do not respond to conservative treatment. A careful history of which medications were tried, and at what doses, will allow a thorough conservative trial. Surgical intervention can be quite effective, and should be considered when appropriate.

Injection with 95 percent alcohol for neurolysis may provide temporary relief. The duration of relief may be a few months up to two years. However, repeat injections are often necessary, and the duration of relief decreases with repeated injections (57). Injections can be painful, and are generally uncommonly performed (63). Injection of the gasserian ganglion has potential serious complications, which include blindness and facial paralysis.

Based on the proposed etiology of TN in MS, such as plaques near the trigeminal root-entry zone in the pons, rhizotomy is considered by most to be the treatment of choice for patients with MS and TN (54). Nondestructive surgical procedures, such as relieving vascular compression, are not believed applicable in patients with demyelination as the etiology (64) for TN. Rhizotomy involves cutting the trigeminal sensory roots. There is selective destruction of trigeminal nociceptive pain fibers such as the unmyelinated C fibers and poorly myelinated A delta fibers, with preservation of the myelinated fibers responsible for touch and motor function (65).

Percutaneous radio frequency trigeminal rhizotomy has been shown to be effective in patients with TN and MS (64). In the general TN population, 99 percent of patients achieve immediate pain relief postoperatively, with only 20 percent pain recurrence within 7 to 9 years and 25 percent by 14 years (64). Pain recurrence rates in MS may be higher (66). All patients experience facial anesthesia if the procedure is effective. Rarely, a painful dysesthesia may develop years after the operation. Other complications include corneal ulceration and motor paresis.

Percutaneous retrogasserian glycerol rhizotomy (PRGR) is an alternative for patients with MS. There is a reduced chance for postoperative trigeminal sensory loss, less associated deafferentation pain, and PRGR does not require physiologic localization (67). PRGR may be useful for individuals who cannot undergo general anesthesia (68). Pain relief may not be immediate, but is expected within the first few weeks. Kondziolka et al. (67) reported on fifty-three patients with MS and TN and found that using PRGR resulted in 59 percent pain relief at 36 months, and a 30 percent rate of repeat operation. The mechanism of action of the glycerol is not known, but the authors propose osmotic and neurolytic effects. Complications from PRGR may include headache and postoperative sensory loss.

The third percutaneous technique that may be useful for TN in patients with MS is mechanical balloon compression. Under general anesthesia, a balloon catheter is inserted to the entrance to Meckel's cave and inflated (63). This technique is not selective. Pain relief was seen in 92 percent in one series, with a recurrence rate of 26 percent (69). Side effects may include dysesthesias and trigeminal motor weakness. Major side effects may include subarachnoid hemorrhage, hydrocephalus, hypotension, and bradycardia (63).

Gamma knife radiosurgery, a relatively new noninvasive treatment, has recently been evaluated for both the general TN population and individuals with MS and TN (70,71). This minimally invasive procedure uses stereotactic radiosurgical treatment to the trigeminal system under local anesthesia. Early studies indicate that approximately 80 percent of patients obtained significant relief (72). Long-term follow-up studies are needed. Facial paresthesias may develop. Results may be worse for patients who have had a prior surgical intervention.

Optic Neuritis

Optic neuritis (ON) is an inflammation of the optic nerve. It is found in MS and in autoimmune disorders or infectious etiologies. *Papillitis* refers to inflammation of the intraocular portion. *Retrobulbar neuritis* refers to orbital involvement, in which the disc is normal in appearance. *Neuroretinitis* refers to involvement of the retina and disc.

Visual loss and central scotoma, usually monocular, as well as changes in color vision are all common. Pain is often reported in patients with MS and retrobulbar neuritis, usually presenting as a tender globe and pain with eye movement. Marcus–Gunn phenomenon may be present on physical examination. Ophthalmoscopic examination may reveal hemorrhages on the retina or disc, and disc edema. Over time, ON atrophy occurs; this results in pallor of the disc.

Findings from the Optic Neuritis Treatment Trial demonstrate that corticosteroids are an effective treatment, and that such treatment may reduce the rate of new MS attacks (73). The probability of developing MS after an episode of ON is 30 percent, and the presence of brain MRI abnormalities at the time of ON diagnosis is a predictor of future development of MS (74). Although early studies suggested the presence of pain with ON was associated with MS (75), more recent studies have not been supportive (74).

Visual disturbance in MS is very common. Difficulty with focusing, diplopia, eye fatigue, and nystagmus are common in patients with MS. Patients with eye pain must be evaluated thoroughly, and those found to have ON should be considered for steroid treatment. Orbital pain in MS should not be overlooked: it should be part of the review of systems for individuals with MS and visual or eye difficulties.

Headaches

Headache (HA) is common in patients with MS. The age of most patients, gender, and familial heritage is common to both. Early studies on HA in MS, which were poorly controlled retrospective reviews, indicated a wide range of frequency, from 0 to 38 percent (76). More recently, HA was found to be associated with 52 percent of MS patients in comparison to 14 percent of patients initially suspected of having MS who, in fact, did not (76). The headaches did not appear to associate with any clinical features of MS. In this study, the incidence of HA at the onset of MS was 6 percent, consistent with other reports, and not supportive of cause and effect.

The association with MS and migraine headache is well recognized: migraine was found in 27 percent in an early study and in 21 percent in a more recent study (76,77). Migraine headaches may be seen with relapses, and may be the presenting symptom for patients ultimately diagnosed with MS (78). The classic migraine occurs with an aura, usually visual, and often unilateral HA. Photophobia and visual symptoms such as flashes are seen by some. Common migraine does not have an aura. In both, the pain can last a few days. The pathogenesis of migraines in MS is unclear. Although for many years it was thought that demyelination was the culprit, more recent evidence suggests other alternatives. 5 HT is thought to be involved in the pathogenesis of migraines, because it increases permeability of the blood–brain barrier, and may therefore play a role in MS (78). Further studies are needed.

There are many other potential causes of HA that are totally independent of MS. For example, vascular abnormalities, muscle strain, trauma (e.g., TBI, whiplash), cervical joint dysfunction, collagen vascular diseases, raised intracranial pressure (e.g., subarachnoid hemorrhage, etc.), and referred pain (e.g., glaucoma, sinusitis, TMJ, etc.) all must be considered. The approach in evaluating patients with MS with HA is similar to that in the general population. A careful history should include the type and severity of pain and its frequency. Exacerbating and associated factors may help differentiate a tension HA from, for example, cluster HA, cervical HA, and migraines.

Cluster HAs are more common in men, are usually unilateral, severe, occur at night, and last up to two hours. This should be differentiated from TN. Tension HA, the most common type, is described as an ache or band of pain around the head. Stress is often a precipitating factor.

Some important features more prevalent in patients with MS might include musculoskeletal problems and spasticity, which can cause HA. The impact of psychological condition, cognitive status, and patient and family stressors can be paramount. A careful history to identify migraines in particular is important, as well as an understanding of the possibility that migraine HAs may precede exacerbations of MS for some. Tension HAs are the most common HA in general, and are often seen in those with MS. General treatment principles include psychologic support for the patient and family. Relaxation, coping strategies, biofeedback, and stress reduction are all important. Specific pharmacologic intervention is dependent on the specific type of HA. For example, for migraines, a selective 5 HT receptor agonist (e.g., sumatriptan), or ergotamines or analgesics may abort an attack. Tricyclic antidepressants may help tension HA and provide prophylaxis for migraines and cervical HA.

Painful Tonic Seizures

Painful tonic seizures (PTS), or dystonic spasms, are sudden episodes of uncontrollable painful positions or spasms usually preceded by pain; PTS may include ataxia, dysarthria, falling, and—rarely—pelvic pain (79,80). Approximately 17 percent of people with MS have PTS at some point in the course of their illness (81). Episodes may last from a few seconds to 3 minutes, usually occur many times a day, and have no associated loss of consciousness (79). The spasms of PTS differ from true spasticity—which is a velocity-dependent increase in tone and PTS usually includes sensory disturbances. PTS are triggered by movement, tactile stimulation, or hyperventilation, or may occur spontaneously (7,43).

The pain of PTS may be intense, burning, tingling, radiating, focal, or bilateral and is usually significant enough for individuals to seek relief. It is often associated with hyperhydrosis, flushing, and piloerection (81). Although the pathophysiology of PTS is unclear (82), it may involve ephaptic transmission among demyelinated axons (79).

L'Hermitte's sign is a pain or tingling sensation caused by passive flexion of the neck; this pain radiates down the spine and sometimes to the legs. It occurs in MS and in other disorders such as spinal cord injury. The etiology is unclear, but may be related to the increased sensitivity of demyelinated fibers to stretch. L'Hermitte's sign may also be related to PTS: individuals with MS and L'Hermitte's sign more commonly have PTS.

The treatment of PTS usually involves the use of anticonvulsant medications.

Spasticity

Spasticity is a frequent and often painful problem for people with MS. It impacts on every aspect of quality of life and function. It is defined as a velocity-dependent increase in tone and involves muscle stiffness, involuntary muscle movement, and increased reflexes. Painful spasms interfere with sleep, hygiene, mobility, self-care, and daily function. It can make the controlled movement of already weak muscles even more difficult. However, some individuals with MS use the stiffness of the muscles created by spasticity to actually compensate for weakness. For example, someone with weak legs might use the stiffness to help with mobility. The same individual might have a harder time functioning if their legs were flaccid and unsupportive. Therefore, the treatment of spasticity must be prefaced by a detailed functional history. Management of the pain from spasticity should be considered in concert with the spasticity's impact on function.

The spasticity seen in MS may fluctuate with the course of the disease, and may be different day to day. It is necessary to evaluate overall trends in tone, rather than provide antispasticity treatment based on point in time. All potentially noxious stimuli, including psychological stresses, can adversely affect spasticity. Urinary tract infections, ingrown toenails, pressure sores, tight legbags all increase spasticity. A careful physical and history that includes a review of bowel and bladder function may identify causes or exacerbating factors which, if treated, may decrease the pain from spasticity.

Treatment of spasticity in MS is indicated when spasticity interferes with function or quality of life. Initial treatment and maintenance includes good general care, proper skin care, pressure relief, effective management of neurogenic bowel and bladder, and avoidance of any noxious stimuli. Proper seating, posture, positioning, and the appropriate use of orthotics is important. Active and passive range-of-motion exercises may give temporary relief. Topical cold may be helpful, with the added benefit of decreasing heat in MS patients who are heat intolerant (83).

The pharmacologic treatment of spasticity and the pain it causes in MS is well documented. Baclofen is generally used as the first drug of choice for patients with MS. It is most effective for spasticity of spinal origin (84). It inhibits the release of excitatory neurotransmitters. Side effects include sedation in higher doses. Additionally, it can cause motor weakness, which can be troublesome to the patient with significant spasticity and weakness. Baclofen should not be stopped abruptly.

Tizanidine, an alpha-2 agonist and imidaziline derivative, has been used successfully in the United States for the last few years and in Europe for many years. It is very effective for the treatment of spasticity in MS and other diseases, shows promise in providing comparable or superior results to baclofen (85), and is well tolerated. The fact that it does not cause as much muscle weakness as other medications offers a significant advantage. Side effects include sleepiness and dry mouth. Tizanidine may also provide nonopiate analgesia secondary to its effects on alpha-2 receptors and polysynaptic pathways: this is currently an area of active research.

Diazepam and other benzodiazepines may be used to treat MS spasticity. These work by increasing presynaptic inhibition (86), but their effects on alertness, attention, and memory may be particularly troublesome for the individual with MS. Dantrolene works as an antispasticity agent by inhibiting the release of calcium from the sarcoplasmic reticulum (83). It is effective in MS (87), but can cause significant drug-induced weakness. Other side effects such as potential liver toxicity, drowsiness, and lethargy make dantrium a second- or third-line choice. Clonidine has been shown to be effective in MS (88) and acts centrally as an alpha-2 agonist. In addition to the oral preparation, it can be applied transdermally, which provides a number of advantages including ease of application, improved compliance, and steady-state blood levels.

If the spasticity is focal, then it may not need systemic treatment with an oral agent. For example, spasticity of the elbow may cause painful elbow flexor spasms and threaten range of motion and function. Selective nerve block or motor point blocks may be very effective in relieving the spasm and pain. Botulinum toxin type-A may be injected directly into the spastic muscle (89). Botulinum toxin type-A has been shown to be safe and effective, and avoids systemic side effects. Botulinum toxin type B can also treat focal spasticity.

In patients with MS and severe pain or spasticity poorly treated with conservative means and oral medications, intrathecal baclofen (IB) is the treatment of choice. It can control the most severe spasticity and improve function (90). After implantation of the pump, computer telemetry allows precise titration and dosing. The programmer can adjust the amount and timing of the dose to provide the greatest control of pain and spasms while preserving and improving function. It generally spares cognitive function, which is particularly helpful in patients with MS who have cognitive compromise. Although generally more effective for the lower extremities, it may help upper extremity pain and spasms as well, although some individuals may need additional oral agents to control upper extremity spasticity.

Surgical options for people with MS who are not candidates for IB include dorsal entry root zone (DERZ) ablation, neurectomy, and rarely myelotomy.

Somatic Musculoskeletal Pain

Pain may arise secondary to problems in body systems other than the nervous system. This is often true for the musculoskeletal systems because of a number of conditions. In MS, problems with weakness and spasticity can result in musculoskeletal changes affecting posture and body positioning. This can cause strain on the bones, joints, ligaments, tendons, muscles, nerves, vasculature, and other connective tissue, resulting in abnormal tensile and compressive forces (7). In patients with MS, postural abnormalities can result in low back pain in 10 to 15 percent of cases, and in 20 to 25 percent when radicular symptoms are included (5,6). The etiology of low back pain is often difficult to pinpoint but can be attributed to progressive degenerative changes along the spine including arthritic spondylosis, stenosis, and scoliosis with segmental instability, which may be attributed to a degenerative cascade (4,91,92). This is seen more often as the functional impact of MS increases as measured by Expanded Disability Scale (EDSS), where the average score of patients with back pain was 2 points higher than patients with simple dysesthesias (5.3 vs. 3.3 points) (5,7). Ambulatory status is diminished with increased seated positioning, including wheelchair use. Torso positioning may be affected by both weakness and spasticity. Contractures may arise because of decreased mobility and spasticity. Pressure ulcers can also develop as a result, causing potential pain and even aggravating spasticity. Muscle disturbances most often include spasms, which have the worst pain symptoms, are likely neurogenic in origin and typically occur in more involved MS patients (EDSS~6.0) (5). Less severe muscle problems include fibromyalgia or myofascial pain syndromes, which are somatic disorders. These may be associated with sleep dysfunction and psychologic disorders involving mood, and anxiety. In these cases, spasticity may be related to prolonged sustained postures with increased muscle tension and it can respond to exercise activities and stretching (93). Findings implicating local tissue hypoxia and reduction in adenosine triphosphate (ATP) levels as well as the ragged red fibers that may be associated with mitochondrial disorders have been noted (94).

Physical limitations and postural abnormalities result in stresses being placed on other anatomic regions, resulting in subsequent problems such as compression in the upper extremity at the hand–wrist, causing median-carpal tunnel syndrome (CTS) or ulnar entrapment at Guyon's canal, ulnar CTS at the elbow, and shoulder–scapular dysfunction affecting the suprascapular nerve and possible TOS (thoracic outlet compression syndrome). Postural abnormalities can affect the sciatic and peroneal nerves in the lower extremity. Problems may also arise because of compensatory changes in body mechanics and overuse syndromes adopted to adapt to deficits caused by MS. Overuse syndromes result in tissue pathology caused by overloading from increased force or repetitive stress and cumulative microtrauma. When these forces exceed the adaptive and regenerative capacities of the tissue, then inflammatory changes occur, resulting in the release of chemotactic and vasoactive substances. Resultant pathology includes arthritic changes, calcific tendinitis, and tenosynovitis with swelling (95). These forces can also cause compression phenomenon such as compartment syndromes and entrapment neuropathies, which can also occur secondary to normal adaptive changes and hypertrophy. The most common examples are upper extremity CTS and the forearm interosseous syndromes at the pronator and supinator muscles.

Because of the ongoing and progressive problems confronting patients with MS, most of these painful disorders fit into the chronic category and are usually secondary in nature. Understanding the basis of these disorders allows some contributing factors to be addressed and some of the symptoms to be alleviated, thereby improving a patient's quality of life. Aside from these ongoing problems, there can be the potential acute pain with injuries such as falls and strains that may result from weakness or sensory deficits; these are accidental in nature and best addressed in a preventative fashion.

Painful Skin Reactions

The relatively recent understanding that MS is an immunologic disease has led to the development and use of immune modulating agents. Since 1993, interferon beta 1b has been used in the treatment of MS. It has been shown to decrease relapse rates by approximately 30 percent. Delivery is subcutaneous, usually every other day. Cutaneous skin reactions are quite common: injection site reactions (85 percent) and injection site necrosis (5 percent), as well as inflammation, pain, and hypersensitivity may occur (96). These lesions can be very painful. Specific dermatologic findings in patients with MS taking interferon beta 1b who have cutaneous reactions include ulcers, erythematous plaques, and sclerotic firm plaques representing the full spectrum from plaque to ulcer (97). Although the majority of patients tolerate interferon beta 1b, many individuals with MS report painful reactions to the injections.

Cutaneous reactions are less common with interferon 1a, which is also used in MS in an attempt to alter the course of the disease. It is given intramuscularly, usually once a week. Both interferon 1a and 1b can cause muscle aches and flu-like symptoms. Copolymer 1, the most recently approved immunologically based treatment for MS, is a chain of four amino acids that cross-react with myelin basic protein. Like the interferons, it acts on the immune system, is given by injection (subcutaneous), and may cause minor injection reactions. Brief, self-limiting postinjection reactions of flushing and chest pain have been reported.

The patient with MS reporting pain should be questioned about medication use and examined to exclude injection site reactions if they are being treated with injectable immunomodulation agents.

CONCLUSIONS

MS is a relatively common disease of the central nervous system that causes impairment and disability in many ways. The keystone of a successful approach to pain management in MS is an understanding of the multitude of symptoms and painful conditions that MS either causes or is associated with. A careful history and physical examination should explore the many MS-specific issues that can be painful in their own right, such as trigeminal neuralgia, or cause pain secondarily, such as spasticity. Pain in MS should be considered one of the "hidden symptoms" of MS. Caregivers should be active in seeking the pain symptoms and identifying pain issues, mindful of the functional and psychological impact of pain, complete in investigating the many potential causes of pain, and aggressive in its treatment. This leads to impressive gains in function and quality of life for those with MS.

REFERENCES

1. Aring CD. Pain in MS. *JAMA* 1973; 223(5):547.
2. Loeser JD. Concepts of pain. In: Stanton-Hicks M, Boaz R (eds.), *Chronic Low Back Pain*. New York: Raven Press, 1982; p. 146.
3. Fields HL. *Pain*. New York: McGraw-Hill, 1987; pp. 62–73, pp. 102–103.
4. Moulin D. Pain in MS. In: Portnoy R (ed.), *Pain Mechanisms and Syndromes*. Neurologic Clinics 1989; 7(2):321–331.
5. Moulin D, Foley K, Ebers G. Pain syndromes in MS. *Neurology* 1988; 38:1830–1834.
6. Clifford D, Trottier J. Pain in multiple sclerosis. *Arch Neurol* 1984; 41:1270–1272.
7. Vermote R, Ketelaer P, Carton H. Pain in MS patients. *Clin Neurol Neurosurg* 1986; 88(2):88–93.
8. Bradley L, Haile J, Jaworski T. Assessment of psychologic status. In: Turk D, Melzack R (eds.), *Handbook of Pain Assessment*. New York: Guilford Press, 1992; chap. 12.
9. Melzack R, Katz J. The McGill Pain Questionnaire. In: Turk D, Melzack R (eds.), *Handbook of Pain Assessment*. New York: Guilford Press, 1992; chap. 10.
10. Casey KL. Pain and central nervous system disease: A summary and overview. In: Casey KL (ed.), *Pain and Central Nervous System Disease*. New York: Raven Press, 1991; pp. 1–11.
11. Irving GA, Wallace MS. Central pain. In: *Pain Management for the Practicing Physician*. New York: Churchill Livingstone, 1997; pp. 109–114.
12. Swerdlow M. Review: Anticonvulsant drugs and chrnoic pain. *Clin Neuropharmacology* 1984; 243(1):51–82.
13. Espir M, Millac P. Treatment of paroxysmal disorders in multiple sclerosis with carbamazepine. *J Neurol Neurosurg Psychiat* 1970; 33:528–31.
14. Davar G, Maciewicz RJ. Deafferentation pain syndromes. *Neurol Clin* 1989; 289–304.
15. Loeser JD. The management of tic douloureux. *Pain* 1977; 3:155–162.
16. Rowbotham MC. Chronic pain: Theory to practical management. *Neurology* 1995; 45(Suppl. 9): p.S8.
17. Tasker RR, deCorvalho G, Dostrovsky J. The history of central pain syndromes, with observations concerning pathophysiology and treatment. In: Casey KL (ed.), *Pain and*

Central Nervous System Disease: The Central Pain Syndromes. New York: Raven Press, 1991; pp. 31–58.

18. Bonica JJ. Introduction: Semantic, epidemiologic and educational issues. In: Casey KL (ed.), *Pain and Central Nervous System Disease: The Central Pain Syndromes.* New York: Raven Press, 1991: pp. 13–29.

19. Sist T, Filadora V, Miner M, Lema M. Gabapentin for idiopathic trigeminal neuralgia: Report of two cases. *Neurology* 1997; 48:1467–1471.

20. Gonzales G. Central pain: Diagnosis and treatment strategies. *Neurology* 1995;45(Suppl. 9):S11–16.

21. Boivie J, Leijon G. Clinical findings in patients with central poststroke pain. In: Casey KL (ed.), *Pain and Central Nervous System Disease: The Central Pain Syndromes.* New York: Raven Press, 1991; pp. 65–75.

22. Galer B. Neuropathic pain of peripheral origin: Advances in treatment. *Neurology* 1995; 45(Supl. 9):S17–25.

23. Waxman SG, Ritchie JM. Hyperexcitability of pathologically myelinated axons in MS. In: Waxman SG, Ritchie, JM (eds.), *Demyelinating Diseases: Basic and Clinical Electrophysiology.* New York: Raven Press, 1981; pp. 289–297.

24. Ramirez-Lassepas M, Tulloch J, Quinones M, Snyder B. Acute radicular pain as a presenting symptom in MS. *Arch Neurol* 1992; 49:255–58.

25. Fields HL. *Pain.* New York: McGraw Hill, 1987; pp. 82–95.

26. Rowbotham M. Chronic pain: Theory to practical management. *Neurology* 1995; 45(Supl. 9):S5–10.

27. Maciewicz R, Bouckoms A, Martin J. Drug therapy of neuropathic pain. *Clin Journ Pain* 1985; 1:39–49.

28. France RD, Krishnan KR. Psychotropic drugs in chronic pain. In: France, Krishnan (eds.), *Chronic Pain.* Washington, D.C.: American Psychiatric Press, 1988.

29. Spiegal K, Kalb R, Pasternak GW. Analgesic activity of tricyclic antidepressants. *Ann Neurol* 1983; 13:462–465.

30. Malseed RT, Goldstein FJ. Enhancement of morphine analgesia by tricyclic antidepressants. *Neuropharmacology* 1979; 18:827–829.

31. Block B. Antidepressants in the tx of pain. *Resident and Staff Physician* 1993; 39(2):49–52.

32. Sindrup SH, et al. The SSRI paroxetine is effective for treatment of diabetic neuropathy symptoms. *Pain* 1990; 42:135–144.

33. Fields H. Introduction to pharmacologic approaches to Rx of chronic pain. Fields HL, Liebeskind J (eds.). Seattle: IASP Press 1994; pp 1–10.

34. Max M. Antidepressants as analgesics in pharmacologic approaches to treatment of chronic pain. In: Fields HL, Liebeskind JC (eds.), Bristol-Myers Squibb Symposium on Pain Research. IASP Press 1994; p. 229–246.

35. Rudick RA, Goodkin DE, Ransohoff RM. Pharmacotherapy of MS. *Clev Clinic J Med* 1992; 59(3):275–276.

36. Campbell RWF. Mexilitene. *N Engl J Med* 1987; 316:29–34.

37. Tanelian DL, Brose WG. Neuropathic pain can be relieved by drugs that are use- dependent sodium channel blockers: Lidocaine, carbamazepine and mexiletene. *Anesthesiology* 1991; 74(5):949–951.

38. Awerbuch GI, Sandyk R. Mexiletene for thalamic pain syndrome. *Intern J Neuroscience* 1990; 55:129–133.

39. Dejgard A, Peterson P, Kastrup J. Mexiletene for treatment of chronic painful diabetic neuropathy. *Lancet* 1988; 2(9):9–11.

40. Stracke H, et al. Mexiletene in the treatment of diabetic neuropathy. *Diabetes Care* 1992; 15:1550–1554.

41. Houtchens MK, et al. Open label gabapentin tx for pain in MS. *Multiple Sclerosis* 1997; 3:250–253.

42. Herman RM, et al. Intrathecal baclofen suppresses central pain in patients with spinal lesions. *Clin Journal of Pain* 1992; 8:338–345.
43. Anderson PB, Goodkin DE. Current pharmacologic treatment of MS symptoms. *West J Med* 1996; 165:313–317.
44. Thompson AJ. MS: Symptomatic treatment. *J Neurol* 1996; 243:559–565.
45. United Kingdom Tizanidine Trial Group. Trial of tizanidine in the treatment of spasticity caused by MS. *Neurology* 1994; 44:S70–78.
46. Byas-Smith MG, Max MB, Muir J, Kingman A. Transdermal clonidine compared to placebo in painful diabetic neuropathy. *Pain* 1995; 60:267–274.
47. Maze M, Tranquilli W. Alpha-2 adrenoreceptor agonists: Defining the role in clinical anesthesia. *Anesthesiology* 1991; 74:581–605.
48. Chiba S, Michiko M, Hiroyuki. Amantadine tx for refractory pain and fatigue in MS. *J Canadien Sciences Neurologiques* 1992; 2:309.
49. Rosenberg GA, Appenzeller O. Amantidine, fatigue and MS. *Arch Neurol* 1988; 45:1104–1106.
50. Kumar K, Nath R, Wyant G. Treatment of chronic pain by epidural spinal cord stimulation. *J Neurosurg* 1991; 75:402–407.
51. Young RF. Evaluation of dorsal column stimulation in the treatment of chronic pain. *Neurosurgery* 1978; 3(3):373–378.
52. Nelson RM, Currier DP. *Clinical Electrotherapy*. Norwalk, Conn.: Appleton & Lange, 1987.
53. NIH Consensus Conference. Acupuncture. *JAMA* 1998; 280(17):1518–1524.
54. Hooge JP, Redekop WK. Trigeminal neuralgia in multiple sclerosis. *Neurology* 1995; 45:1294–1296.
55. Brisman R. Trigeminal neuralgia and multiple sclerosis. *Arch Neurol* 1987; 44:379–381.
56. Friedman CE. Trigeminal neuralgia in a patient with multiple sclerosis. *J Endodontics* 1989; 15(8):370–380.
57. Bayer DB, Stenger TG. Trigeminal neuralgia: An overview. *Oral Surg Oral Med Oral Path* 1979; 48(5):393–399.
58. Jensen TS, Rasmussen P, Reske-Nielsen ER. Association of trigeminal neuralgia with multiple sclerosis: Clinical and pathological features. *Acta Neurol Scanda* 1982; 65:182–189.
59. Reder AT, Arnason BG. Trigeminal neuralgia in multiple sclerosis relieved by a prostaglandin E analogue. *Neurology* 1995; 45:1097–1100.
60. Meaney JF, Watt JW, Eldridge PR, Whitehouse GH, Wells JC, Miles JB. Association between trigeminal neuralgia and multiple sclerosis: role of magnetic resonance imaging. *J Neurology Neurosurgery Psychiatry* 1995; 59:253–259.
61. Yang J, Simonson TM, Ruprecht A, Meng D, Vincent SD, Yuh WT. Magnetic resonance imaging used to assess patients with trigeminal neuralgia. *Oral Surgery Oral Medicine Oral Pathology* 1996; 81:343–350.
62. Davies AN. Trigeminal neuralgia managed by a change in lifestyle. *J Palliative Care* 1997; 13(2):50–51.
63. Brisman R. Surgical treatment of trigeminal neuralgia. *Sem Neurology* 1997; 17(4):367–372.
64. Brett DC, Ferguson GG, Ebers GC, Paty D. Percutaneous trigeminal rhizotomy. treatment of trigeminal neuralgia secondary to multiple sclerosis. *Arch Neurol* 1982; 39:219–221.
65. Taha JM, Tew J. Treatment of trigeminal neuralgia by percutaneous radiofrequency rhizotomy. *Neurosurgery Clin N Am* 1997; 8(1):31–39.
66. Broggi G, Franzini A. Radiofrequency trigeminal rhizotomy in treatment of symptomatic non–neoplastic facial pain. *J Neurosurg* 1982; 57:483–486.
67. Kondziolka D, Lunsford D, Bissonette D. Long–term results after glycerol rhizotomy for multiple sclerosis related trigeminal neuralgia. *Can J Neurologic Sci* 1994; 21(2):137–140.

68. Jho HD, Lunsford D. Percutaneous retrogasserian glycerol rhizotomy: Current technique and results. *Neurosurgery Clin N Am* 1997; 8(1):63–74.

69. Brown JA, Gouda JJ. Percutaneous balloon compression of the trigeminal nerve. *Neurosurgery Clin N Am* 1997; 8(1):53–61

70. Kondziolka D, Lunsford LD, Habeck M, Flickinger JC. Gamma knife radiosurgery for trigeminal neuralgia. *Neurosurgery Clin N Am* 1997; 8(1):79–85.

71. Young RF, Vermeulen SS, Grimm DO, Blasko J, Posewitz A. Gamma knife radiosurgery for treatment of trigeminal neuralgia: idiopathic and tumor related. *Neurology* 1997; 48:608–614.

72. Kondziolka D, Perez B, Flickinger JC, Habeck M, Lunsford D. Gamma knife radiosurgery for trigeminal neuralgia. *Arch Neurol* 1998; 55:1524–1529.

73. Beck RAW, Clearly PA, Tribe, JD, et al. The Effect of corticosteroids for acute optic neuritis on the subsequent development of multiple sclerosis. *N Engl J Med* 1993; 329:1764–1769.

74. Optic Neuritis Study Group. The 5-year risk of multiple sclerosis after optic neuritis. *Neurology* 1997; 49:1404–1413.

75. Bradley WG, Whitty CWM. Acute optic neuritis: prognosis for development of multiple sclerosis. *J Neurol Neurosurg Psychiatry* 1968; 31:10–18.

76. Brown S, Rolak LA. Headaches and multiple sclerosis: A clinical study and review of the literature. *J Neurol* 1990; 237:300–302.

77. Sandyk R, Awqerbuch GI. The co–occurrence of multiple sclerosis and migraine headache: the serotininergic link. *Intern J Neuroscience* 1994; 76:249–257.

78. Waktins SM, Espir M. Migraine and multiple sclerosis. *J Neurol Neurosurg Psychiatry* 1969; 32:35–37.

79. Honig LS, Wasserstein PH, Adornato BT. Tonic spasms in multiple sclerosis. *West J Med* 1991; 6(154), 723–726.

80. Miro J, Garcia–Monco C, Leno C, Berciano J. Pelvic pain: An undescribed paroxysmal manifestation of multiple sclerosis. *Pain* 1988; 32:73–75.

81. Shibasaki H, Kuroiwa Y. Painful tonic seizure in multiple sclerosis. *Arch Neurol* 1974; 30:47–51.

82. Watson CP, Chiu M. Painful tonic seizures in multiple sclerosis; localization of a lesion. *Le Journal Canadien des sciences neurologiques* 1979; 6(3):359–366.

83. Katz RT. Management of spasticity. *Am J Phys Med Rehabil* 1988; 67(3):108–116.

84. Young RR, Dewaine PJ. Drug therapy: spasticity. *NEJM* 1981; 304(2):96–99.

85. Robinson KM, Whyte J. Pharmacological management. In: *The Practical Management of Spasticity in Children and Adults.* Ed: Glenn and Whyte. 1990. Lea and Febiger, Philadelphia 1990; 1–26.

86. Costa E, Guidott A. Molecular mechanisms in the receptor action of benzodiazepines. *Annu Rev Pharmacol Toxicol* 1979; 19:537–545.

87. Gelenberg AJ, Poskanzer DC. The effect of dantrolene sodium on spasticity in muscle sclerosis. *Neurology* 1973; 23:1313–1315.

88. Maynard FM. Early clinical experience with clonidine in spinal spasticity. *Paraplegia* 1986; 24:175–182.

89. Simpson DM. Clinical trials of botulinum toxin in the treatment of spasticity. Muscle and Nerve 1997; suppl 6:169–175.

90. Azouvi P, Manc M, Thiebaut JB, Denys P, Remy-Neris O, Bussel B. Intrathecal baclofen administration for control of severe spinal spasticity: functional improvement and long term follow up. *Arch Phys Med Rehabil* 1996; 77(1):35–39.

91. Kirkaldy–Willis WH, et al. Pathology and pathogenesis of lumbar spondylosis and stenosis. *Spine* 1978; 3:419.

92. Kirkaldy–Willis WH, Farfan HF. Instability of the lumbar spine. *Clin Orthop* 1982; 165–170.

93. Waylonis GW. Fibromyalgia. In: *PM&R State of the Art Reviews*. Hanley and Belfus 1992; 6(2):253–257.
94. Henriksson KG, Bengtsson A. Muscular changes in fibromyalgia. *Advances in Pain Research and Therapy*. Raven Press 1990; 17:258–67.
95. Lubbers LM, Wilson C, Gordon C. CTD of the upper extremity. In: *PM&R State of the Art Reviews*. Hanley and Belfus 1992; 6(2):233–243.
96. Physicians Desk Reference 1999.
97. Elgart GW, Sheremata W, Ahn YS. Cutaneous reactions to recombinant human interferon beta 1b: the clinical and histologic spectrum. *J Am Acad Dermatol* 1997; 37:553–558.

8 | Management of Pain Associated with Peripheral Neuropathy

Jaywant J. Patil, M.D.

The exact prevalence of painful polyneuropathy is unknown, although many physicians, regardless of their specialties, frequently encounter this problem. The pain that accompanies polyneuropathy has a significant negative impact on a patient's quality of life, because it decreases activity and causes depression and suffering (1). The impact of pain on functional status in a patient with polyneuropathy has not been studied and there is a scarcity of information regarding rehabilitative interventions to improve pain in this patient population. This chapter reviews the pathophysiology, causes, diagnosis, and management of pain in patients with polyneuropathy.

PATHOPHYSIOLOGY

The exact pathophysiologic processes that initiate and maintain pain in patients with peripheral neuropathy are not known. Many pathologic processes may incite initial pain and others may contribute to the persistence of chronic pain.

Several pathophysiologic processes may be involved in any one disease or in any one patient. For example, a diabetic patient may have small-fiber neuropathy with allodynia to warming, whereas another patient may have allodynia to cooling. Based on experimental work on animals, various mechanisms have been postulated to cause pain in patients with peripheral neuropathy. Either the peripheral, autonomic, or central nervous system may be the site of abnormal function following lesions of the peripheral nerves, and all levels of the nervous system may play a role in the development and persistence of pain in these patients.

According to Devor and Rappaport (1990) ectopic discharges are generated at the site of a peripheral nerve fiber and its dorsal root ganglion. This causes the peripheral nerve to become abnormally sensitive to mechanical stimuli and results in abnormal electrical discharges (2). It has been reported that there is an upregulation of sodium channels at these sites of ectopic discharges in animal models. Sodium channel antagonists such as mexiletine have been shown to reduce ectopic discharges and mechanosensitivity (3,4). Not only the injured nerves fibers but regenerating axons may also have an increase in mechanosensitivity. There may also be "ephaptic crosstalk" (a chemical or electrical communication) between afferent fibers of the normally isolated nerves or between fibers from the peripheral nervous system and the sympathetic nervous system (5). It also has been postulated that increased sensitization of peripheral nerve receptors by various stimuli can contribute to hyperalgesia and that certain chemicals like potassium, bradykinin, prostaglandins, and others may play a role in sensitizing high-threshold nerve nociceptive receptors (6).

An altered pain modulatory mechanism at the spinal cord level has also been hypothesized. Selective damage to the large myelinated fibers may result in disinhibition at the spinal cord level—the so-called "gate control" theory (7). This disinhibition then facilitates the perception of pain. However, some of the painful polyneuropathies show no evidence of large-fiber involvement, and some neuropathies with large-fiber lesions have no associated pain.

The brain is an integral part of the pain modulating system, sending fibers directly to the dorsal horn gate, which results either in amplification or dampening of the ascending pain signals from the dorsal horn (8). Animal studies have shown that there is reorganization and enlargement of the receptive fields in the spinal cord as well as in the somatosensory cortex following peripheral nerve injury. These changes can be demonstrated histologically as well as biochemically (6). There is also evidence that cellular and gene expression changes occur within the central nervous system (CNS) following peripheral nervous system injury (9).

The sympathetic nervous system may also play a role in peripheral neuropathic pain. The development of abnormal communication between afferent fibers and the sympathetic nervous system has been postulated (4). Animal models have shown that injured neurons are sensitive to adrenergic activity (4). Higher norepinephrine levels in patients with painful diabetic polyneuropathy have also been reported. Galer (1997) found that 37 percent of patients who had painful diabetic polyneuropathy had clinical findings similar to RSD (10), perhaps pointing to a similar pathophysiology (11).

It is also believed that pain can be mediated from the primary afferent fibers in the peripheral nerves and the nerve roots. These afferent fibers release aspartate and glutamate, which are excitatory amino acids, along with a variety of neuropeptides, substance P, and endogenous opioids within the different layers of the dorsal horn (12). Inhibitory amino acids such as gamma-amino butyric acid (GABA), glycine, monoamine neurotransmitters, and other peptides become involved in the spinal stage of pain transmission. The descending pathways, on the other hand, contribute to the nocioceptive inhibitory monoamine that modulates pain signals both directly and indirectly. These inhibitory properties arise from the cerebral cortex and the hypothalamus and project into the periaqueductal gray matter in the midbrain. Finally, these fibers project onto the dorsal horn of the spinal cord where they modulate the activities of different neurons (13). Recent studies have shown that long-standing changes in the neuronal activity of the spinal cord are brought about by the activation of N-methyl-D-aspartate (NMDA) receptors, oncogenes, and second messengers (14). It has also been found that input of pain signals in one dermatome can spread to other segments, thus producing painful sensations in a wider area. This leads to changes in the input in the spinal thalamic and spinal reticular systems, which eventually leads to changes in the representational mapping within the somatotopic organizations in the thalamus (14). For example, painful signals can sensitize spinal neurons through the activation of NMDA receptors and lead to enhancement of the pain response. These pain signals may then fail to trigger the GABA-producing neurons of the thalamus, which normally have a descending inhibitory effect on the dorsal horn (15). These changes in the thalamus can subsequently cause pain sensation independent of the afferent input. They can also produce pain as a result of afferent input not previously associated with pain sensation.

CLASSIFICATION OF PERIPHERAL NEUROPATHY

There are various ways to classify polyneuropathies. For example, Adams and Victor classify neuropathic syndromes based on their clinical presentations (see Table 8.1), such as ascending-type motor paralysis, subacute motor sensory paralysis, chronic relapsing polyneuropathy, chronic sensory motor polyneuropathy, mononeuropathies and multiple neuropathies, and genetically determined neuropathies (16). Others have classified neuropathies based on the underlying etiology and pathology. The healthcare professional must be aware of the fact that for any given disease there may be several types of clinical presentations arising from differing underlying pathologies (17).

Table 8.1. Classification of Neuropathic Syndromes Based on Clinical Presentation

Ascending motor paralysis associated with sensor disturbance
    Landry–Guillain–Barré Syndrome
    Chronic inflammatory demyelinating polyneuropathy
    Porphyric neuropathy

Subacute motor sensory paralysis
    Alcoholic peripheral neuropathy
    Type I and Type II diabetes mellitus

Chronic relapsing polyneuropathy
    Polyarteritis nodosa

Chronic sensorimotor polyneuropathy
    Neuropathies associated with elevated cryoglobulins
    Neuropathy secondary to carcinoma

Genetically determined neuropathies
    Fabry disease
    Charcot–Marie–Tooth disease
    Dejerine–Scottas disease

Mononeuropathies

DIAGNOSIS

Clinicians are required to establish the presence of peripheral neuropathy and its cause and to determine the appropriate treatment and management. In patients with classic symptomatology, the clinical diagnosis of polyneuropathy is most often made by history and examination of the neurologic system. At times the typical manifestations are lacking or are difficult to ascertain. In such cases ancillary studies such as nerve conduction studies, electromyography, and quantitative sensory testing may be required to confirm clinical and subclinical polyneuropathy and to document the patient's progress over time. A number of laboratory procedures such as biochemical testing and examination of cerebrospinal fluid, sural nerve, and muscle biopsy are carried out to determine the underlying etiology and pathology.

History and Clinical Examination

A number of sensory, motor, and trophic symptoms and signs are typical of peripheral neuropathy. Sensory symptoms are the most troublesome of all neuropathic symptoms. In patients with diabetic polyneuropathy the symptoms tend to be symmetric and initially involve the lower limbs.

Sensory symptoms may include a tingling, electriclike sensation, numbness, and pain. Some patients have tingling and numbness only, whereas others may have severe pain. The quality of pain may be described as aching, sharp, cutting, or crushing sensations. A tingling and burning sensation, induced by tactile stimuli, may radiate and persist after the stimulus is withdrawn. Although the patient's reaction to these stimuli may seem to indicate hypersensitivity (hyperesthesia), the sensory threshold is actually raised and only the response is exaggerated. Paraesthesias and dysesthesias are more common in alcoholic peripheral neuropathy (beriberi) and in patients with diabetes mellitus; these patients describe severe burning pain in the feet.

Sensory loss tends to affect the distal segments of the extremities, in the legs more so than in the arms. As the disease worsens, sensory loss spreads to more proximal parts of the limbs.

A patient may present with a history of weakness with or without sensory symptoms. The weakness most often starts in the feet and legs and later may involve the upper limbs. In its milder form, only the lower legs are involved. Weakness usually is symmetrical, except for some patients with Landry-Guillain-Barré syndrome and patients with diabetic amyotrophy, where there is asymmetrical weakness involving the proximal muscles. The weakness usually progresses slowly and leads to muscle atrophy. Atrophy is the product of denervation and disuse. In chronic neuropathies the paralysis and atrophy parallel one another. It has been suggested that the largest and longest nerves are more vulnerable and that a "dying back" phenomenon is involved.

Tendon reflexes are usually diminished or absent in patients with peripheral neuropathy. In small-fiber neuropathies, however, one may occasionally observe retained reflexes. In most polyneuropathies fasciculation is not an important finding. However, there may be evidence of myokymia.

Patients may present with poor balance that manifests as ataxia. This is caused by proprioceptive loss with retention of a reasonable amount of motor function. In some patients with diabetes mellitus, ataxia without weakness may be confused with tabes dorsalis.

Deformity and trophic changes involving the feet and spine are seen in a number of chronic polyneuropathies. These deformities are more common when the polyneuropathy begins in childhood. Foot deformities are common and may be found in 30 percent of patients with an early childhood form of hypertrophic hereditary sensory polyneuropathy. Asymmetrical weakness of the paravertebral muscles leads to kyphoscoliosis. Talipes equinus deformity is the result of weak pretibial and peroneal muscles and unopposed action of the posterior tibialis. The intrinsic foot muscle weakness allows the long extensors of the toes to dorsiflex the proximal phalanges and the long flexors to increase the arch, shorten the foot, and pull the distal phalanges into flexion, thus resulting in a claw foot.

Electrodiagnostic Testing

Electromyography and nerve conduction studies are used to detect the involvement of large peripheral nerve fibers. These tests are helpful in differentiating between demyelinating and axonal neuropathy. Patients may have a mixed polyneuropathy that involves both the myelin sheath and axons. Electrodiagnostic tests are also helpful in defining whether the patient has purely motor or sensory neuropathy. Electrodiagnostic tests may be completely normal in patients with painful polyneuropathy involving the small nerve fibers. It is recommended that at least three limbs should be examined, and the nerve conduction studies should include both sensory and motor nerves. Needle EMG of the appropriate muscles should be carried out to document the presence or absence of cell membrane instability. In patients where a diagnosis of polyneuropathy is suggested and the routine EMG and nerve conduction studies are normal, quantitative sensory testing may be helpful in correctly diagnosing a small-fiber painful polyneuropathy.

Quantitative Sensory Testing

Quantitative sensory testing (QST) provides a sensitive measure of both large and small nerve fiber function and is also useful in documenting abnormal sensory processing and perception (1). Verdugo and Ochoa (1992) suggest that QST should be incorporated into the routine neurologic assessment (18). In a consensus report by the Peripheral Neuropathy Association, it is recommended that QST be used in the evaluation of neuropathy (19). QST is a noninvasive procedure that takes 15 to 60 minutes to complete. Large-fiber function is measured by vibration detection threshold, which has been reported to be a sensitive measure of subclinical diabetes polyneuropathy (20). QST can also evaluate small fiber function by a variety of measures. It is believed that warm detection threshold most likely measures the function of unmyelinated C-fibers and that cold detection threshold evaluates myelinated A-delta fibers. QST may also provide information regarding abnormal perceptions provoked by thermal stimuli, such as thermal allodynia.

PAIN ASSESSMENT

The assessment of pain has been described in Chapter 2. It is important to understand the various types of neuropathic pain that a patient may experience. Make note of the patient's description of pain because not all pain patients have the same pain experiences. There are various pain scales for use in assessing the severity of pain. However, use of a pain measure specific to neuropathic pain, such as the Neuropathic Pain Scale, may be more helpful in defining pain in these patients (21).

It is also very important to know how the pain affects the patient's functional status with specific reference to work, activities of daily living (ADLs), ambulation, sleep, leisure activities, social responsibilities, mood, and sexual functioning. For example, proximal muscle weakness contributes to difficulty in ambulating and negotiating stairs. Weakness of distal muscles giving rise to foot drop may result in frequent falls. A patient may complain of difficulty in rising from a chair or commode. A patient may present with poor fine-motor dexterity and difficulty in grooming resulting from weakness of the upper extremities. Cranial nerve involvement may result in problems with swallowing, speaking, and chewing. Poor balance may be secondary to sensory deficits. A patient may experience difficulty in performing activities of daily living because of his inability to feel objects.

Many of these patients are depressed and may have a poor quality of life. These key assessments—the pain qualities, allodynia, hyperalgesia, and functional status—are not only important at initial consultation, but are also important features to follow in subsequent visits to evaluate the treatment outcomes.

Dyck et al. (1985) and Feldman et al. (1994) have developed evaluation procedures to identify the presence and severity of neuropathy (22,23). Dyck and his colleagues used the Index of Pathology, which combines reduction in myelinated fiber density with abnormalities detected in surviving teased-fiber myelinated nerve fibers (22). It is reported that clinical assessments using the Neuropathy Symptom Scale, Neurologic Disability Score, and Nerve Conduction studies produce valid discrimination between neuropathy and absence of neuropathy. The investigators proposed four stages : Stage 0, no evidence of neuropathy; Stage 1, asymptomatic neuropathy; Stage 2, symptomatic neuropathy; and Stage 3, disabling neuropathy (22). According to Thomas (1997), the Index of Pathology does not include an evaluation of unmyelinated axons, and teased-fiber studies fail to sample small myelinated fibers adequately (17). Methods described by Feldman et al. (1994) to evaluate peripheral neuropathy include a brief questionnaire and screening examination. If the patient scores above a threshold level, he or she is then assessed by the Michigan Diabetic Neuropathy Score (MDNS) (23). MDNS combines a quantified neurologic evaluation, which concentrates on the abnormalities that occur in diabetic polyneuropathy, and a battery of nerve conduction studies. Patients are categorized into four stages: 0, no neuropathy; 1, mild neuropathy; 2, moderate neuropathy; and 3, severe neuropathy. The Feldman et al. method is simpler and has a good correlation with the Mayo Clinic classification (23). Another approach for the assessment of sensory polyneuropathy is to perform serial sural nerve biopsies. Although this assessment has been incorporated into a number of treatment trials, the approach is invasive.

ETIOLOGY OF PAINFUL POLYNEUROPATHY

Once a diagnosis of peripheral neuropathy is made, it is important to diagnose the underlying etiology so that attempts can be made to improve symptoms, reverse the nerve dysfunction, and prevent further damage. There are many causes for painful neuropathy, and it is not within the scope of this chapter to describe all of them. Some of the causes include metabolic diseases such as diabetes mellitus and uremia. Other causes include nutritional deficiencies, such as thiamine deficiency, which may cause a painful polyneuropathy. Thiamine deficiency is commonly seen in patients with a history of alcohol abuse and is often secondary to drug toxicity, such as that produced by chemotherapeutic agents and anticonvulsants. Human immunodeficiency virus (HIV) infection is another cause of painful polyneuropathy that may present with a history of "burning feet." Painful polyneuropathy may be a manifestation of paraneoplastic syndromes and systemic vasculitis, including polyarteritis nodosa. Amyloidosis may cause painful polyneuropathy with small nerve fiber and autonomic involvement (24). When no identifiable cause is found, it is important to address the lack of an etiologic diagnosis with the patient. Commonly encountered clinical entities are described in the following sections.

DIABETIC NEUROPATHY

Thomas (1997) has divided diabetic peripheral neuropathy into five classes (17):

• *Hyperglycemic neuropathy,* which includes minor sensory symptoms, reduced nerve conduction velocity, and resistance to ischemic conduction failure. It is more likely caused by nerve hypoxia and is rapidly reversible.

• *Symmetric polyneuropathy*, which is most common in this category, is predominantly sensory and autonomic. It is usually of insidious onset and involves the distal lower limbs first. There is relatively minor motor involvement; a distal axonopathy of dying-back may represent the underlying pathogenic basis and it is largely irreversible. Autonomic neuropathy is usually associated with sensory neuropathy.

• *Acute painful diabetic neuropathy* merits a separate and distinct syndrome (17). In these patients there is a history of marked weight loss and severe unremitting burning pain distally in the lower limbs. The symptoms are worse at night and are associated with unpleasant contact hyperesthesia in the legs. Motor function is usually preserved. Archer (1983) has described the natural history of acute painful neuropathy in diabetic patients (25).

• *Focal and multifocal lesions* giving rise to cranial, thoracoabdominal, and limb neuropathies, including proximal limb motor neuropathy (diabetic amyotrophy), may be seen in older diabetic patients (17). Some of these neuropathies may have an ischemic basis. The third, sixth, and seventh cranial nerves may be involved. The onset of dysfunction in the third nerve is often acute and is accompanied by pain (26). Girdle pain may be caused by truncal neuropathy and at times is associated with focal weakness of the anterior abdominal wall musculature (27,28).

• *Diabetic amyotrophy* (first described by Garland [29], also known as Garland's amyotrophy) often presents with subacute onset of weakness and wasting of the bilateral proximal lower limb muscles. It is accompanied with moderate to severe pain around the hip and lower back. Weakness is asymmetrical and the condition is usually not associated with sensory deficits. This is considered to be a purely motor neuropathy. Its occurrence is independent of sensorimotor neuropathy, and it is common in middle age or later in life. Occasionally it may occur in young individuals with long-standing diabetes mellitus. Controversy and confusion have surrounded diabetic amyotrophy over the years. However, the syndrome of diabetic amyotrophy has a characteristic clinical picture that can be clinically differentiated from common diabetic distal polyneuropathy or mononeuropathy multiplex (30). In a study by Llewelyn and colleagues (1998) four of 15 patients with proximal diabetic neuropathy showed changes of microvasculitis in biopsy specimens of the intermediate cutaneous nerve of the thigh and sensory branch of the femoral nerve (31). In one patient similar changes were found in a quadriceps muscle biopsy specimen. The authors concluded that secondary vasculitic or other inflammatory reactions might contribute to some forms of diabetic neuropathy (31). The site of lesioning in these patients remains controversial. According to Chokroverty, diabetic amyotrophy may be caused by proximal intramuscular crural neuropathy (distal neuronitis), which in some patients resembles mononeuropathy multiplex (30). The condition is self-limiting and improvement occurs in most cases, athough the symptomatic period may be prolonged.

Although diabetic peripheral neuropathy is a common complication of both type I and type II diabetes mellitus, its exact prevalence is not known (32,33). According to Galer, the frequency of neuropathy in diabetes varies widely, from 16 to 61 percent among studies, depending on the criteria used to define neuropathy (32). A recent Diabetes Control and Complications Trial reported a 69 percent reduction of neuropathy in patients using intensive insulin therapy (34). The frequency of pain in insulin-dependent and noninsulin-dependent diabetic patients is reported to be 11.6 percent and 32.1 percent respectively.

GUILLAIN-BARRÉ SYNDROME

Guillain-Barré syndrome (GBS) is an acute inflammatory polyneuropathy. It is a relatively uncommon condition with a reported incidence of 1 or 2 cases per 100,000 population (35). However, with the virtual elimination of poliomyelitis it has become the most common cause of acute generalized paralysis (36). It is generally regarded as a predominantly motor neuropathy with some sensory symptoms. In more than 50 percent of GBS cases, there is an antecedent history of upper respiratory tract infection, usually of viral etiology (37). Some authorities recognize an association of GBS with cancer, lymphoma, sarcoidosis, and a number of endocrine disorders (38,39). Paraesthesias in the toes is often the first neurologic symptom, followed within hours or days by weakness of the legs (40). The motor symptoms progress for about two weeks and recovery begins 2 to 4 weeks after the progression stops. Although a majority of patients make a good recovery, complete recovery often takes months to years. A significant proportion of these patients may require lengthy hospitalization and prolonged assistance from others to carry out activities of daily living (40). Pain or paraesthesia in GBS has been reported in 7 to 75 percent of patients (37,41–43). In their review article, Pentland and Donald (1994) describe various types of pain and pain syndromes in patients with GBS (40).

Ropper and Shahani (1984) describe the clinical features of 29 patients with GBS (44). In their study, 55 percent of patients reported low back and proximal leg pain early in the course of illness, and in 72 percent the pain was present at some time during the first month. Patients describe the pain as similar to severe muscle strain after lifting a heavy weight incorrectly. It may also take the form of severe cramping pain. The most common sites include the hamstrings, quadriceps, and gluteal areas. The pain is often reported to be worse at night. However, there was no formal assessment of pain intensity or disability (44).

In a prospective study of 55 patients with GBS, Moulin et al. (1997), report that 49 patients (89.1 percent) described pain during the course of their illness (45). Pain preceded weakness by a mean of 6.1 days in 16 patients, and both pain and weakness appeared simultaneously in seven patients. Twenty-six of these 49 patients described pain that was either distressing, horrible, or excruciating. The most common pain syndromes were a deep aching back, leg pain, and dysesthetic extremity pain. Thirty-seven patients (67.3 percent) described deep aching or throbbing pain in the lower back region with radiation into the buttocks, thighs, and occasionally calves. A straight leg raising test was positive in 32 of these patients. Eleven patients (20 percent) reported dysesthetic pain—a feeling of burning, tingling, or shocklike sensation—involving the lower legs and at times the upper limbs. Myalgic-rheumatic extremity pain was present in about nine percent of the subjects and was associated with joint stiffness. During follow-up there was an increase in the number of patients having dysesthetic and myalgic pain. Pain intensity on admission correlated poorly with neurologic disability on admission and throughout the period of the study. On a disability grading scale, 49 patients were moderately disabled or worse at the time of admission, and at 24 weeks follow-up 13 patients remained moderately disabled (45).

CHRONIC INFLAMMATORY DEMYELINATING POLYNEUROPATHY (CIDP)

Although the syndrome known as chronic inflammatory demyelinating polyradiculoneuropathy has no known etiology, several investigators have described its broad clinical features and electrodiagnostic findings (46-48). CIDP is believed to be immune-mediated, and it accounts for approximately 20 to 30 percent of initially undiagnosed peripheral neuropathies (49). It is common in people between 40 and 60 years of age. There are several possible clinical presentations: (*a*) slow monophasic; (*b*) chronic relapsing, in which there are fluctuations of weakness or improvement over weeks or months; (*c*) continuous but stepwise progression; and (*d*) slowly progressive. Most patients have both motor and sensory symptoms involving the upper and lower limbs. Motor weakness affects both proximal and distal muscles. Sensory symptoms and signs may be present in both the hands and feet. Paresthesias, dysesthesias, and burning or aching pain have been described.

Various authors have reported response to treatment interventions such as plasma exchange and intravenous gammaglobulin (50–52). Gorson et al. (1997) have recently summarized the clinical features and response to treatment in 67 consecutive patients with and without a monoclonal gammopathy (51). Average follow-up was 28 months after the onset of first symptoms. There were several variant presentations that conformed to the clinical and electrophysiologic definitions of CIDP. In 58 percent of patients, the most common clinical presentation was weakness and numbness. Pain was present in 42 percent of patients. Conduction block was the most common EMG abnormality, detected in at least one nerve in 73 percent of patients. Only 31 percent of patients had a pure demyelinating neuropathy, and the majority had some degree of axonal change. Patients were treated with three modalities that included plasma exchange, IVIg, and steroids therapy. Overall, 66 percent responded to one of the three treatment modalities (51).

In CIDP, there is usually segmental demyelination, remyelination, and the presence of perivascular mononuclear cell infiltrates. Nerves are generally hypertrophied. During an exacerbation of the disease there is usually evidence of axonal loss.

Chronic inflammatory demyelinating polyneuropathy is thought to be the most common treatable neuropathy seen in most neuromuscular clinics in North America. It is important to identify this condition not only because it is treatable, but also because some of these patients have an underlying systemic illness such as occult malignancy, HIV-1 infection, or plasma cell dyscrasias (53). The most helpful diagnostic feature suggestive of an acquired demyelinating neuropathy is abnormal temporal dispersion or partial conduction block. Reduction in the amplitude of the CMAP of more than 50 percent following proximal and distal stimulation reflects some degree of conduction block. Changes in the temporal dispersion and increases exceeding 15 percent over short segments and 20 percent over long segments indicate abnormality (54). An abnormal median sensory with normal sural response occurs more commonly in acute inflammatory demyelinating polyneuropathy (AIDP) than in CIDP.

HUMAN IMMUNODEFICIENCY VIRUS (HIV) INFECTION

Various clinical presentations of HIV infection may be encountered. (See Chapter 14 for a detailed discussion of pain management in HIV.) Hewitt et al. (1997)

have described various pain syndromes and their etiologies in ambulatory AIDS patients (55). In 28 percent of 151 patients, pain was considered to be caused by polyneuropathy. The most common pain diagnosis in their study was headache, reported by 46 percent of the patients (55).

When using electrodiagnostic testing, even in the absence of symptoms, some patients infected with HIV-1 show evidence of peripheral nerve disease. Symptoms of axonal neuropathy may occur in patients with AIDS and usually consist of burning and painful paresthesias in the feet more so than in the hands. Examination shows a greater loss of sensory function than of motor function; and the loss is more distal than proximal.

Polyneuropathy may present as (a) distal symmetric polyneuropathy; (b) inflammatory demyelinating polyneuropathy; (c) mononeuropathy multiplex (d); progressive polyradiculopathy; or (e) autonomic neuropathy. The most common presentation is one of distal symmetric polyneuropathy (56,57).

In the study by Tagliati et al. (1999), 38 percent of 251 HIV-infected patients were diagnosed with distal symmetrical polyneuropathy (DSP) (57). In this study the most common clinical features were nonpainful paresthesias (71 percent), abnormalities of pain and temperature perception (71 percent), and reduced or absent ankle reflexes (66 percent). Patients with DSP were significantly older and had lower CD4 lymphocyte counts than those without DSP. The authors conclude that a combination of factors, including immunosuppression, nutritional status, and age contribute to distal peripheral nerve dysfunction. To characterize further, Bouhassira and colleagues (1999) compared quantitative sensory testing (QST) and electrodiagnostic parameters in patients with painful or painless DSP (58). These investigators conclude that patients with DSP have thermal, mechanical, and electrophysiologic deficits, suggestive of both small and large peripheral nerve fiber involvement. Conversely, patients with painful neuropathy present with static mechanical allodynia or hyperalgesia, suggestive of a selective alteration in the processing of mechanoreceptive signals, which might have a significant role in the pathophysiology of spontaneous and evoked pain in these patients (58).

Bradley and Verma described painful vasculitis in two patients with HIV-1 infection (59). The patients were in the B2 stage of HIV infection and presented with a subacute onset of painful neuropathy. Electrophysiologic studies revealed predominantly axonal sensorimotor neuropathy. Sural nerve biopsy in both cases showed a necrotizing vasculitis. DSP usually manifests in patients with other symptoms and signs of AIDS (59). It may also be associated with the neurotoxic drugs administered in attempts to control HIV. Patients may present with symptoms and signs similar to CIDP. The occurrence of progressive polyradiculopathy is usually seen in patients with advanced HIV disease (56).

ALCOHOLISM AND NEUROPATHY

Although the precise incidence of alcoholic polyneuropathy is unknown, it is one of the most common forms of peripheral disease. Alcoholic polyneuropathy invariably occurs in the setting of long-standing, serious alcoholism and secondary nutritional deficiency. The majority of patients with alcoholic polyneuropathy report substantial weight loss prior to or concomitant with the evolution of the peripheral neuropathy.

A history of excessive alcohol consumption over many years invariably leads to a generalized, predominantly axonal sensorimotor peripheral neuropathy (60). Polyneuropathy may have an acute or subacute onset. Patients present with symptoms of paresthesias, a distressing burning sensation or a sharp lancinating pain around the feet, and muscle weakness. In some patients the onset is insidious, with slow progression of clinical signs. The symptoms of alcoholic neuropathy are worse and signs are more pronounced in the lower limbs. In long-standing cases, the upper limbs may also become involved, predominantly the hands. The exact etiology is not known. The nutritional deficiency of thiamine, pyridoxine, and pantothenic acid is reported to be in a greater degree responsible for this condition than the actual toxic effects of alcohol (61). This form of neuropathy may be associated with gastrointestinal disturbances that impair the absorption of these vitamins. Wallerian degeneration is the primary abnormality, with small degrees of secondary demyelination. Lower extremity sensory nerve conduction studies are abnormal early in the disease process, and these abnormalities may be present in asymptomatic patients. H-reflex latency may become prolonged and later become absent. Brainstem and visual evoked potentials (VEPs) are reported to be abnormal, suggesting involvement of central portions of the cranial nerves (62,63). According to Hillbom (1984), abstaining from alcohol consumption and eating a balanced diet may reverse of some of the symptoms over a course of several years (64).

ENTRAPMENT NEUROPATHIES

Entrapment neuropathies are focal neuropathies secondary to the compression phenomena. They are commonly seen in patients with a history of diabetes mellitus, hypothyroidism, and other conditions that produce a tendency to retain fluid. Some of the common entrapment neuropathies like carpal tunnel syndrome and meralgia paresthetica are associated with burning, tingling, and painful dysesthesias.

PAINFUL MONONEUROPATHY

Painful mononeuropathies may result from injury to the nerve, vascular problems, or from inflammatory or neoplastic lesions. Injury to the nerve does not always result in chronic pain. Those with symptoms of mononeuropathy describe the pain as aching, burning, electrical, sharp, or stabbing. There may be hyperesthesia, hyperalgesia, or associated allodynia over the painful site. Usually there is local tenderness because of an underlying neuroma. Posttraumatic neuroma and pain secondary to compression are probably the two most common causes of traumatic painful neuropathies.

Brachial neuritis is an example of an inflammatory neuropathy affecting the brachial plexus. This condition is preceded by an upper respiratory viral infection and presents with the acute onset of pain around the shoulder, neck, and arm. The patient may also have other sensory symptoms. The condition is associated with muscle weakness. It is a self-limiting condition; however, the patient may be left with considerable weakness. Management of brachial neuritis includes a range of exercises and local physical modalities. Attempts should be made to maintain strength. A short course of oral steroids may help to relieve pain and minimize morbidity. Once the pain is under control, a strengthening exercise program should be prescribed.

GENERAL MANAGEMENT OF NEUROPATHIES

The general management of patients with painful neuropathies includes a comprehensive assessment regarding the diagnosis, etiology, severity of pain, complications resulting from weakness and sensory loss, functional status, and social and psychological status. Vocational needs should also be assessed. It is important to anticipate complications that may be expected during the acute and chronic stages of polyneuropathies so that measures can be taken to prevent or minimize these complications and the resulting pain. These complications may include muscle weakness resulting from disease and disuse, muscle tightness, deformities, and functional impairments.

Muscle Weakness

Most patients with painful neuropathies have muscle weakness of varying degree and are prone to develop joint contractures. Patients with poor balance and foot drop may have a history of falls, which results in more pain problems. Weakness, although present in most polyneuropathies, varies in its presentation. If not managed well, it may affect the rehabilitation outcome. Distal weakness in lower limbs manifests itself in gait abnormalities and poor balance, whereas distal weakness in upper limbs manifests in poor fine motor control. Proximal weakness interferes with gait, transfer activities, and gross movement. Attempts should be made to maintain and improve strength with appropriate exercise programs. It is important to prevent contractures by prescribing range-of-motion exercises. If balance cannot be improved with an exercise program, the patient should be prescribed an assistive device. In some instances, strengthening exercises may be harmful to these patients. In particular, progressive resistive exercises can cause more harm than good if they cause fatigue (65). Low-intensity exercise may be beneficial for maintenance of strength gains in those patients with grade four or better strength.

SOFT TISSUE TIGHTNESS

Soft tissue tightness may occur as a result of polyneuropathy. Tightness may develop early during the course of the illness (within the first few weeks) and may contribute to the pain experienced by these patients. Muscle tightness appears in the muscles crossing two joints and may effect any joint. Tightness usually results in a flexion contracture. Asymmetrical muscle weakness and tightness may produce a malalignment of body segments and progressive deformities. Malalignment may be the result of inappropriate equipment prescription. Frequent areas of soft tissue tightness are the ankle plantar flexion, foot inversion, knee flexion, hip flexion and hip internal rotation, and finger and elbow flexion. Proper positioning, frequent postural changes, selective stretching, and appropriate bracing of the involved joints can prevent postural abnormalities. Fixed malalignments may need corrective surgical procedures and mechanical stretching with serial casts and dynamic bracing. An aggressive approach must be taken when these deformities interfere with functional activities.

Bracing

If the neuropathic pain is associated with muscle weakness, especially when involving the dorsiflexors of the ankles, bracing options should be considered and discussed with the patient. Depending on the degree of weakness and sensory loss, one can consider appropriate static or dynamic ankle–foot orthosis (AFO). There are wide varieties of AFOs, but these can be separated into metal, polypropylene, and hybrid metal and plastic styles. The best orthosis is one that can balance the floor reaction forces to provide the most efficient gait and reduce deforming forces. Comfort and correct fit are very important in preventing complications such as ulcerations caused by ill-fitting orthoses. An AFO with an anterior stop acts like the plantar flexors to stabilize the knee by enhancing knee extension. Although it increases knee stability, it could also cause a hyperextension that may produce knee pain. A posterior stop replaces weak dorsiflexion and prevents equinus in the swing phase. Excessive posterior stop may cause a knee flexion at heel strike, putting the knee into an unstable position. The knee may buckle and create a balance problem and/or fall. Thus, it is very important to assess the strength of various muscle groups across the ankle and knee joints. For practical purposes, a metal orthosis with double uprights is the preferred choice in a patient with fluctuating edema and insensate limbs. Metal orthoses can be fabricated with a soft leather shoe and soft inner lining to avoid skin irritation. If fluctuating edema is a major problem, a total contact orthosis with an anterior panel might control edema in the limb. When prescribing a metal orthosis it is important to avoid skin contact with the metal brace at the ankle to prevent possible ulceration. Because metal braces are heavy and cumbersome, a plastic AFO can be prescribed in patients with no significant sensory loss. Plastic AFO are lightweight, simple to put on and take off, and less expensive than metal AFOs. It is important for the patient or his caregiver to inspect the skin on a regular basis for any signs of skin irritation and skin breakdown. Patient preference is also taken into account in the choice of plastic or metal orthosis.

Physical Modalities

The local application of superficial heat, cold, hydrotherapy, and transcutaneous electrical stimulation (TENS) can be tried in selected conditions such as brachial neuritis and postherpetic pain. The role of these modalities in patients with polyneuropathy has not been systematically studied. Caution should be used when applying local modalities such as heat and cold in patients with sensory deficits.

PAIN MANAGEMENT IN NEUROPATHIES

Currently, the management of the pain is identical for all painful polyneuropathies (8), although, biofeedback, relaxation exercises, and meditation may significantly improve psychological and physical functioning, drug therapy remains the most effective approach to relieve pain in these patients. A variety of pharmacologic agents have been shown to be safe and effective in relieving pain in patients with polyneuropathy. These include tricyclic antidepressants, anticonvulsants, and local anesthetic and antiarrhythmic drugs. Sympatholytic drugs and opioids may also help some patients. Topical agents, such as lidocaine and capsaicin, may prove to be beneficial in the management of several peripheral neuropathic pain syndromes.

The current mode of pharmacotherapy employs sequential drug trials, because significant individual variability exists within the same class of pharmacologic agents (8). Moreover, there is no target dose for any drug. Titration is required to achieve an optimum dose that achieves the most pain relief with the fewest side effects. Patient education is very important regarding the titration process and the various limiting side effects for each class of these drugs. Galer (1998) has provided "Guidelines for Pharmacotherapy" (see Figure 8.1) for the management of neuropathic pain and also has outlined an algorithm to treat the pain associated with polyneuropathy (1,8). According to the author "successful pain medication must result in all of the following: significant pain relief, tolerable side effects, and increased activity and function of the patients. Furthermore, a drug that significantly alleviates pain but causes significant cognitive side effects or sedation is no better than one that produces no pain relief at all."

Tricyclic Antidepressants

Although tricyclic antidepressants (TCAs) do not provide good analgesia or may have side effects that limit the effective dose, drugs such as amitriptyline and desipramine are still the first line of drugs used to treat pain secondary to polyneuropathy (1). In patients with painful diabetic polyneuropathy, the relief of pain is independent of the effect on depression (66–68). These drugs may relieve constant burning and deep pain as well as lancinating pain. It is believed that the mechanism of action is to enhance neurotransmission within the CNS and influence the brain stem-dorsal horn modulating systems (12). TCAs act at a variety of receptor sites, which may explain the significant variability in response experienced by individual patients. Most of the side effects are caused by the anticholinergic properties of TCAs, and the drugs should be prescribed with caution in elderly patients. The recommended initial dose is 10 to 25 mg at bedtime. The dose is increased every week until adequate pain relief is achieved or intolerable side effects develop. Failure of one TCA should not preclude the use of a different

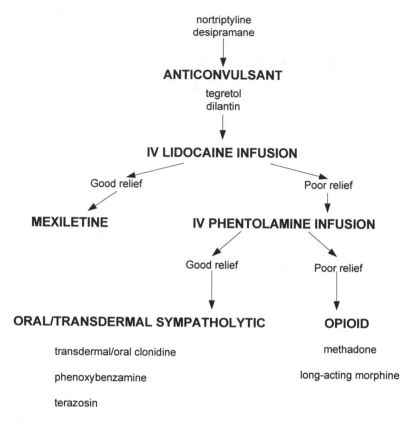

Figure 8.1. Pharmacotherapeutic algorithm. (From Galer, In: Seminars In *Neurology* Volume 14, Page 241.)

TCA. TCAs should not be prescribed to patients with a history of closed-angle glaucoma, prostatic hypertrophy, or acute myocardial infarction.

Anticonvulsants

Phenytoin and carbamazepine are reported to be beneficial in painful polyneuropathies (69,70). The dose–response relationship has not been assessed with reference to pain relief, and some patients may experience pain relief at serum levels that are below the therapeutic range for treating epilepsy (1).

Local Anesthetic and Antiarrhythmics

Local anesthetics and antiarrhythmics such as intravenous lidocaine infusion and oral mexiletine are effective analgesic agents in neuropathic pain syndromes (71–73). Intravenous lidocaine requires continuous supervision and monitoring for cardiac arrhythmias and blood pressure. It is recommended that resuscitative equipment be available (1). Intravenous lidocaine has been used as a predictor of response to oral mexiletine.

Sympathetic Agents

Sympathetic agents such as intravenous phentolamine infusion, oral terazosin, and transdermal clonidine are reported to relieve neuropathic pain (74–76). The side effects of these agents include transient nasal congestion, dizziness, flushing, nausea, vomiting, and abdominal pain. Sympathetic agents should not be prescribed to patients with a history of cardiovascular or cerebrovascular disease (76).

Other Drugs

In patients with painful polyneuropathy, Sindrup et al. (1999) report pain relief with tramadol, an analgesic drug that acts directly on opioid receptors and indirectly on monoaminergic receptor systems (77). The dose of tramadol slow-release tablets was titrated to at least 200 mg/day up to a maximum of 400 mg/day. Tramadol was found to be significantly superior to placebo (77). Boucher et al. (2000) reported the beneficial effects of glial cell line-derived neurotrophic factor (GDNF) to both prevent and reverse sensory abnormalities that developed in neuropathic pain models without affecting pain-related behavior in normal animals (78). According to these investigators, GDNF reduces ectopic discharges within sensory neurons after nerve injury; these findings provide a rational basis for the use of GDNF as a therapeutic treatment for neuropathic pain states (78).

PAIN MANAGEMENT IN SPECIFIC CONDITIONS

Painful Polyneuropathy in Patients with HIV Infection

In two patients with HIV infection, Bradley et al. (1996) reported rapid relief of pain with prednisone therapy followed by arrest of the neuropathic process in vasculitic neuropathy (59). In one patient, the shooting pain resolved dramatically with a 60 mg/day dose, and the tenderness and hyperpathia became progressively better in about three weeks. When the prednisone was stopped, there was a recurrence of pain and difficulty in walking that necessitated restarting prednisone therapy at 20 mg/day. The pain remained under control with a continued dose of 10 mg/day. The second patient responded to a similar dose and was pain-free with a continued dose of 20 mg/day. The authors conclude that vasculitic neuropathy must be considered among the treatable causes of painful neuropathy in HIV-1 infected individuals (59).

Chronic Painful Diabetic Peripheral Neuropathy

Pfeifer and colleagues describe a treatment algorithm based on the anatomic site and neuropathophysiologic source of the neuropathic pain (79). Seventy-five diabetic patients with chronic painful distal symmetrical peripheral neuropathy of more than 12 months duration were treated. Fifty-three of these patients received treatment with imipramine (with or without mexiletine) for deep pain, capsaicin for superficial pain, and stretching exercises and metaxalone (with or without piroxican) for muscular pain. Twenty-three patients received no treatment. A significant pain improvement was noted in the treated group but not in the untreated group. Twenty-one patients who received treatment became pain-free and 66 percent reported improvement. Tsigos et al. (1995) measured cerebrospinal fluid levels of beta-endorphin in painful and painless diabetic polyneuropathy (80). Reduced concentrations of beta-endorphin were found in patients with painful polyneuropathy when compared to the control subjects. These investigators conclude that the results may explain why opioid analgesics are of little, if any, help in alleviating diabetic neuropathic pain (80).

Levodopa was reported to relieve pain in a double-blind placebo controlled study in patients with symmetrical diabetic polyneuropathy (81). An experimental group of 14 patients received 100 mg of levodopa, plus 25 mg of benserazide, three times a day for 28 days; 11 patients received identical placebo capsules. The investigators conclude that the results seem promising, indicating that levodopa may be a choice for the control of pain in neuropathies for which there are few alternative treatments (81).

Simeonov and colleagues studied the therapeutic efficiency of Milgamma® (a mixture of benfothiamine and cyanobalamine) in patients with painful diabetic neuropathy (82). Patients received two Milgamma® tablets (each tablet containing 50 mg benfothiamine and 0.25 mg cyancobalamine) QID for three weeks followed by one Milgamma, tablet three times a day for nine weeks. The control group received a vitamin B complex treatment regimen using Neurobex®. A statistically significant relief of neuropathic pain was achieved in all patients treated with Milgamma® tablets, whereas the sensory symptom improvement was insignificant in the Neurobex®-treated patients. The authors conclude that these results underscore the importance of Milgamma® tablets as an indispensable element in the therapeutic regimen of patients with painful diabetic polyneuropathy (82).

In a randomized, double-blind, placebo-controlled, 8-week trial, Backnoja and colleagues (1998) evaluated the effect of gabapentin monotherapy (titrated from 900 to 3,600 mg/day, or to a maximum tolerated dosage) on pain associated with diabetic peripheral neuropathy (83). The primary outcome measure was daily pain severity, and secondary measures included quality of life and mood states. The authors conclude that gabapentin monotherapy appears to be efficacious for the treatment of the pain and sleep interference associated with diabetic peripheral neuropathy, and that gabapentin exhibits positive effects on mood and the quality of life (83).

Dejgard (1988) reported the beneficial effects of mexiletine in patients with diabetic painful polyneuropathy (71). The usual starting dose is 150 mg once or twice a day. The dose is then titrated for optimum results. The dose may be increased to 1,200 mg a day. The most common side effect is upper gastrointestinal distress; taking drug with food or using an antacid may minimize this side effect. Because mexiletine may cause chest pain and palpitation, it should not be prescribed in patients with a history of atrioventricular conduction block and cardiac arrhythmias.

Zeigler et al. (1992) conclude that there might be a subset of patients with diabetic polyneuropathy who respond to 0.3 mg/day transdermal clonidine patches (76).

Results from clinical trials on the use of capsaicin in painful diabetic peripheral neuropathy has been conflicting (84–86). In a randomized controlled trial of 0.075 percent capsaicin in diabetic patients with painful neuropathy, Chad et al. (1990) report no beneficial effects (84), whereas the Capsaicin Study Group report improvement in diabetic patients receiving capsaicin when compared to a placebo group (85). In the Capsaicin Study Group, investigators at 12 sites enrolled 277 patients with painful peripheral polyneuropathy or radiculopathy in a 12-week double-blind controlled study. Either 0.075 percent capsaicin cream or a placebo vehicle cream was applied to the painful areas four times a day. Statistically significant differences showing improvement in favor of capsaicin versus the placebo were noted in the areas of pain intensity, walking, sleeping, working, and participating in recreational activities. The investigators conclude that the results suggest that topical capsaicin is effective for reducing pain in patients with painful diabetic neuropathy, producing subsequent improvement in daily activities and thus enhancing the quality of the patient's life (85).

Guillain–Barré Syndrome

Although GBS is a self-limiting disease, in the initial stages of onset it is associated with marked motor weakness that may lead to contractures and muscle and joint pain. It is important to prevent these complications through correct positioning and the appropriate splinting of paralyzed limbs. The use of pressure-relieving mattresses may prevent discomfort from pressure areas (87). Other methods advocated by Hughes and colleagues (1981) include the use of cold or warm pads and gentle massage that can also bring considerable relief in some cases (87). Regular passive range-of-motion exercises may prevent musculoskeletal stiffness and pain (88). Drug therapy should start with simple analgesics and nonsteroidal antiinflammatory agents (NSAIDs). If required, other drugs, such as those described above, can be tried. A single intramuscular injection of methylprednisolone was successful in alleviating severe muscle pains within 2 hours in some patients (44). Hughes et al. also report considerable success with opiates.

Pentland and Donald (1994) advocate caution with the use of narcotic agents in a condition in which the need for analgesics may be prolonged (40). The authors conclude that the nature of pain experiences are various and the proliferation of remedies for pain in GBS is a testament to the lack of a foolproof method, but fortunately most patients' pain resolves spontaneously with time (37).

The mainstay of treatment for acute GBS is plasma exchange and gamma-globulin infusion, both directed at the assumed underlying pathogenic process (89). Kuwabara and colleagues (2001) compare the effects of intravenous immunoglobulin therapy (IVIg) and plasmapheresis for the IgG anti-GM1-positive subtype of GBS (90). Clinical and electrophysiologic recoveries were analyzed in

24 patients (10 with IVIg and 14 with plasmapheresis). The patients treated with IVIg had significantly lower Hughes grades scores 1, 3, and 6 months after onset and a higher probability to regain independent locomotion at 6 months. The authors conclude that IVIg therapy may be a more efficacious treatment than plasmapheresis (90).

CONCLUSIONS

The management of pain associated with peripheral neuropathy can be very challenging. A good understanding of the etiology and pathophysiology of the neuropathic process is crucial to the proper treatment and management of neuropathic pain. The management of such pain is often achieved through multiple treatment modalities.

REFERENCES

1. Galer BS. Painful polyneuropathy: Diagnosis, pathophysiology, and management. *Seminars in Neurology* 1994; 14:237–246.
2. Devor M, Rappaport ZH. Pain and the pathophysiology of damaged nerve. In: Fields HL (ed.), *Pain Syndromes in Neurology*. London: Butterworths, 1990; pp 47–85.
3. Fields HL, Rowbotham MC. Multiple mechanisms of neuropathic pain: A clinical perspective. In: Gebhart GF, Hammond DL, Jensen TS (eds.), *Proceedings of the 7th World Congress on Pain*. Seattle: IASP Press, 1994; pp 173–183.
4. Jensen TS. Mechanisms of neuropathic pain. In: Campbell, JN (ed.), *Pain 1996–An Updated Review*. Seattle: IASP Press, 1996; pp 77–86.
5. Loeser JD. Peripheral nerve disorders and peripheral neuropathies. In: Bonica JJ (ed.), *The Management of Pain*. Philadelphia: Lea & Febiger, 1990; pp 211–220.
6. Gershkoff A.M. Pain in neuropathy: State-of-the-art review. In: Walsh NE (ed.), *Physical Medicine and Rehabilitation: Rehabilitation of Chronic Pain* vol 5, No. 1. Philadelphia: Hanley & Belfus, 1991.
7. Melzack R, Wall PD. Pain mechanisms: A new theory. *Science* 1965; 150:971–979.
8. Galer BS. Painful neuropathy: Neuropathic pain syndromes. *Neurologic Clin* 1998; 16:791–811.
9. Coderre TJ, Katz J, Vaccarino AL, et al. Contribution of central neuroplasticity to pathological pain: Review of clinical and experimental evidence. *Pain* 1993; 52:259–285.
10. Tsigos C, Reed P, Weinkove C, White A, Young RJ. Plasma norepinephrine in sensory diabetic polyneuropathy. *Diabetes Care* 1993; 16:722–727.
11. Galer BS, Bruehl S, Harden RN. IASP diagnostic criteria for complex regional pain syndrome (CRPS): A preliminary empirical validation study. *Clin J Pain*, 1997; 14: 48–54.
12. Fields H.L Heinricher MM, Mason P. Neurotransmitters in nociceptive modulatory circuits. *Ann Rev Neuroscience* 1991; 14:219–245.
13. Cross S. Pathophysiology of pain. *Mayo Clin Proc* 1994; 69:375–383.
14. Dubner R. Neuronal plasticity and pain following peripheral tissue inflammation or injury. In: Bond MR, Charlton JE, Woolf CJ (eds.), *Proceedings of the Sixth World Congress on Pain*. Amsterdam: Elsevier 1991; 263–276.
15. Barinaga M. Playing "telephone" with the body's message of pain. *Science* 1992; 258: 1085.
16. Adams RD, Victor M. Diseases of the peripheral and cranial nerves. In: *Principles of Neurology*, Ch.26. New York: McGraw-Hill, 1977.

17. Thomas PK. Classification, differential diagnosis, and staging of diabetic peripheral neuropathy. *Diabetes* 1997; 46:S54–S57.

18. Verdugo R, Ochoa JL. Quantitative somatosensory thermo-test: A key method for functional evaluation of small caliber afferent channels. *Brain* 1992; 115:893–913.

19. Peripheral Neuropathy Association. Quantitative sensory testing: A consensus report from the Peripheral Neuropathy Association. *Neurology* 1993; 43:1050–1052.

20. Ratzmann KP, Raschke M, Gander I, et al. Prevalence of peripheral neuropathy in newly diagnosed type II diabetes. *J Diabetic Complications* 1991; 5:1–5.

21. Galer BS, Jensen M. Development and preliminary validation of a pain measure specific to neuropathic pain: The neuropathic pain scale. *Neurology* 1997; 48:332–339.

22. Dyck PJ, Karnes JL, Daube J, O'Brien P, Service FJ. Clinical and neuropathological criteria for the diagnosis and staging of diabetic polyneuropathy. *Brain* 1985; 108:861–880.

23. Feldman EL, Stevens MJ, Thomas PK, Brown MB, Canal N, Greene DA. A practical two-step quantitative clinical and electrophysiological assessment for the diagnosis and staging of diabetic neuropathy. *Diabetes Care* 1994; 17:1281–1289.

24. Thomas PK, King RHM. Peripheral nerve changes in amyloid neuropathy. *Brain* 1974; 97:395–406.

25. Archer AG, Watkins PJ, Thomas PK, Sharma AK, Payan J. The natural history of acute painful neuropathy in diabetes mellitus. *J Neurol Neurosurg Psychiatry* 1983; 46:491–499.

26. Asbury AK, Aldredge H, Hershberg R, Fisher CM. Oculomotor palsy in diabetes mellitus: A clinico-pathological study. *Brain* 1970; 93:555–566.

27. Sun SF, Streib EW. Diabetic thoracoabdominal neuropathy: Clinical and electrodiagnostic features. *Ann Neurol* 1981; 9:75–79.

28. Boulton AJM, Angus E, Ayyar DR, Weiss R. Diabetic thoracic polyradiculopathy presenting as an abdominal swelling. *Br Med J* 1984; 289:798–801.

29. Garland H. Diabetic amyotrophy. *Br J Clin Pract* 1961; 15:9–13.

30. Chokroverty S. Proximal nerve dysfunction in diabetic proximal amyotrophy. *Arch Neurol* 1982; 39:403–407.

31. Llewelyn JG, Thomas PK, King RH. Epineural microvasculitis in proximal diabetic neuropathy. *J Neurol* 1998; 245:159–165.

32. Galer BS. Diabetic neuropathy. *Amer Pain Soc Bull* October/November 1993; 18–19.

33. Handevidt F. Peripheral neuropathy in persons with diabetes. *Clin Excell Nurse Pract* 2001; 5:17–20.

34. The Diabetes Control and Complications Trial Research Group. The effect of intensive treatment of diabetes on the development and progression of long-term complications in insulin-dependent diabetes mellitus. *N Engl J Med* 1993; 329:977–986.

35. Hughes RAC. Chronic inflammatory demyelinating polyneuropathy. In: Hughes RAC (ed.), *Guillain-Barré Syndrome*. London: Springer-Verlag, 1990, 205–246.

36. Ropper AH. The Guillain-Barré syndrome. *N Engl J Med* 1992; 326:1130–1136.

37. Winer JB, Hughes RAC, Anderson MJ, Jones DM, Kangro H, Watkins RPF. A prospective study of acute idiopathic neuropathy. II. Antecedent events. *J Neurol Neurosurg Psychiatry* 1988; 51:613–619.

38. Hughes RAC, Winer JB. Guillain-Barré syndrome. In: Mathews WB, Glaser GH (eds.), *Recent Advances in Clinical Neurology*, vol 4. Edinburgh: Churchill Livingstone, 1984; 19–49.

39. Ropper AH, Wijdicks EFM, Shahani BT. Electrodiagnostic abnormalities in 113 consecutive patients with Guillain-Barré syndrome. *Arch Neurol* 1990; 47:881–887.

40. Pentland B, Donald SM. Pain in the Guillain-Barré syndrome: A clinical review. *Pain* 1994; 59:150–164.

41. Greenwood RJ, Hughes RAC, Bowden AN, et al. Controlled trial of plasma exchange in acute inflammatory polyradiculopathy. *Lancet* 1984; 1:877–879.

42. Ropper AH, Wijdicks EFM, Truax BT. *Guillain-Barré Syndrome*. Philadelphia: FA Davis, 1991.
43. Winer SJ, Evans JG. Guillain-Barré syndrome in Oxfordshire: Clinical features in relation to age. *Age Aging* 1993; 22:164–170.
44. Ropper AH, Shahani BT. Pain in Guillain-Barré syndrome. *Arch Neurol* 1984; 41:511–514.
45. Mouline DE, Hagen N, Feasby TE, Amireh R, Hahn A. Pain in Guillain-Barré syndrome. *Neurology* 1997; 48:328–331.
46. Barohn RJ, Kissel JT, Warmolts JR, Mendell JR. Chronic inflammatory demyelinating polyneuropathy: Clinical characteristics, course, and recommendations for diagnostic criteria. *Arch Neurol* 1989; 46:878–884.
47. Bromberg MB. Comparison of electrodiagnostic criteria for primary demyelination in chronic polyneuropathy. *Muscle Nerve* 1991; 14:968–976.
48. Simmons Z, Albers JW, Bromberg MB, Feldman EL. Presentation and initial clinical course in patients with chronic inflammatory demyelinating polyneuropathy: Comparison of patients without and with monoclonal gammopathy. *Neurology* 1993; 43:2202–2209.
49. Dimitru, D. General polyneuropathy. In: *Electrodiagnostic Medicine*, 1st ed., Philadelphia: Hanley & Belfus, 1995, pp 763.
50. Simmons Z, Albers JW, Bromberg MB, Fledman EL. Long term follow-up of patients with chronic inflammatory demyelinating polyneuropathy without and with monoclonal gammopathy. *Brain* 1995; 118:359–368.
51. Gorson KC, Allam G, Ropper AH. Chronic inflammatory demyelinating polyneuropathy: Clinical features and response to treatment in 67 consecutive patients with and without monoclonal gammopathy. *Neurology* 1997; 48:321–328.
52. Choudhary PP, Huges RAC. Long-term treatment of chronic inflammatory demyelinating polyradiculoneuropathy with plasma exchange or intravenous gammaglobulin. *QJM* 1995; 88:493–502.
53. Cornblath DR, Asbury AK, Albers JW, et al. Report from an ad hoc subcommittee of the American Academy of Neurology AIDS Task Force Research criteria for the diagnosis of chronic inflammatory demyelinating polyneuropathy (CIDP). *Neurology* 1991; 41:617–618.
54. Brown WF, Feasby TE. Conduction block and denervation in Guillain-Barré polyneuropathy. *Brain* 1984; 107:219–239.
55. Hewitt DJ, McDonald M, Portenoy RK, Rosenfeld B, Passik S, Breitbart W. Pain syndromes and etiologies in ambulatory AIDS patients. *Pain* 1997; 70:117–123.
56. Simpson DM, Olney RK. Peripheral neuropathies associated with human immunodeficiency virus infection. *Neuro Clin* 1992; 10:685–711.
57. Tagliati M, Grinnell J, Godbold J, Simpson DM. Peripheral nerve function in HIV infection: Clinical, electrophysiological, and laboratory findings. *Arch Neurol* 1999; 56:84–89.
58. Bouhassira D, Attal N, Willer JC, Brasseur L. Painful and painless peripheral sensory neuropathies due to HIV infection: A comparison using quantitative sensory evaluation. *Pain* 1999; 80:265–272.
59. Bradley WG, Verma A. Painful vasculitic neuropathy in HIV-1 infection: Relief of pain with prednisone therapy. *Neurology* 1996; 47:1446–1451.
60. Windebank AJ. Polyneuropathy due to nutritional deficiency and alcoholism. In: Dyck PJ, Thomas PK, Griffin JW, et al. (eds.), *Peripheral Neuropathy*, 3rd ed. Philadelphia: WB Saunders, 1993, pp 1310–1321.
61. Victor M. Polyneuropathy due to nutritional and alcoholism. In Dyck PJ, Thomas PK, Lambert EH (eds.), *Peripheral Neuropathy*. Philadelphia: WB Saunders, 1975; pp 1030.
62. Chan Y-W, McLeod JG, Tuck RR, et al. Brain stem auditory evoked responses in chronic alcoholics. *J Neurol Neurosurg Psychiatry* 1985; 48:1107–1112.
63. Chan Y-W, McLeod JG, Tuck RR, et al. Visual evoked responses in chronic alcoholics. *J Neurol Neurosurg Psychiatry* 1986; 49:945–950.

64. Hillbom M, Wennberg A. Prognosis of alcoholic neuropathy. *J Neurol Neurosurg Psychiatry* 1984; 47:699–703.

65. Herbison G, Jaweed MM, Ditunno JR. Exercise therapies in peripheral neuropathies. *Arch Phys Med Rehab* 1983; 64:201–205.

66. Max MB, Culname M, Schafer SC, et al. Amitriptyline relieves diabetic neuropathy pain in patients with normal or depressed mood. *Neurology* 1987; 7:589–596.

67. Max MB, Lynch SA, Muir et al. Effects of desipramine, amitriptyline, and fluoxetine on pain in diabetic neuropathy. *N Engl J Med* 1992; 326:1250–1256.

68. Gomez-Perez FJ, Rull JA, Dies H, et al. Nortriptyline and fluphenazine in the symptomatic treatment of diabetic neuropathy: A double blind cross-over study. *Pain* 1985; 23:395–397.

69. Chadda VS, Matghaur MS. Double-blind study of the effects of diphenylhydantoin sodium on diabetic neuropathy. *J Assoc Physician India* 1978; 26: 403–406.

70. Wilton TD. Tegretol in the treatment of diabetic neuropathy. *South Afr Med J* 1974; 48:869–872.

71. Dejgard A, Petersen P, Kastrup J. Mexiletine for treatment of chronic diabetic neuropathy. *Lancet* 1988; 2:9–11.

72. Rowbotham MC, Reisner-Keller LA, Fields HL. Both intravenous lidocaine and morphine reduce the pain of postherpetic neuralgia. *Neurology* 1991; 41:1024–1028.

73. Galer BS, Miller KV, Rowbotham MC. Response to intravenous lidocaine differs based upon clinical diagnosis and site of nervous system injury. *Neurology* 1993; 43:1233–1235.

74. Raja SN, Treede RD, Davis KD, Campbell JN. Systemic alpha-adrenergic blockade with phentolamine: A diagnostic test for sympathetically maintained pain. *Anesthesiology* 1991; 74:691–698.

75. Galer BS, Lipton RB, Kaplan R, Kaplan JG, Arezzo JC, Portenoy RK. Bilateral burning foot pain: Monitoring of pain, sensation and autonomic sympathetic function during successful treatment with sympathetic blockade. *J Pain Symptom Management* 1990; 6:92–97.

76. Zeigler D, Lynch SA, Muir J, Benjamin J, Max MB. Transdermal clonidine versus placebo in painful diabetic neuropathy. *Pain* 1992; 48:403–408.

77. Sindrup SH, Andersen G, Madsen C, Smith T, Brosen K, Jensen TS. Tramadol relieves pain and allodynia in polyneuropathy: A randomized, double-blind, controlled trial. *Pain* 1999; 83:85–90.

78. Boucher TJ, Okuse K, Bennett DL, Munson JB, Wood JN, McMahon SB. Potent analgesic effects of GDNF in neuropathic pain states. *Science* 2000; 290:124–127.

79. Pfeifer MA, Ross DR, Schrage JP, Gelber DA, Schumer MP, Crain GM, Markwell SJ, Jung S. A highly successful and novel model for treatment of chronic painful diabetic peripheral neuropathy. *Diabetic Care* 1993; 16:1103–1105.

80. Tsigos C, Gibson S, Crosby SR, White A, Young RJ. Cerebrospinal fluid levels of beta endorphin in painful and painless diabetic polyneuropathy. *J Diabetes Complications* 1995; 9:92–96.

81. Ertas M, Sagduyu A, Arac N, Uludag B, Ertekin C. Use of levodopa to relieve pain from painful diabetic polyneuropathy. *Pain* 1998; 75:257–259.

82. Simeonov S, Pavlova M, Mitkov M, Mincheva L, Troev D. Therapeutic efficacy of Milgamma in patients with painful neuropathy. *Folia Med (Plovdiv)* 1997; 39:5–10.

83. Backonja M et al. Gabapentin for the symptomatic treatment of painful neuropathy in patients with diabetes mellitus: A randomized controlled trial. *JAMA* 1998; 280(21):1831–1836.

84. Chad DA, Aronin N, Lundstrom R, et al. Does capsaicin relieve the pain of diabetic neuropathy? *Pain* 1990; 42:387–388.

85. Capsaicin Study Group. Effect of treatment with capsaicin on daily activities of patients with painful diabetic neuropathy. *Diabetic Care* 1992; 15:159–165.

86. Low PA, Opfer-Gehrking TL, Dyck PJ, Litchy WJ, O'Brien PC. Double-blind, placebo-controlled study of the application of capsaicin cream in chronic distal painful polyneuropathy. *Pain* 1995; 62:163–168.

87. Hughes RAC, Kadlubowski M, Hufschmidt A. Treatment of acute inflammatory polyneuropathy. *Ann Neurol 9* (Suppl.) 1981; 125–133.

88. Soryal I, Sinclair E, Hornby J, Petland B. Impaired joint mobility in Guillain-Barré syndrome: A primary or secondary phenomenon? *J Neuol Neurosurg Psychiatry* 1992; 55:1014–1017.

89. Ropper AH: The Guillain-Barré syndrome. *N Engl J Med* 1992; 326:1130–1136.

90. Kuwabara S, Mori M, Ogawara K, Hattori T, Oda S, Koga M, Yuki N. Intravenous immunoglobulin therapy for Guillain-Barré syndrome with IgG antibody. *Muscle Nerve* 2001; 24:54–58.

9 | Pain Associated with Poliomyelitis

Carlos Vallbona, M.D.

Acute poliomyelitis has been successfully eradicated from the American continent since 1991 (1), but it still occurs in some parts of the world—most notably on the Asian subcontinent. In addition, every year in the United States eight to ten cases of acute poliomyelitis may occur in children after receiving the oral Sabin vaccine or, more exceptionally, in unvaccinated children who have been in close contact with a vaccinated person during the excretion phase of the live vaccine virus.

In 1987, there were an estimated 1.634 million survivors of poliomyelitis in United States, of which 0.641 million had residual paralysis (2). Patients with paralytic polio are at risk of developing post-poliomyelitis syndrome (PPS). The current prevalence of PPS is estimated at 100,000 to 300,000. Synonyms for PPS include *progressive neuromuscular disease*, *progressive post-polio muscular atrophy*, and *late sequelae of poliomyelitis*.

Post-polio symptoms were reported in the nineteenth century by Carriere and Lepine (3), and by Raymond and Charcot in 1875 (4). C.S. Potts described "progressive muscular atrophy" in 1903 (5). A few other publications before 1980 reported on the late effects of poliomyelitis as summarized (6) in the article by Alter et al. (1982).

Currently, in the United States, numerous survivors of poliomyelitis—contracted years ago—consult specialists in physical medicine and rehabilitation because of a constellation of symptoms, which are typical of PPS. PPS is a well recognized clinical entity, which has generated an abundance of scientific literature since the 1980s. (A recent Medline search yielded 220 references from 1981 to 2001; 34 of these publications included *pain* as a keyword.) The clinical manifestations of PPS are either very specific (e.g., increasing muscle weakness on previously affected or unaffected muscles, muscle fasciculations) or somewhat unspecified (e.g., fatigue, pain).

PAIN IN POLIOMYELITIS

During the acute stage of poliomyelitis, a great majority of patients present with excruciating pain, regardless of the extent of the muscle involvement. This pain occurs in practically all muscle groups, not only those that eventually become per-

Table 9.1. Prevalence of Joint and Muscle Pain in Subjects with Paralytic Poliomyelitis

	Joint Pain	Muscle Pain
Codd et al., 1985	74%	48%
Halstead et al., 1985	71%	71%
Chetwynd et al., 1993	60%	52%
Agre et al., 1989	77%	86%
Ramlow et al., 1992	42%	38%
Halstead et al., 1987	80%	79%

manently paralyzed, but in those that show complete or incomplete recovery of muscle function after the acute phase. Such pain probably is caused by severe myofasciitis secondary to the muscle breakdown that occurs as a result of anterior horn-cell neurolysis.

The pain reported by post-polio patients falls generally into two major pathophysiologic categories: myofascial, which can be elicited in various muscle groups; and arthritic, which is evident on active or passive mobilization of several joints (7). The initial Halstead et al. report on post-polio syndrome (1985) indicated that the prevalence of pain among polio survivors who responded to a questionnaire was 75.5 percent (8). Subsequent reports confirm that the types of pain experienced by post-polio patients are multiple, but mostly include diffuse muscle and joint pain (7,9–11). The prevalence of pain in patients with paralytic polio is reported from 42 percent to 80 percent (12–17) (see Table 9.1). In our experience with over 1,200 patients diagnosed with PPS at The Institute for Rehabilitation and Research (TIRR) Post-Polio Clinic, Houston, Texas, pain is reported by practically all patients.

Joint pain, muscle pain, muscle cramps, and back pain are common complaints in postpoliomyelitis patients (14–17). Knee and shoulder joint pains are common sites for pain in these patients. Pain in the joints is thought to be the result of degenerative arthritis, caused in part by age but more because of the long-standing asymmetrical load placed on specific joints because of the paresis or paralysis of scattered skeletal muscle groups. This paresis or paralysis is a permanent sequela of poliomyelitis. Frequently, pain is reported not only in the joints of the affected extremities but also in the low back area, the cervical column, and the sacroiliac joint. Much less common, because of the low prevalence of bulbar poliomyeltiis survivors, is pain in the temporo-mandibular joint which might be detected in those patients who in the acute phase of polio had involvement of the muscles of mastication innervated by the V cranial nerve.

JOINT PAIN

Knee Pain

Knee pain is more common in patients with genu recurvatum and in those who either have no orthoses or ill-fitting orthoses. Many of these patients have a lurching gait pattern, using a forward weight shift to move the center of gravity anterior to the axis of the knee joint to assist with knee extension. In patients with foot drop, a side-to-side gait pattern is implemented to circumduct the leg. For example, in the study by Perry and Flemming (1985), 54 of 193 patients had problems with genu recurvatum (18). Of these 54 patients, 40 (74 percent) reported knee pain. This problem was essentially resolved with the fitting of an appropriate orthosis. Waring et al. (1989) reported similar findings. A significant reduction in knee pain is achieved in subjects receiving an appropriate orthosis (19).

Shoulder Pain

Agre et al. (1989) reported that about 30 percent of 79 patients with a history of poliomyelitis had shoulder pain (16). Patients with significant lower limb weakness, who either ambulate with assistive devices or use a wheelchair and need frequent in and out transfers, are more prone to shoulder pain secondary to degenerative joint disease and rotator cuff problems.

Back Pain

Back pain is a common complaint in patients with a history of poliomyelitis. Back pain is usually multifactorial in nature. Two factors that may contribute to the problem of back pain include scoliosis and biomechanical stresses placed on the back during ambulation and transfer activities. A poorly fitted seating system may aggravate back pain. A careful assessment is needed to identify the causative factors. Pain originating from sacroiliac joints may be described as diffuse low back pain; it can be readily localized through palpation of specific painful spots located in the subcutaneous tissue adjacent to one or both sacroiliac joints. A recent analysis of patients evaluated at the TIRR Post-Polio Clinic yielded a prevalence of sacroiliac pain of 80 percent in women and 50 percent in men. In the majority of patients, sacroiliac pain is elicited bilaterally but with different intensity at each side.

Muscle Pain

Muscle pain may either be related to muscle overuse or to myofascial pain. Muscle overuse pain can be diagnosed from the patient's history. In these patients muscle pain is aggravated with activity and relieved by rest. It is not uncommon for patients to experience muscle overuse pain in the lower limb that was not involved with poliomyelitis. This is probably caused by excessive stresses secondary to poor gait patterns or owing to lack of the use of an appropriate orthosis.

The muscular pain of PPS can be objectively elicited by palpating the reported sore muscles and identifying discrete painful spots or specific trigger points associated with referred pain. The atlas of trigger points included in Travell and Simons is of great aid in the search for such trigger points (20,21). Symptomatic cervical arthritis may be accompanied by a considerable degree of tightness of the neck muscles, causing painful spots in the sternocleidomastoid, scalenus, and trapezius areas.

Muscle cramps in the legs are a common occurrence in post-polio patients, especially in those who have new weakness of the previously unaffected muscle groups or those who were affected in the initial stage but recovered to almost complete function in the early stages of convalescence. Cramps may be the consequence of excessive physical activity, but they may equally occur in patients who have adopted a more sedentary lifestyle as a result of PPS.

PATHOPHYSIOLOGY OF JOINT PAIN IN POLIOMYELITIS

The underlying factors that produce osteoarthritic pain are not well understood in either the post-polio or general population. Only a portion of patients with radiographic signs of osteoarthritis (OA) presents with pain (22–25), whereas others with typical symptoms of degenerative joint disease may not show radiologic changes. Postulated direct causes of OA-related pain include synovial inflammation, stretching of nerve endings in the joint capsule, ischemia in the subchondral bone, muscle spasm, stress or depression, and sleep deprivation (26). Other factors leading to pain are thought to be associated with fragmentation of cartilage (shedding of surface layers of cartilage), crystal or enzyme release from cartilage, inflammatory mediators, torn or degenerated menisci, and changes in synovial fluid (27). In approximately 50 percent of patients with radiographically assessed mild to moderate OA, synovitis may be a factor in reported pain, although it is not a predictor of such pain (27). In advanced OA, most patients with joint pain have synovitis (27).

Studies in post-polio patients show a decreased blood flow in the extremities most affected by paralysis, but this decreased blood flow is sometimes detected in apparently unaffected extremities (28). This is not surprising, because it is known that the poliovirus may cause lesions in the neurons of the lateral column of the spinal cord; these lesions send impulses to the sympathetic nerves (29,30). As a result, it has been hypothesized that there is an imbalance between the sympathetic vasoconstrictor and the parasympathetic vasodilator mechanisms, although some studies have not confirmed this hypothesis (31). The impact of autonomic imbalance on blood flow may aggravate the decreased blood flow in atrophied muscles and may explain a patient's intolerance to low environmental temperatures, with associated pain and discomfort (32).

Regardless of the type of pain, it is well demonstrated that post-polio patients have increased sensitivity to nociceptive stimuli (33), so it is not surprising that pain is reported so often by polio survivors.

MANAGEMENT OF PPS

It is important to review several general recommendations that are made to PPS patients because of their potential contribution to the alleviation of pain. Many patients do not receive optimum support for their unstable joints. It is desirable that a thorough assessment of gait abnormalities and a comprehensive muscle strength examination be carried out. Appropriate orthoses should be prescribed. A common example of orthotically correctable gait patterns are the forward weight shift and the side-to-side pattern (in patients with footdrop) described earlier (19). In patients who ambulate relatively long distances with crutches and complain of shoulder pain, the use of a wheelchair and of a motorized scooter can be quite helpful in controlling pain. Appropriate modification of transfer techniques may be helpful. In some cases a lift device is indicated to prevent excessive stresses on the shoulder.

Some poliomyelitis patients have difficulty sleeping because of muscle, back, or joint pain. These patients may benefit from the use of a tricyclic antidepressant (TCA).

Energy Conservation Program

Curtailment of energy demands is the primary management tool in PPS. Patients who perform physical exercises hoping to strengthen the weakening muscle groups aggravate their weakness and experience even more pain. On the other hand, patients who decrease their level of physical activity slow down the rate of progression of their weakness and eventually notice a reduction of the frequency and intensity of their pain episodes.

An energy conservation program includes decreasing excessive walking or self-propelling of manually operated wheelchairs. The use of a motorized tri-wheeler for ambulation at the workplace, home, supermarkets, shopping malls, and airports is strongly recommended. Tri-wheelers are preferable to electric wheelchairs because of their maneuverability, especially at home. Patients who either work or stay at home should have periods of rest, especially in the afternoon and preferably lying down on a sofa or reclining chair. Even if the patient does not fall asleep, the supine or semisupine position can be very relaxing and provide much needed preservation of energy.

Selective Exercise Program

The role of exercise is to prevent contractures and to increase muscle strength: Appropriate exercise programs must be prescribed to prevent the deleterious effects of inactivity and immobilization. Range-of-motion exercises are prescribed to prevent contractures. Precautions should be taken not to overstretch the weak muscles. Attempts should be made to maintain proper posture and correct or minimize gait abnormalities.

Some controversy exists as to the beneficial effects of muscle strengthening programs. Earlier studies yielded conflicting results, some reporting beneficial outcomes (34,35), and others indicating that exercise was detrimental (36–38). It appears that the key difference among these studies has to do with the intensity of the exercise program (32). Recent studies report increased muscle strength, improved general well-being, and improvements in the activities of daily living without adverse affects (39–42).

Although some of these studies report benefit from exercising unaffected muscle groups, the problem is in identifying such groups either in the trunk or in partially affected extremities and ensuring that the selective exercise of seemingly unaffected muscles be done without activating adjacent muscles that were definitely affected by poliomyelitis. The ubiquitous dissemination of the polio virus throughout the lower motor neurons of the spinal cord in the acute stage may have left residual damage even in muscle groups that were unaffected in the acute stage or had recovered their function during early convalescence.

Weight Reduction

Because of the relatively sedentary life style imposed by extensive residual paralysis, many post-polio patients have increased their body weight. Adoption of energy conservation techniques after the diagnosis of the PPS may aggravate weight problems. Low-fat consumption and adherence to the prudent heart diet advocated by the American Heart Association may be beneficial. Halstead (1998) recognizes the value of the proteins contained in lean mean because they may help increase the energy level in patients with PPS (32).

Correction of Posture and Gait Deviations

Ambulatory patients should adopt adequate postures that minimize the biomechanical consequences of paralysis and the stresses caused by the uneven forces of gravity on one or several joints. This posture correction may be achieved through lightweight orthotic devices (either AFO or KAFO) that stabilize the lower extremities during ambulation. Patients who have poor sitting posture should use simple devices such as a lumbar roll or an inflatable low back support while seated. The use of a custom-made corset may be too restrictive in some patients but quite helpful in others. Upper extremity involvement may require elbow or wrist supports such as those used by typists to prevent fatigue and typical carpal tunnel pain.

Analgesics

Complaints of excruciating pain by post-polio patients may require the prescription of analgesics and, in the case of degenerative joint disorders, antiinflammatory drugs. The pharmacologic management of pain in these patients is a major challenge and is discussed in greater detail later.

Special Precautions with Drugs or Substances Affecting the CNS

Post-polio patients may report enhanced responses to sedatives or other medications or substances (e.g., alcohol) that act on the central nervous system (CNS). This is probably caused by the overall decrease in neuronal population and lean body mass with a concomitant greater availability of drug levels per unit of neuronal population. At the TIRR Post-Polio Clinic we usually recommend that sedatives or psychotropic drugs be administered at doses of about 50 to 60 percent of those usually prescribed for persons of similar age or body weight. These considerations are particularly relevant to post-polio patients who need to undergo surgery under general anesthesia (43).

MANAGEMENT OF PAIN IN ACUTE POLIOMYELITIS

The pharmacologic management of the excruciating pain of acute-stage poliomyelitis is limited to the administration of analgesics, especially antiinflammatories. The administration of opioids should be used only in exceptional circumstances.

Because the pain may persist for several days or weeks throughout the convalescent phase, it is important to institute other appropriate measures to alleviate the pain as soon as the febrile period is over. The most common approach is bed rest and the application of hot packs to all muscle groups. These constitute the hallmark of the old Sister Kenny treatment. As soon as the patient is able to be moved out of bed, whirlpool therapy with hot water is indicated at least twice a day.

To prevent the eventual development of contractures during the earliest stages of the acute phase of the illness, all joints must be kept in a neutral position with appropriate lightweight splints. As soon as the patient can tolerate it, institution of gentle range-of-motion (ROM) exercises and manual muscle stimulation is very important to facilitate recovery of function and preserve joint mobility.

MANAGEMENT OF PAIN IN PATIENTS WITH PPS

Currently, the widely recommended pain treatment for PPS consists of a decrease in physical activity, application of traditional modalities of physical therapy, administration of muscle relaxants (at doses approximately 50 percent below those recommended for young adults), and analgesics or antiinflammatory agents (at normally prescribed doses). The effectiveness of the majority of pharmacologic agents, including the newly developed cyclooxygenase inhibitors, is generally poor in our post-polio population.

Although the cyclooxygenase inhibitors are apparently well tolerated (44), virtually all drug treatments for arthritic pain are known to have side effects that may result in other health problems for the patient. The risks for side effects with pure analgesics, such as acetaminophen, are fairly low (45,46), but the use of aspirin or NSAIDs has been associated with gastritis or ulceration of the gastrointestinal tract, often independent of dosage or frequency of treatment (47–49).

Adjuvant antidepressants, muscle relaxants, or anticonvulsant drugs may have fewer side effects than analgesics but their use in conjunction with other drugs to manage pain may increase the potential for adverse drug reactions, particularly in the elderly. As stated earlier, all drugs with neurotropic action (including sedatives and antihistaminics) should be prescribed at lower dosages than recommended for the general adult population. A prudent approach is to start with doses approximately 25 to 50 percent lower than those recommended for young adults who do not have PPS.

Although some suggest that the problem of opioid drugs has been exaggerated, fear of drug dependency and addiction often inhibits practitioners from prescribing these drugs to manage chronic pain, particularly in elderly patients (50). Tramadol, a centrally acting synthetic analgesic with opioid activity may be useful at doses of 50 mg (exceptionally, 100 mg) three or four times daily. Even though it is less addicting than traditional opioids, it has the potential to cause psychologic and physical dependency, and it is not recommended for patients who are already dependent on opioids.

Muscle cramps are difficult to control, but may be significantly decreased through the administration of clonazepam at a dose of 0.5 to 1 mg at bedtime; this dose can be repeated 4 hours later, if needed. Quinine water or tablets of quinine sulfate have not been effective in the TIRR post-polio patient population.

Other techniques for managing the pain of PPS include traditional physical modalities (e.g., heat, cold), direct neural pathway interventions (e.g., nerve blocks, trigger point injections, transcutaneous electrical nerve stimulation [TENS]), mobilization and manipulation, and surgical treatment (51). Unfortunately, many interventions (e.g., inactivity, surgical intervention, narcotic medications) that are effective in treating acute pain are not effective in managing chronic pain. Also, when used improperly, as in the case of too much current with TENS therapy, these treatments can exacerbate pain rather than relieve it (52).

Nontraditional therapeutic tools, such as relaxation and meditation, hypnotherapy, acupuncture, biofeedback (BF), and cognitive-behavioral therapy (CBT) are increasingly used in the general population. The benefits of acupuncture, when administered by a well-trained practitioner, have been documented in managing some types of pain (e.g., back pain), with results thought to be caused by the release of humoral substances, such as bradykinins, substance P, and leukotreines (53). Although there is some evidence of the efficacy of several behavioral and relaxation interventions in the treatment of chronic pain, available data are insufficient to conclude that one technique is usually more effective than another for a given condition (54). Cognitive-behavioral therapy (CBT) is cited by the National Institutes of Health (NIH) as being more effective than placebo and routine care in dealing with OA-related pain (54). Both relaxation and biofeedback (BF) are considered effective in treating many types of chronic pain, although OA and related conditions were not specifically mentioned in the NIH report. Hypnosis appears to be most beneficial in treating cancer-related pain and some other conditions, including irritable bowel syndrome, oral mucositis, temporomandibular disorders, and tension headaches (54).

There is no evidence in the scientific literature that any of these approaches are superior to others in the management of pain in PPS. Several of our post-polio patients have reported equivocal and disappointing results with acupuncture and other behavioral approaches such as meditation, yoga, or biofeedback. However, this does not negate the proven beneficial effect of these techniques as mood elevators and stress control helpers.

MAGNETIC FIELDS TO CONTROL PAIN

The limited success of pain control in post-polio patients prompted us to explore alternative methods of pain management. Static and fluctuating electromagnetic fields have been applied with apparent successful pain relief in a variety of orthopedic conditions, most commonly traumatic bone fractures or surgical osteotomies

(55–57). As early as 1938, Hansen reported on a study of the effectiveness of electromagnetic fields (which had "a carrying power of from 8.5 to 14 kg") applied for a period of 1 to 15 minutes duration (58). Twenty-three out of twenty-six patients with complaints of "sciatica," "lumbago," and "arthralgia" reported a rapid and significant relief of their pain. The study was not double masked, but the author reported no pain reduction in two patients to whom the electromagnetic device was applied without the electricity being turned on (58).

The therapeutic application of magnets appears to offer promise in alleviating chronic articular or musculoskeletal pain. However, there is a paucity of data from clinically sound studies of magnet therapy. One proponent, George J. Washnis (1998), has published a fairly comprehensive book on clinical applications of magnets, but he provides very few references of well-conducted clinical trials (59). As Washnis notes, federally supported research on the therapeutic benefits of magnets has recently started, but few reported results are available in the scientific literature. Lawrence, Rosch, and Plowden (1998) also cite several studies, but few were randomized double-masked clinical trials (60). Washnis also cites a number of studies that report good results from use of magnet therapy for fibromyalgia, postoperative healing, traumatic injury (gunshot wound to the hand), and soft tissue damage (ligament tear) to the hand (59). Unfortunately, many of these studies were supported by commercial vendors whose products were used in the studies, raising questions about the appropriateness of the methods used and the objectivity of the interpretation of results. With the exception of our own research, none of the research cited by Washnis or Lawrence and colleagues could be found in refereed journals.

Pulsating Electromagnetic Fields

Pulsating electromagnetic fields (PEMF) have been in use as therapeutic modalities for at least 40 years (61). A well recognized and standard use of PEMF is for enhancing the rate of healing in nonunion fractures (62,63). PEMF also have been shown to be effective in treating osteoarthritis of the knee and spine (64,65). The biological phenomenon that is responsible for alternations in wound healing rates and chronic disease processes upon exposure to PEMF is not well understood. However, both human and animal studies indicate that increased peripheral blood flow results from such exposure (66,67). One study found that human exposure to PEMF resulted in changes in fibroblast concentration, fibrin fibers, and collagen at wound sites, which was attributed to increased blood flow (68). Most recently, researchers reported good results in both an open and double-masked placebo-controlled study of PEMF in treating migraine headaches (61). The small sample sizes (eleven patients in the open study and twelve in the controlled study) preclude generalizing the results (61). A study by Richards et al. (1998) reports the benefits obtained in the management of multiple sclerosis patients (69). The therapeutic application of electromagnetic shocks have been well researched and were reported by several authors in a special issue of *CNS Spectrum*, edited by George (70).

An excellent overview of the biological effects of electromagnetic fields may be found in a two-volume publication edited by Carpenter and Ayrapetyan (71,72). The body of literature continues to grow and is built on further efforts to scientifically document the impact of magnetic fields on biological systems (73–79). The safety of application of these electromagnetic fields is attested by the World Health Organization, which reported "the available evidence indicates the absence of any adverse effects on human health due to exposure to static magnetic fields up to two Tesla" (1 T = 10,000 gauss) (80).

Static Magnetic Fields

Holcomb (1991) is a pioneer in the use of static magnetic fields to control pain. He acquired considerable experience with the use of static magnetic fields generated by a block of four magnets of alternating polar configurations (Magnabloc®). His early experience reporting significant relief of back pain in a double-masked trial dates from 1991 (75), but no new data on the use of the Magnabloc® have been reported in the peer-reviewed literature. In attempting to clarify the mechanism of pain relief, McLean (1995), a collaborator with Holcomb, demonstrated that under the influence of a magnetic field, it is possible to block the action potentials produced by stimulating cultured sensory neurons (78). A more recent paper by Weintraub (1999) reports on a single-masked, active-placebo crossover study of a static magnetic insole of multipolar configuration that was considered effective in controlling foot pain in diabetic neuropathy patients (77). Mann (1999) reports the benefits of static magnetic fields in a randomized study to evaluate wound healing and pain control in patients who underwent liposuction (81).

On the other hand, Borsa et al. (1998) report on a lack of protective pain relief with static magnets in a single-masked study of healthy athletes who were instructed to keep a device (active or placebo) in the nondominant arm for several hours after repetitive strenuous muscular activity of the same arm (82). It should be noted that the exercise in these subjects produced a very small increase in pain scores, and it is not surprising that static magnetic fields applied to those subjects may not have produced detectable changes. Certainly, the pain scores of all Borsa's subjects are not comparable to the pain intensity exhibited by untreated patients with chronic musculoskeletal problems. Hong et al. (1982) performed a double-masked evaluation of a loose, magnetized necklace on the cervical pain manifested by otherwise healthy young persons (83). Although he did not observe any effect, contrary to the benefit reported by Nakagawa (1976) with an identical device (84), Hong admits that the distance between the loose necklace and the painful neck structures may have interfered with the close delivery of a sufficiently intense magnetic field (85). In a more recent study, Callacott et al. (2000) reports that static magnetic fields applied to patients with chronic deep back pain failed to produce significant benefits, but the authors admitted that the distance between the magnet surface and the pain area may have interfered with the penetration of the magnetic field (86).

Static magnets for the management of pain are widely available in various con-figurations, sizes, and types of magnetized material (i.e., rigid, flexible, made with metal or with various alloys). The most important issue is the configuration of the magnet according to two prototypes: dipole or multipole.[1] Claims are made by manufacturers about the superiority of one prototype versus the other.

Investigators of Baylor College of Medicine's Departments of Family and Community Medicine, Physical Medicine and Rehabilitation, and Molecular Biology and Biophysics conducted a randomized double-masked clinical trial of magnet therapy in the treatment of arthritic or muscular pain in patients diag-nosed with PPS (87). The study was designed to test the efficacy of using static magnets of known surface strengths (measured in gauss) to treat localized pain. A total of fifty patients participated. Of these, twenty-nine received a magnetized device applied over a painful spot and twenty-one received a nonmagnetized device of identical appearance. A specific localized area of pain was selected for treatment. An active pain response was grossly elicited by finger palpation and then more precisely identified by firm application of a blunt object approximately 1 cm in diameter. In nonpainful areas, the blunt object elicits a sense of pressure, but no pain. Each subject was asked to grade the pain at the response point using a 10-point visual analog scale (VAS), with a subjective rating of 1 being least painful and a rating of 10 being most painful. If palpation elicited pain in more than one area, then the area with the most painful score (i.e., closest to 10 on the scale) was selected.

Each patient with an attached device was required to remain in the immediate clinic area in whatever position was most comfortable for him or her (e.g., sitting, standing, or walking) for 45 minutes. After this interval, and prior to removing the device from the skin, the patient was asked to describe any sensations felt while the device had been in place. After removal, each patient was asked to use the same 10-point scale in subjectively rating the amount of pain felt upon palpa-tion of the treated point by the research clinician. Although exact pressures applied with the blunt instrument before and after "treatment" were not mea-sured, efforts were made to use the same amount of pressure in eliciting responses to palpation. No systematic follow-up of patients was done after the treatment visits, but in many cases follow-up information was obtained during later clinic visits.

Following each treatment, the device code and the scores obtained before and after each individual treatment were entered into a database for subsequent analy-sis using standard descriptive analytic methods. The pre- and posttreatment pain score results are summarized in Table 9-2.

---

[1] We use the term "dipole or dipolar" to refer to magnets that have one pole of the magnetic field applied over the skin (most manufacturers label this pole as "N" because it attracts a North-seeking compass nee-dle), and the other pole not attached to the skin. Confusion exists because manufacturers usually refer to these magnets as "unipolar." The term "multipole or multipolar" refers to magnets which, at the surface applied over the skin, deliver magnetic fields from multiple alternating North or South poles in a concen-tric ring or grid pattern. Manufacturers usually refer to these magnets as "bipolar."

Table 9.2. Pre-Treatment and Post-Treatment Pain Scores

Measure	Active Magnetic Device	Inactive Device	Significance
Number of subjects	29	21	N/A
Pre-treatment pain score (mean ± SD)	9.6 ± 0.7	9.5 ± 0.8	NS
Post-treatment pain score (mean ± SD)	4.4 ± 3.1	8.4 ± 1.8	$p < .0001$
Change in score (mean ± SD)	5.2 ± 3.2	1.1 ± 1.6	$p < .0001$

Source: Vallbona C, Hazelwood CF, Jurida G. Response of pain to static magnetic fields in post-polio patients: A double-blind pilot study. *Arch Phys Med Rehab* 1997; 78:1200-1203.

Those patients who reported at least a three-point decrease in pain after treatment were categorized as "improved." The three-point decrease was selected because it represented the average placebo effect (plus 1.6 standard deviation). Patients who reported a decrease in pain of less than three points following treatment were categorized as "not improved." The results are summarized in Table 9-3.

The results of this pilot study suggest that static magnetic fields may indeed provide measurable relief for people who have localized muscoloskeletal pain. The study was done on a group of patients who are representative, with respect to demographic characteristics, of the larger patient population seen in the post-polio clinic. Additional studies should look more closely at magnet configuration, surface strength, and other magnetic field properties as factors in pain relief, and should include more systematic follow-up of patients to determine how long any beneficial effects may last following an active treatment session.

The magnetized devices were effective in controlling pain over the applied area within 45 minutes, but we did not systematically assess the duration of effect beyond the post-magnet treatment. Anecdotal evidence gathered from some of our experimental patients indicates that pain relief lasted for several hours, days, and even weeks (one patient, who had been randomized to receive the magnetized device, reported to be pain free two years after his participation).

After having demonstrated the effectiveness of static magnetic fields in PPS through a randomized double-blind clinical trial, we offer an open-label treat-

Table 9.3. Proportion of Subjects Reporting Pain Improvement by Magnetic Activity of the Treatment Device

Measure	Active Magnetic Device (n = 29)	Inactive Device (n = 21)
Pain improved	N = 22 (76%)	N = 4 (19%)
Pain not improved	N = 7 (24%)	N = 17 (81%)

$X2$ (1 df) = 20.6 $(p < .0001)$

Source: Vallbona C, Hazlewood CF, Jurida G. Response of pain to static magnetic fields in post-polio patients: A double-blind pilot study. *Arch Phys Med Rehab* 1997; 78:1200–1203.

ment with magnets to Post Polio Clinic of The Institute for Rehabilitation and Research patients who have elective painful spots. We use the same criteria as that of our randomized study and apply either multipolar or dipolar magnets over one or several painful spots if the intensity of perceived pain exceeds a score of 5 points on the McGill pain scale. If there is a significant effect, it is usually noticed within 30 minutes, at which time we remove the device. To those patients who exhibit a benefit we recommend that they acquire similar magnetic devices and use them on a PRN basis. We have not yet carried out a systematic post-treatment interview of all these patients, but there seems to be a general pattern of satisfaction at the time of a subsequent follow-up. The overwhelming majority of patients are very pleased with the PRN use of magnets for periods that vary from a few hours to a few days. Muscular pain seems to respond much more rapidly and for longer periods of time than articular pain. Patients who use magnets may use them as a complement to other medication, but in general their need for pharmacologic treatment is much less when using magnets. A few of our patients have reported that over a period of several months, the magnetic fields seem to lose effectiveness, but they have seldom stopped using the magnets altogether. Only a few patients have reported benefit from sitting or sleeping on magnetized pads, but we have not carried out any scientific evaluation of these devices in our patient population.

We do not have a clear explanation for the significant and rapid pain relief observed in the post-polio patients who participated in our study. It is possible that the effect could result from a local or direct change in pain receptors, but it is also possible that there was an indirect central response in pain perception at the cerebral cortical or subcortical areas, or a change in the release of enkephalins or opioids at the reticular system. If the magnetic fields have an impact on the sub-cortical level of the brain, it is possible that the application of a magnetic device in one painful area may benefit, to a greater or lesser extent, the pain elicited in other trigger points. Bruno has pointed out that poliomyelitis lesions exist in various areas of the brain of survivors, and he believes that these lesions may explain the hypersensitive response to painful stimuli that he has observed in post-polio patients (88). This should not be interpreted to mean that the relief of pain produced by magnetic fields that we observed in our study was specific for post-polio patients, because similar responses to magnetic fields have been reported in patients without identifiable lesions of the CNS (89).

CONCLUSIONS

Pain in the acute stage of poliomyelitis is excruciating and requires application of hot packs to relieve muscle spasm and facilitate recovery of muscle function. Analgesics should be used if needed.

The institution of an integral plan of management for PPS is important to facilitate control of pain. The plan that we use in the Post-Polio Clinic of TIRR includes adherence to an energy conservation program, a selective exercise program (only if possible), weight reduction, correction of posture and gait deviations, and the administration of analgesics (acetaminophen, nonsteroidal antiinflammatories [NSAIDs], cyclooxygenates inhibitors, and muscle relaxants).

Despite these general and well-accepted modalities of treatment, the management of pain in PPS patients represents a major challenge because it seems to be refractory to the majority of measures that are available.

REFERENCES

1. Bulletin of the World Health Organization. Emerging infectious diseases: Memorandum from a WHO meeting. Reprint No. 5540, 1994; 72 (6): 845–50.
2. Halstead LS, Wiechers DO, Rossi CR. Late effects of poliomyelitis: A national survey. In: Halstead LS, Wiechers DO (eds.), Late effects of poliomyelitis. Miami: Symposia Foundation; 1985; pp. 11–31.
3. Cornil Lepine. Sur un cas de paralysie generale spinale anterieure subaigue, suivi d' autopsie. *Gaz Med* (Paris) 1875; 4:127–29.
4. Raymond M (with contribution by Charcot, JM). Paralysie essentiele de l'Enfance: Atrophie musculaire consecutive. *Gaz Med* (Paris) 1875; 225.
5. Potts CS. A case of progressive muscular atrophy occurring in a man who had acute poliomyelitis nineteen years previously. *Univ Penn Med Bull* 1903; 16:31.
6. Alter M, Kurland LT and Molgaard CA. Late progressive muscular atrophy and antecedent poliomyelitis. In: Rowland LP (ed.), *Advances in Neurology: Human Motor Neuron Diseases*, Vol 36. New York: Raven Press, 1982; pp 301–309.
7. Smith LK, Mabry M. Part one: poliomyelitis and the post-polio syndrome. In: Umphred D (ed.), *Neurologic Rehabilitation*. 3rd ed. St. Louis: C.V. Mosby Co.; 1995. pp. 571–587.
8. Halstead LS, Wiechers DO, Rossi CR. Late effects of poliomyelitis: A national survey. In: Halstead LS, Wiechers DO (eds.), *Late Effects of Poliomyelitis*. Miami: Symposia Foundation; 1985; pp. 11–31.
9. Agre JC. The role of exercise in the patient with post-polio syndrome. *Ann NY Acad Sci* 1995; 753:321–24.
10. Jubelt B, Drucker J. Post-polio syndrome: An update. *Semin Neurol* 1993; 13:283–290.
11. Maynard FM. Managing the late effects of polio from a life-course perspective. *Ann NY Acad Sci* 1995; 753:354–60.
12. Ramlow J, Alexander M, Laporte R, et al. Epidemiology of the post-polio syndrome. *Am J Epidemiol* 1992; 136: 769–784.
13. Codd MB, Mulder DW, Kurland LT, et al. Poliomyelitis in Rochester, Minnesota 1935–1955: Epidemiology and long-term sequelae: a preliminary report. In: Halstead LS, Weichers DO (eds.), *Late Effects of Poliomyelitis*. Miami: Symposia Foundation 1985; pp.121–134.
14. Halstead LS, Rossi CD. Post-polio syndrome: Results of a survey of 539 survivors. *Orthopedics* 1985; 8:845–850.
15. Chetwynd J, Hogan D. Post-polio syndrome in New Zealand: A survey of 700 polio survivors. *N Z Med J* 1993; 106:406–408.
16. Agre JC, Rodriquez AA, Sperling KB. Symptoms and clinic impression of patients seen in post-polio clinic. *Arch Phys Med Rehabil* 1989; 70:367–370.
17. Halstead LS, Rossi CD. Post-polio syndrome: Clinical experience with 132 consecutive outpatients. *Birth Defects* 1987; 23: 13–26.
18. Perry J, Fleming C. Polio: Long-term problems. *Orthopedics* 1985; 8: 877–881.
19. Waring WP, Maynard F, Grady W, et al. Influence of appropriate lower extremity orthotic management on ambulation, pain, and fatigue in a post-polio population. *Arch Phys Med Rehabil* 1989; 70:371–375.

20. Travell JG, Simmons DG. *Myofascial Pain and Dysfunction: The Trigger Point Manual*, Vol 1, The Upper Extremities. Baltimore: Williams and Wilkins; 1983.

21. Travell JG, Simmons DG. *Myofascial Pain and Dysfunction: The Trigger Point Manual*, Vol 2, The Lower Extremities. Baltimore: Williams and Wilkins; 1992.

22. Carman WJ. Factors associated with pain and osteoarthritis in the Tecumseh community health study. *Sem Arthritis Rheum* 1989; 18 (suppl 2):10–13.

23. Felson DT, Naimark A, Anderson J, et al. The prevalence of knee osteoarthritis in the elderly: The Framingham osteoarthritis study. *Arthritis Rheum* 1987; 30:914–18.

24. Hochberg MC, Lawrence RC, Everett DF, et al. Epidemiologic associations of pain in osteoarthritis of the knee: Data from the National Health and Nutrition Examination Survey and the National Health and Nutrition examination–I epidemiologic Follow-up Survey. *Sem Arthritis Rheum* 1989; 18(suppl 2):4–9.

25. Lawrence JS, Bremmer JM, and Bier F. Osteoarthrosis: Prevalence in the population and relationship between symptoms and X-ray changes. *Ann Rheum Dis* 1966; 25:1–24.

26. Altman RD and Dean D. Introduction and overview: Pain in osteoarthritis. *Sem Arthritis Rheum* 18 (suppl 2):1–3.

27. Myers SL. Relationship of joint pain to synovial inflammation in osteoarthritis. In: Baker JR, Brandt KD (eds.), *Reappraisal of the Management of Patients with Osteoarthritis*. Springfield, N.J.: Scientific Therapeutics Information, Inc., 1993.

28. Bruno RL, et al. Motor and sensory functioning with changing ambient temperature in post-polio subjects: Autonomic and electrophysiological correlates. In: Halstead LS, Wiechers DO (eds.), *Late Effects of Poliomyelitis*. Miami: Symposia Foundation, 1985; p. 95–108.

29. Kottke FJ, Stillwell GK. Studies on increased vasomotor tone in the lower extremities following anterior poliomyelitis. *Arch Phys Med* 1951; 32:401–407.

30. Smith E, Rosenblatt P, Limauro A. The role of the sympathetic nervous system in acute poliomyelitis. *J Pediatr* 1949; 34: 1–11.

31. Abramson DI, Flachs K, Freiberg J et al. Blood flow in extremities affected by anterior poliomyelitis. *Arch Intern Med* 1943; 71:391–96.

32. Halstead LS, ed. *Managing Post-polio Syndrome*, Washington, D.C.: NHR Press, 1998.

33. Bruno RL, Frick NM, Cohen J. Polioencephalitis, stress, and the etiology of post-polio sequelae. *Orthopedics* 1991; 14:1269–1276.

34. DeLorme TL, Schwab RS, Watkins AL. The response of the quadriceps femoris to progressive resistance exercise in poliomyelitis patients. *J Bone Joint* [Am] 1948; 30:834–747.

35. Gurewitsch AD. Intensive graduated exercises in early infantile paralysis. *Arch Phys Med Rehabil* 1950; 31:213–218.

36. Hyman G. Poliomyelitis. *Lancet* 1953; 1:852.

37. Mitchell GP. Poliomyelitis and exercise. *Lancet* 1953; 2:90–91.

38. Knowlton GC, Bennett RL. Overwork weakness in partially denervated skeletal muscle. *Clin Orthop* 1958; 38:18–20.

39. Einarsson G, Grimby G. Strengthening exercise program in post-polio subjects. *Birth Defects* 1987; 23:275–283.

40. Einarsson G. Muscle conditioning in late poliomyelitis. *Arch Phys Med Rehabil* 1991; 72:11–14.

41. Fillyaw MJ, Badger GH, Goodwin GD, et al. The effects of long-term non-fatiguing resistance exercise in subjects with post-polio syndrome. *Orthopedics* 1991; 14:1253–1256.

42. Agre JC, Rodriquez AA, Franke TM, et al. Low-intensity alternate day exercise improves muscle performance without apparent adverse affect in post-polio patients. *Am J Phys Med Rehabil* 1996; 75:50–58.

43. Calmes SH. Anesthesia concerns for the polio survivor. *Polio Network News* 1997; 1–2.

44. Hawkey CJ. COX–2 inhibitors. *Lancet* 1999; 353: 307–314.

45. Diamond AW and Coniam SW. *The Management of Chronic Pain* (2nd edition). Oxford, U.K.: Oxford University Press, 1997.

46. Bradley JD, Brandt KD, Katz, BP, et al. Comparison of antiinflammatory dose of ibuprofen, and an analgesic dose of ibuprofen and acetaminophen in the treatment of patients with osteoarthritis of the knee. *N Engl J Med* 1991; 325:870–891

47. Max MB. Antidepressants and analgesics. In: Fields HL, Liekeskind JC (eds.), *Progress in Pain Research and Management*. Seattle: IASP Press, 1994.

48. Lanas A, Sekar MC, Hirschowitz BI. Objective evidence of aspirin use in both ulcer and nonulcer upper and lower gastrointestinal bleeding. *Gastroenterology* 1992; 103:862–869.

49. Allison MC, Howatson MG, Torrance CJ, Lee FD, et al. Gastrointestinal damage associated with the use of nonsteroidal antiinflammatory drugs. *N Engl J Med* 1992; 327:749–54.

50. American Geriatrics Society. Chronic Non-Cancer Related Pain in Elderly People: A Clinical Practice Guideline (January 19, 1997 Draft). New York: The American Geriatrics Society Panel on Chronic Pain, 1997.

51. Grabois M, VanDeventer J. Chronic pain. In: Garrison SJ (ed.), *Handbook of Physical Medicine and Rehabilitation Basics* (1st ed). Philadelphia: J.B. Lippincott Company, 1995.

52. Irving GA, Wallace MS. *Pain Management for the Practicing Physician*. New York: Churchill Livingstone, 1997.

53. Long SP, Kephart W. Myofascial pain syndrome. In: Ashburn MA, Rice LJ (eds.), *The Management of Pain*. New York: Churchill Livingstone, 1998.

54. National Institutes of Health. Integration of behavioral and relaxation approaches into the treatment of chronic pain and insomnia. Technology assessment conference statement 1995; Oct. 16–18; 1–34.

55. Becker RO. The perils of electromedicine, the promise of electromedicine. In: *Cross Currents*. New York: Putnam, 1990.

56. Becker RO, Selden G. *The Body Electric: Electromagnetism and the Foundation of Life*. New York: William Morrow and Company, 1985.

57. Miner WK, Markoll R. A double blind trial of clinical effects of pulsed electromagnetic fields in osteoarthritis. *J Rheumatol* 1993; 20:456–460.

58. Hansen KM. Some observation with a view to possible influence of magnetism upon the human organism. *Acta Med Scanda* 1938; 97:339–364.

59. Washnis GH. *Discovery of Magnetic Health: A Health Care Alternative*. Wheaton, Md.: Health Research Publishers, 1998.

60. Lawrence R, Rosch PJ, Plowden J. *Magnet Therapy: The Pain Cure Alternative*. Rocklin, Calif.: Prima Publishing, 1998.

61. Sherman RA, Robson L, Marden LA. Initial exploration of pulsating electromagnetic fields in treatment of migraine. *Headache* 1998; 38:208–213.

62. O'Connor M, Bentall R, Monahan J. *Emerging Electromagnetic Medicine*. New York: Springer-Verlag, 1990.

63. Bassett A. Therapeutic uses of electric and magnetic fields in orthopedics. In: Carpenter DO, Ayrapetyan S (eds.), *Biological Effects of Electric and Magnetic Fields*, Vol 2, Beneficial and Harmful Effects. San Diego: Academic Press, 1994.

64. Trock DH, Bollet AJ, Markoll R. The effect of pulsed electromagnetic fields in the treatment of osteoarthritis of the knee and cervical spine. Report of randomized, double blind, placebo controlled trials. *J Rheumatol* 1994; 21:1903–1911.

65. Zizic TM, et al. The treatment of osteoarthritis of the knee with pulsed electrical stimulation. *J Rheumatol* 1995; 22:1757–1761.

66. Erdman W. Peripheral blood flow measurements during application of pulsed high frequency currents. *Am J Orthop* 1960; 2:196–197.

67. Fenn JE. Effect of pulsed electromagnetic energy (Diapulse) on experimental hematomas. *Can Med Assoc J* 1969; 100:251–254.

68. Ross J. Biological effects of PEMFs using Dipulse. In: O'Connor M, Bentall R, Monahan J (eds.), *Emerging Electromagnetic Medicine*. New York: Springer-Verlag, 1990.
69. Richards TL, Lappin MS, Lawne FW, et al. Bioelectromagnetic application for multiple sclerosis. *Phys Med Rehabil Clinics N Am* 1998; 9:659–674.
70. George MS. TMS: An issue worthy of a single focus. *CNS Spectrum* 1997; 2:17–18.
71. Carpenter DO, Ayrapetyan S. *Biological Effects of Electric and Magnetic Fields: Beneficial and Harmful Effects*. San Diego:Academic Press, 1994.
72. Carpenter DO, Ayrapetyan S. *Biological Effects of Electric and Magnetic Fields*, Sources and Mechanisms. San Diego: Academic Press, 1994.
73. Tenforde TS, ed. Magnetic field effect on biological systems. Based on the proceedings of the Biomagnetic Effects Workshop held at Lawrence Berkeley Laboratory, University of California, 1978; April 6–7.
74. Adey WR, Chopart A. Cell surface ionic phenomena in transmembrane signaling to intracellular enzyme systems. In: Blank M, Findl E (eds.), *Mechanistic Approaches to Interactions of Electromagnetic Fields with Living Systems*. New York: Plenum Press, 1987; 365–387.
75. Holcomb RR, Parker RA, Harrison MS. Biomagnetics in the treatment of human pain, past, present, future. *Environmental Medicine* 1991; 8:24–30.
76. McLean MJ, Holcomb RR, Wamil AW, Pickett JD. Effects of steady magnetic fields on action potentials and sodium currents of sensory neurons in vitro. *Environmental Medicine* 1991; 8:36–45.
77. Weintraub MI. Alternative medicine magnetic biostimulation in painful diabetic peripheral neuropathy: A novel intervention, a randomized, double-placebo crossover study. *Am J Pain Management* 1999; 9:8–17.
78. McLean MJ, Holcomb RR, Wamil WA, et al. Blockage of sensory neuron action potentials by a static magnetic field in the 10 mt range. *Bioelectromagnetics*, 1995; 16:147–151.
79. Adey WR. Tissue interactions with non-ionizing electromagnetic fields. *Physiol Rev* 1981; 51:435–514.
80. United Nations Environment Programme M. The International Labor Organization. World Health Organization, 1987
81. Man D, Man B, Plosker H. The influence of permanent magnetic field therapy on wound healing in suction lipectomy patients: A double-blind study. *Plast Reconstr Surg* 1999; 104 (7): 2261–2266; discussion 2267–2268.
82. Borsa PA, Liggett C. Flexible magnets are not effective in decreasing pain perception and recovery time after muscle microinjury. *J Athletic Training* 1998; 33:150–155.
83. Hong CZ, Lin JC, Bender LF, Schaeffer JN, Meltzer RJ, Causin P. Magnetic necklace: Its therapeutic effectuveness on neck and shoulder pain. *Arch Phys Med Rehabil* 1982; 63:462–466.
84. Nagakawa K. Magnetic field deficiency syndrome and magnetic treatment. *Japan Med J* 1976; 27–45.
85. Hong CZ. Static field influence on human nerve function. *Arch Phys Med Rehabil* 1987; 68: 162–164.
86. Collacott EA, Zimmerman JT, White DW, Rindone JP. Bipolar permanent magnets for the treatment of chronic low back pain. A pilot study. *JAMA* 2000; 283:1322–1325.
87. Vallbona C, Hazelwood CF, Jurida G. Response of pain to static magnetic fields in postpolio patients. A double-blind pilot study. *Arch Phys Med Rehab* 1997; 78: 1200–1203.
88. Bruno RL, Frick NM, Cohen J. Polioencephalitis, stress and the etiology of polio sequelae. *Orthopedics* 1991; 14:1269–1276.
89. Hansen KM. Some observations with a view to possible influence of magnetism upon the human organism. *Acta Med Scanda* 1938; 97:339–364.

10 | Pain Management Post Amputation

Alberto Esquenazi, M.D.

The International Association for the Study of Pain defines pain as an unpleasant sensory and emotional experience associated with actual or potential tissue damage or described in terms of such damage. Pain in the amputee patient may not always fall within this description. The pain in the patient with an amputation can be divided into four possible categories. These are postsurgical pain, residual limb pain, prosthetic pain (caused most frequently by standing and ambulating with the prosthesis), and phantom pain (pain perceived as coming from the amputated body part). Each one of these pain categories is described as separate entities, but overlap of the different types of pain may occur.

Pain may originate in regions of the body other than the site of amputation and be referred to the amputated limb. Such pain may be cardiogenic, neuropathic, or radiculopathic in origin. Systemic diseases such as diabetes, ischemia, or arthritis can also be the cause of pain and should be ruled out prior to attempting treatment of pain. With a wide variety of pain sources and treatment options available, treatment of pain in the amputee must begin with accurate diagnosis. Once the nature of the patient's pain has been clarified, appropriate interventions can proceed to allow the patient to function comfortably.

ACUTE POSTSURGICAL PAIN

Postsurgical pain is the sharp, localized pain experienced by the patient at the surgical site in the postoperative period (generally 1 to 3 weeks following the amputation). Movement of the limb, swelling, or pressure in the area of the wound exacerbates the pain. The pain is to be expected as part of the surgical trauma to bone, nerve, and soft tissues and is usually self-limited, gradually resolving as the edema decreases and the amputation wound heals.

Management of Acute Postsurgical Pain

Pain in this period can be controlled with medications and through the use of physical modalities. Recently, acute postsurgical analgesia is frequently provided

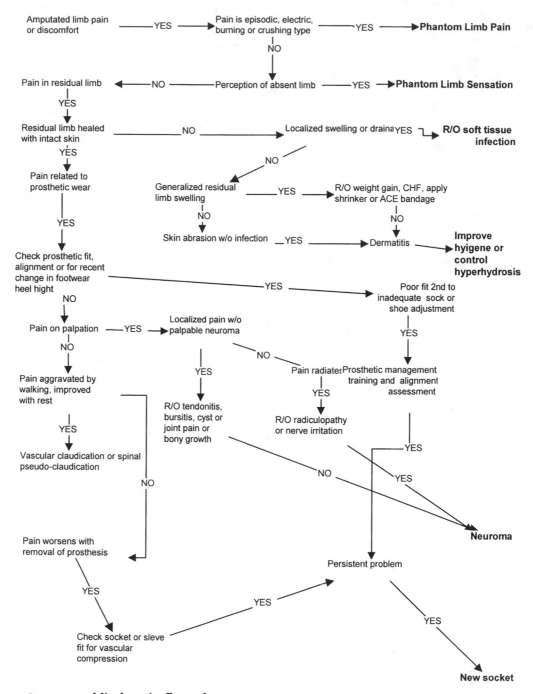

Amputated limb pain flow chart

through the use of epidural medication. Often this approach provides excellent sensory analgesia for several days following the surgery. The advent of patient controlled analgesia (PCA) also provides a better analgesic approach. There is some evidence to indicate and refute the concept that adequate perioperative pain control decreases the incidence of phantom pain (1,2,3).

Switching to oral analgesic medication typically occurs on postoperative day three or four in conditions of primary wound healing. Oral medications commonly used to relieve postoperative pain include narcotics, acetaminophen, and nonsteroidal antiinflammatory drugs (NSAIDs), such as ibuprofen and indomethacin. For the first week following the amputation, relatively high doses of medications may be given (e.g., 3,250 mg per day of acetaminophen, 50 mg per day of oxycodone, or 600 mg per day of propoxyphene). Thereafter, lower doses are needed. This medication usually can be discontinued within four weeks following the amputation surgery, when soft tissue healing has occurred.

Acute postsurgical pain is better controlled with the application of a postoperative rigid dressing (4). This dressing promotes the control of edema and pain and encourages residual limb maturation; it may reduce the time from amputation to prosthetic fitting. The immediate postoperative rigid dressing (IPORD) as proposed by Burgess (5) reduces the likelihood of developing flexion contractures, but should only be used for clean, uninfected wounds. Other popular dressing methods include the removable rigid dressing proposed by Wu (6) that, while permitting frequent wound inspection and care, provides adjustable compression for swelling control. These dressings provide protection from trauma to the residual limb during rehabilitation or in the case of a fall, which is possible after amputation, when the patient attempts to stand and walk, unaware that the limb is not there any more. Other options for edema control include the use of soft elastic bandages and subsequent pneumatic compression, which frequently reduces pain. The Unna® boot dressing is also very effective in providing edema control and promoting wound healing (7). All wound dressings must be applied carefully (tighter distally and looser proximally) to avoid a tourniquet effect and to promote edema reduction, which contributes to wound healing and reduces pain.

Physical interventions can also provide significant pain control. The residual limb should be elevated above heart level for one to two hours several times each day to reduce local edema. Although elevation should be used to control edema and limit pain, full range of motion of the limbs must be maintained and contractures (hip, knee, and elbow flexion in particular) prevented. Ice may help control edema in the nonischemic limb. Galvanic and electrical stimulation can also be helpful interventions in reducing pain and postacute inflammation. The painful postsurgical limb must be evaluated for other causes of pain, particularly infection and ischemia. The presence of localized heat, swelling, erythema, or drainage may indicate local pathology such as wound hematoma, infection, or dehiscence. Changes in skin color or skin temperature reduction accompanied by pain may indicate an acute ischemic episode.

Postoperative pain can be vastly decreased by beginning pain treatment before surgery. This so called *pre-emptive analgesia* is expected to stop pain from starting by blocking the nervous system's usual response to pain. It is believed that the trauma of surgery may cause the nerves in the spinal cord to "wind-up," which can heighten sensitivity and result in enduring pain after surgery.

PHANTOM LIMB, PHANTOM PAIN

Gaston Leroux in his 1911 masterpiece *The Phantom of the Opera* wrote:

> "The Opera ghost really existed. He was not, as long believed, a creature of the imagination of the artists, the superstition of the managers, or a product of the absurd and impressionable brains of the young ladies of the ballet... Yes, he existed in flesh and blood, although he assumed the appearance of a real phantom; that is to say a spectral shade." (8)

Pain in the healed residual limb is less common and often more difficult to diagnose and treat. Pain is part of a protective warning system. Under certain conditions, this essential warning system becomes overactive and the signal to the brain may be amplified, sustained, and disproportionally enhanced by bizarre overtones to a point that may be disabling. In such cases, the protective mechanism of pain may become a life-distorting force that interferes with functional activities (9). Fortunately, such severe pain is infrequently seen in the amputee.

Some amputees feel pain in the absent limb portion (phantom limb pain). Phantom limb pain begins in the acute postamputation period, generally subsides, and is seldom a long-term problem. However, in a few patients with a limb amputation, this pain becomes problematic, thus resulting in a chronic pain syndrome that may be refractory to treatment (1). Only a small group reports varying degrees of pain, from unpleasant tingling to excruciating stabbing or squeezing, or electric or cold sensations. These sensations are more commonly associated with mangled limb injuries or episodes of sustained severe pain prior to limb amputation, as seen in chronic ischemia or delayed amputation following war injuries and attempts at limb salvage after severe trauma.

In our experience and that of other centers a large proportion of patients report the presence of phantom limb sensation or awareness. Phantom limb sensation is the feeling that all or a part of the amputated limb is still present. This sensation is felt by as many as 97 percent of acquired amputees. However, phantom limb sensation usually disappears or decreases sufficiently over time so as not to interfere with prosthetic fitting and day-to-day activities (8). Phantom limb sensation is not often bothersome and when appropriate may be useful during the phase of myoelectric prosthetic training. A telescoping phenomenon, or the sensation that the phantom foot or hand has moved proximal toward the stump, commonly occurs over time.

A smaller percentage of patients experience long-term pain, whereas others have recurrent pain later in life. When pain persists for more than 6 months, the prognosis for spontaneous improvement is poor and it can be extremely difficult to treat successfully (1,8,9). Parkes reports that phantom limb pain experienced 13 months after amputation correlated with seven factors (10):

- rigid or compulsively self-reliant personalities;
- two or more people living at home;
- illness of over one year's duration before amputation;
- persistent illness with threat to life or a limb after surgery;
- pain in the stump or phantom pain after the first month following amputation surgery;
- persistent residual limb complications; and
- unemployment or retirement at 13 months post amputation.

This pain is often described as a cramping or contorted posture of the missing limb. If a painful wound was present prior to the amputation, the phantom pain may mimic the pain of that lesion. Such pain may alter lifestyle and become the focus of a patient's existence. Perceived pain intensity is closely related to anxiety level, depression, and other personal factors (1,9,11). Prosthetic fitting problems also can intensify phantom pain.

The traditional explanation for phantom limb and phantom pain is that the remaining nerves in the amputated limb continue to generate impulses that flow through the spinal cord and the thalamus to the somatosensory areas of the cerebral cortex. Another theory suggests that phantom pain is caused by changes in the flow of signals through the somatosensory circuit in the brain, while yet another suggests that phantom pain arises from excessive, spontaneous firing of spinal cord neurons that have lost their normal sensory input from the body (11). Phantom pain may result from reactivation of a nociceptive engram in certain cerebral structures that existed before amputation. Carlen (13), in his study of young soldiers who underwent war-related amputations, reported a 67 percent incidence of phantom limb pain in the first few months. Jensen (14) studied a group of patients with nontraumatic amputations who had pain before surgery. He found a high, but decreasing over time, incidence of phantom limb pain that affected as many as 72 percent of patients in the first weeks post amputation and 59 percent of patients after 2 years. Of interest are the findings made by Back (15), who evaluated patients with pre-amputation pain to whom he administered a three-day preoperative lumbar epidural block. Patients reported less phantom pain than a control group with similar characteristics and pain levels who were not provided with epidural blocks. Clearly, the etiology of the phantom limb phenomenon is more complex than present theories would suggest and treatment can be complex. An important issue to discuss with the patient is the relationship between phantom pain and tension, anxiety, stress, and depression (16, 17).

Phantom limb pain, phantom limb sensation, and residual limb pain must be differentiated for the amputee to effectively determine the best treatment modalities.

Management of Phantom Limb Pain

Sherman (1980) described more than sixty different treatments for phantom limb pain (12). Although a particular treatment may be effective for one patient, it may not benefit another because of the multiple differences in the mechanisms of pain production. Phantom limb pain is difficult to treat, causing frustration for patients and clinicians alike. Conservative treatment for phantom pain should begin with tactile stimulation and biofeedback. Other modalities commonly used to diminish this pain are ultrasound, percussion, vibration, massage, acupuncture, biofeedback, hypnosis, relaxation techniques, and transcutaneous electrical nerve stimulation (TENS). Winnem (18,19) and others have reported the use of TENS applied to the residual limb in an area proximal to the pain or in the nerve distribution of the perceived pain source. The use of TENS on the contralateral limb to reduce pain in the phantom limb has been reported by Caravelli (20) (see Figure 10.1).

A patient may often achieve some pain control by using brain imagery or biofeedback to activate the muscles and nerves of the residual limb, thus creating the feeling of movement in the phantom limb, for example, wiggling the toes or bending the ankle of a lower-limb amputation.

Pharmacologic agents are used frequently to treat phantom pain, with inconsistent results (8,12). Management of phantom limb pain may include the use of narcotic medications only during the immediate postoperative period. The use of narcotics, synthetic narcotics, or other potentially addictive substances may be used in the case of new episodes of acute severe pain but are contraindicated beyond the immediate postoperative phase or as a long-term treatment intervention.

Medications that are used to diminish and control phantom pain include analgesics, neuroleptics, anticonvulsants, tricyclic antidepressants, beta-blockers, and sodium channel blockers. These medications should be used in a prescribed order. For problematic pain each drug should be tried at the maximally tolerated dose before changing to another medication. In some instances, combinations of medications may need to be administered for optimal pain control.

Regional neurologic blockade has had some success, especially if sympathetic nervous overflow appears to be a significant component of the pain. Injection near

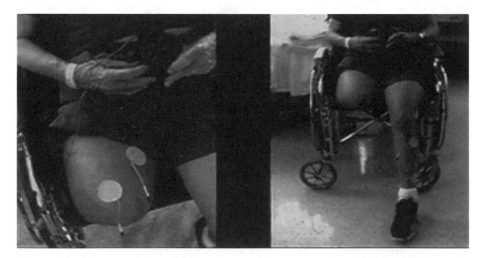

Figure 10.1. (a) TENS for phantom pain applied to the residual limb; (b) TENS for phantom pain applied to the opposite limb.

or into a neuroma can also be useful. More invasive procedures for pain control include sympathectomy, neuroma excision, sensory branch neurectomy, dorsal root rhizotomy, electrical spinal cord stimulation, and sensory thalamic stimulation. Great variability in the success of these interventions has been reported. Surgical techniques have been attempted in refractory cases, but one should note that in general nonsurgical interventions are far more successful than surgical ones in the management of phantom limb pain (12).

PAINFUL RESIDUAL LIMB

Residual limb pain is defined as pain in the residual limb that does not descend into the missing limb portion (10,11). This pain can frequently be traced to extrinsic or intrinsic causes such as reactive hyperemia, dermatitis, ischemia, inappropriate surgical beveling of the bones, ectopic bone, reflex sympathetic dystrophy, and other mechanical causes.

The pain may also be related to neuroma formation or be the result of physical changes in the residual limb. A common source of pain is related to the pressures caused by an ill-fitted prosthesis.

Examination of the painful limb includes inspection (looking specifically for deformity, discoloration, masses, fluctuance, heat, joint instability, tissue mobility, trauma, and swelling) and evaluation of strength and range of motion. A thorough history is essential, including the character, intensity, location, and duration of the pain as well as identification of the factors that ameliorate or worsen the pain.

Causes of bone and joint pain include arthritis, fracture, osteomyelitis, heterotopic ossification, bony spicules, and, in children under the age of 12, bony overgrowth. Soft tissue causes may include ischemia, abscess, cellulitis, adherent tissue, scar formation, peripheral neuropathy, muscle strain, nerve entrapment, and neuroma.

Management of Painful Residual Limb

Treatment of residual limb pain focuses on the underlying problem. Bony pathology and abscesses require surgical intervention. Ischemic pain generally requires surgical revascularization or the use of medications to improve circulation. Localized injection of analgesic or corticosteroids can be extremely effective for pain caused by arthritis, scar formation, nerve entrapment, adherent tissue, or neuroma. Oral analgesic medications are also used to treat residual limb pain. Topical analgesics, such as capsaicin, are helpful in certain cases of neuropathic pain; other medications may also be effective and appropriate. Topical agents may cause burning and skin rashes.

Physical modalities are generally helpful in residual limb pain as well. Mechanical stimulation, including massage, tapping, and rubbing, reduces local limb sensitivity. Ultrasound, warm compresses, ice packs, electrical stimulation, and TENS are all useful in managing residual pain (11,20). Less frequently, neurolytic procedures (using agents such as phenol, alcohol, or hypertonic saline solution) or nerve blocks (peripheral stellate ganglion block, lumbar sympathetic block) are needed for pain control.

Tricyclic antidepressants such as amitriptyline and nortriptyline, when used at low doses (25 to 75 mg per day), often relieve the dull, aching neuropathic pain symptoms seen frequently as a complication of diabetes (21). For sharp, lancinating neuropathic pain gabapentin (100 mg three times per day and gradually increasing as tolerated) or other anticonvulsant agents such as carbamazepine (200 to 600 mg per day) can be useful as well. Baclofen and mexiletine, an antidysrhythmic drug (150 mg twice daily) have also been used for good pain control. Occasionally, neuroleptics (e.g., thioridazine), benzodiazepines (e.g., clonazepam), or selective serotonin reuptake inhibitors (e.g., sertraline) are used. Side effects from this drug must be monitored and include dizziness, drowsiness, sedation, bradycardia, and hypotension.

PROSTHETIC PAIN

Prosthetic pain is generally more readily diagnosed and easier to treat. The pain is usually mechanical in origin, and is frequently caused by pressure or friction. The patient can point out the location of the pain, and the experienced clinician can identify the corresponding area in the prosthetic socket.

For transtibial amputees, the tibial tubercle, distal anterior tibia, fibular head, and hamstring tendons are common sites of mechanical pain (22). Occasionally the tibial crest or lower pole of the patella may be a source of pain if the socket concentrates pressure in this nonweight bearing anatomic structure. A socket that produces increased pressure or one with inadequate suspension that causes pistoning, bell clapping, and excessive shear over a bony prominence, may result in the development, enlargement, or inflammation of a bursa. The pain will be present primarily in relation to prosthetic wear. A tender, warm, and fluctuating mass is palpable over the bony prominence.

Management in Transtibial Amputees

Prosthetic limb alignment adjustments, such as increasing socket flexion to better expose the weight-bearing surface area of the limb, is sometimes indicated (see Figure 10.2). The use of silicon liners for suspension or cushioning of bony prominences and the use of flexible sockets with fenestrated rigid frames are useful interventions that usually alleviate the pain complaint (see Figure 10.3).

Management in Transfemoral Amputees

For the transfemoral amputee, the common sites for prosthetic-related pressure pain are the adductor tendons and the distal anterior and distal lateral areas of the femur. Occasionally the pubic ramus and the ischium may be sources of pain if the socket concentrates excessive weight bearing over these structures.

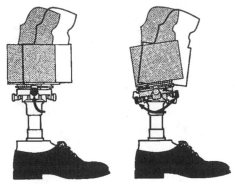

Figure 10.2. Prosthetic alignment modifications.

Alignment and socket modifications are appropriate interventions. When skin breakdown occurs, the amputee should avoid wearing the prosthesis until the wound heals and the cause of the ulceration is corrected. By using crutches or a walker, the lower limb amputee can remain ambulatory in most instances without the use of the prosthesis. If the amputee continues to use an ill-fitting prosthesis, worsening skin ulceration and permanent tissue loss can occur.

Pain can also result from traction on the skin caused by the prosthesis. In this situation, the socket fit must be modified to reduce tension on the skin. This can be accomplished by using a thin sock or sheath made of nylon, silicone, or similar material, which will support the skin and reduce shear and traction. A cotton or nylon pull sock can be used to draw the soft tissue deeply into the socket and suction can be implemented to contain the tissue, thereby reducing shear and traction. A loose fitting socket allows the residual limb to slide to the bottom of the socket, causing distal pressure and pain; complaints of proximal pain may also be present. Additional stump socks, proximal pads, or the use of air-adjustable sockets can provide proximal support to alleviate this problem. If the socket is too tight, generalized residual limb pain and reactive hyperemia results; the patient must use fewer socks or a larger socket to address this problem.

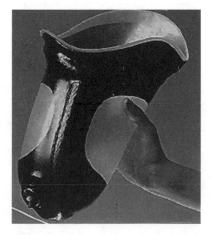

Figure 10.3. Flexible socket construction.

In some cases claudication of vascular origin will produce pain after short-distance ambulation. This pain is not related to socket fit, but could be greatly improved with the provision of a bypass prosthesis that improves the mechanics of walking and reduces the effort of the residual calf muscles. Such a device redistributes weight bearing and reduces the stresses to proximal surfaces through the use of a thigh corset or ischial weight-bearing brim (23). Silicon sleeves may apply pressure that exceeds the capillary pressures of the limb, thus producing pain in patients with relative ischemia. Using a slightly larger silicon sleeve may address this problem.

For the upper-limb amputee, pressure can occur over the distal end and the elbow condyles if the prosthesis does not fit optimally. In the upper-limb amputee, contralateral wrist pain may be caused by an overuse injury, as seen in carpal tunnel syndrome. At times the symptoms may be related to compression of the neurovascular bundle in the axilla when a figure-eight or figure-nine harness is used to suspend or activate a body-powered prosthesis. A carpal tunnel release is ineffective in this situation, but changing the design of the harness to a shoulder saddle or a chest strap may relieve the symptoms.

Skin problems such as dermatitis, cellulitis, or other skin inflammatory problems frequently cause residual limb pain. Treatment of these conditions can be accomplished with improved hygiene, application of topical antiinflammatory agents, or systemic antibiotics if necessary (23). Prosthetic socket modifications to redistribute pressure application are usually effective. Hyperhydrosis is another condition that may result in excessive skin traction, friction, and skin breakdown (24). Frequent sock changes where applicable and the use of high-concentration topical antiperspirants such as Drysol®, if tolerated, play an effective role in the treatment of this condition. For selected patients the use of Botox® injections to paralyze the sweat glands has been effective in controlling hyperhydrosis (25). This treatment approach is preferred when the patient presents this condition as a seasonal problem or in the initial adjustment period when using a silicon liner. Silicon liners and sleeves can, in the first several weeks of use, produce increased perspiration and in some cases result in contact dermatitis. A nylon sock may be used as an interface between the skin and the liner to reduce skin irritation but suspension may be compromised, thus requiring a secondary suspension system.

If the pain seems related to a neuroma, prosthetic modifications to the socket and the alignment or the use of silicon socks or pads may be attempted first. If ineffective, local infiltration with anesthetic with or without steroids may improve the pain. A neuroma is considered a normal development of a nerve ending after transection. However, when a neuroma is entrapped in scar tissue or is set in an exposed location where pressure can be exerted over it, pain may develop. Magnetic resonance imaging (MRI) of the limb will likely reveal the presence of a heterogeneous structure of intermediate intensity surrounded by a rim of low signal intensity on T1 images. Singson and collaborators (26) postulate that this represents collagen matrix and cellular nerve fascicles. MRI may help differentiate between a neuroma and scar tissue, abscess, osteomyelitis, and hematoma as

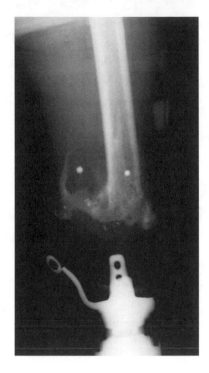

Figure 10.4. Extra bone formation in a transfemoral amputation.

causes of residual limb pain. Neuroma resection with relocation of the terminal end of the nerve deeper into the residual limb may improve the problem (5,12).

Sometimes pain may be caused by the presence of heterotopic ossification, myositis ossificans, or, in children under the age of twelve, bony overgrowth. To assess this, radiographic evaluation should be considered. AP and lateral views of the limb are necessary to better localize the source of the problem. Weight-bearing views of the affected portion of the residual limb in the prosthesis should also be obtained (see Figure 10.4). If available, xeroradiography may provide a more detailed view of the soft tissue contours and the bony structures in relation to the socket (27).

Bony deformities frequently can be accommodated within the socket, but at times surgery must be performed. Lack of distal end contact or distal end "choking" can result in the development of painful edema and if chronic, verrucose hyperplasia formation with exudate (24). This is frequently seen when patients have gained weight or are using more socks than necessary, thus causing loss of distal end contact. Socket replacement or modification to assure total limb contact is the most effective treatment intervention in these cases.

Referred pain from radiculopathy or joint degeneration should also be considered. Electromyography and X-rays help in making the diagnosis of these conditions, and appropriate treatment interventions can be implemented.

Reflex sympathetic dystrophy (RSD) is sometimes present. This syndrome is characterized by burning pain, abnormal vasomotor response, and dystrophy.

RSD does not develop immediately postsurgery, but the symptoms appear gradually until they dominate the clinical picture, which progresses from vascular changes to profound trophic changes and severe joint contractures. In the early stages the residual limb may be swollen and warm with severe hyperesthesias and intolerance to cold. The condition progresses with brawny edema, trophic changes, and contracture. Sympathetic block can be used to temporarily treat this condition and if ineffective, surgical sympathectomy is indicated.

CONCLUSIONS

Pain in the amputated limb that interferes with the functional use of a prosthesis may be caused by several factors, including phantom pain, causalgia, neuroma, and referred pain from other sources in the body. Prosthetic fitting problems and skin, soft tissue, and bone pathology can also result in painful conditions. Several treatment modalities and preventive interventions have been reviewed, including optimizing postoperative pain management techniques, the application of postoperative dressings, and the appropriate use of modalities and medications. Prosthetic modifications and the use of relaxation and mental imaging and the impact of optimal care protocols in controlling pain have also been examined.

REFERENCES

1. Davis R. Phantom sensation, phantom pain and stump pain. *Arch Phys Med Rehabil* 1993; 74:79.
2. Bach S, Noreng M, Tjellden N. Phantom limb pain in amputees during the first 12 months following limb amputation, after preoperative lumbar epidural blockade. *Pain* 1988; 33: 297–301.
3. Elizaga AM, Smith DG, Sharar SR, Edwards T and Hansen S T. Continuous regional analgesia by intraneural block: Effect on postoperative opioid requirements and phantom limb pain following amputation. *J Rehab Res Develop* 1994; 31 (3): 179–187.
4. Mooney V, Harvey JP, McBride E, Snelson, R. Comparison of postoperative stump management: Plaster vs. soft dressings. *J Bone and Joint Surg* 1971; 53-A:241–249.
5. Burgess EM, Romano RL, Zettl JH. The Management of Lower-Extremity Amputations. TR 10–6. Washington, D.C.: U.S. Government Printing Office, August 1969.
6. Wu Y, Keagy RD, Krick HJ, Stratigos JS, Betts HB. An innovative removable rigid dressing technique for below the knee amputation. *J Bone Joint Surg* 1979; 61:A:5,724–29.
7. Ghiulamila RI. Semirigid dressing for postoperative fitting of below knee prosthesis *Arch Phys Med Rehabil* 1972; 53:186–190.
8. Kamen LB, Chapis GJ. Phantom limb sensation and phantom pain. In: Esquenazi A (ed.), *PM&R State of the Art Reviews* 1994; pp73–88.
9. Sherman RA. Phantom pain. In: *Pain: A Psychophysiological Analysis*. New York: Academic Press, 1968.
10. Parkes CM. Factors determining the persistence of phantom pain in amputees. *J Psychosom Res* 1973; 17:97–108.
11. Melzack R. Phantom limbs. *Sci Am*, 1992; pp. 120–126 (April).
12. Sherman RA and Gall GN. A survey of current phantom limb pain treatment in the United States. *Pain* 1980; 8: 85–99.
13. Carlen PL, Wall PD, Nadvorna H, Steinbach T. Phantom limbs and related phenomena in recent traumatic amputations. *Neurology* 1978; 28: 211–217.

14. Jensen TS, Krebs B, Nielsen J, Rasmussen P. Immediate and long-term phantom limb pain in amputees: Incidence, clinical characteristics and relationship to pre-amputation limb pain. *Pain* 1985; 21:267–278.

15. Back S, Noreng MF, Tjeliden NU. Phantom limb pain in amputees during the first 12 months following limb amputation, after preoperative lumbar epidural blockade. *Pain* 1988; 33:297–301.

16. Dise-Lewis J. Psychological adaptation to limb loss. In: Atkins JD, Meier HR III (eds.), *Comprehensive Management of the Upper–Limb Amputee*. New York: Springer-Verlag, 1989; pp. 165–172.

17. Esquenazi A. Geriatric amputee rehabilitation. *Geriatric Clin N Am* 1993, November.

18. Winnem M, Amundsen T. Treatment of phantom limb pain with TENS. *Pain* 1982; 12:299–300.

19. Monga TN, Jaksic T. Acupuncture in phantom limb pain. *Arch Phys Med Rehabil* 1981; 62: 229–231.

20. Carabelli RA, Kellerman WC. Phantom limb pain: Relief by application of TENS to contralateral extremity. *Arch Phys Med Rehabil* 1985; 66:466–467.

21. Max MB, Lynch SA, Muir J, Shoaf SE, Smoller B, Dubner R. Effects of desipramine, amitriptyline, and fluoxetine on pain in diabetic neuropathy. *N Eng J Med* 1992; 326:1250–1256.

22. Lower-Limb Prosthetics, Prosthetics and Orthotics, New York University Post–Graduate Medical School, 1980.

23. Esquenazi A, Vachranukunkiet T, Torres M. A method for continuing bipedal ambulation in below-knee amputees with residual limb complications. *Arch Phys Med Rehabil* 1983; 64: 482.

24. Levy WS. Skin problems of the amputee. In: Bowker JH, Michael JW (eds.), *Atlas of Limb Prosthetics* 2nd ed. St. Louis: Mosby, 1992; pp. 681–688.

25. Neumann M, Bergmann I, Hoffmann U, Hamm H, Reiners K. Botulinum toxin for focal hyperhydrosis: Technical considerations and improvements in application. *Br J Dermatol* 1998; 139:1123–1124.

26. Singson RD, Feldman F, Staron R, Fechtner D, Gonzalez E, Stein J. MRI of postamputation neuromas. *Skeletal Radiol* 1990; 19:259–262.

27. Taft, CB. Radiographic evaluation of stump socket fit. *Artificial Limbs* 1969; 13(2):36–40.

11 Arthritis Pain

P. Michelle Muellner, M.D.
Victoria A. Brander, M.D.

More than any other medical condition, the pain that accompanies joint disease is responsible for the disability that accompanies aging. The National Arthritis Data Workgroup, organized by the National Institutes of Health, estimates a prevalence of self-reported arthritis in people over age 65 to be about 50 percent. Arthritis limits activity in 11.6 percent of people over age 65 (1). The study of pain in arthritis must therefore include special attention to pain measurement and patho-physiology in the elderly, as well as the generalization of treatments to those over 65 whose concomitant medical illnesses may require special attention.

Although the prevalence and incidence of joint disease does increase with age, this is not merely a disease of the old nor is it an inevitable consequence of aging. Arthritis and musculoskeletal disorders are one of the leading causes of disability in people ages 16 to 72.

Because joint disease is so common and disabling, it is also costly. Sixty percent of people with arthritis are of working age. Arthritis cost the U.S. economy $65 billion in medical costs and lost wages in 1992 (2). Arthritis is second only to heart disease as a cause of work disability.

This chapter discusses the pathophysiology of joint pain and gives an overview of pain management principles in two representative rheumatic diseases: osteoarthritis (OA) and rheumatoid arthritis (RA).

PATHOPHYSIOLOGY OF JOINT PAIN

The sensory nervous system consists of peripheral receptors, afferent nerve fibers and their cell bodies, the second order neurons that receive input from the primary fibers at the level of the dorsal horn of the spinal cord, the ascending white matter tracts, the third order neurons that originate in the thalamus, and their projections to sensory cortex.

Sensory receptors include such specialized units as the various cutaneous, sub-cutaneous, muscle, and skeletal mechanoreceptors (Meissner's, Merkel's, pacin-ian, Ruffini's) and the less specialized bare nerve endings, or nociceptors. The nociceptors are further characterized as mechano- and thermonociceptors and polymodal nociceptors. There does not seem to be transduction or filtering of the original stimulus at the level of the nociceptor, as there is with other sensory receptors. Pain-sensitive structures in the joint include the capsule, ligaments and tendons, periosteum, synovium, subchondral bone, blood vessels, and periarticular structures, but not the cartilage (3).

At the level of the afferent nerve, there are four different categories, grouped in descending order of fiber diameter, conduction velocity, and extent of myelination. These include groups I, II (Ab), III (Ad), and IV (C). Impulses, such as those stimulated by touch, pressure, vibration, or proprioception in skin, subcutaneous tissue, muscle, or connective tissue, are carried mainly by the larger Aa and C fibers. The unmyelinated C fibers make up three-quarters of the fibers in the peripheral nerve in general and possibly more in articular nerves; however, whereas all nociceptors transmit via C fibers, not all C fibers are associated with nociceptors. Overall, 2 percent of C fibers carry sympathetic efferent signals, but in joints the figure is closer to 50 percent.

Afferent fibers carrying nociception enter the dorsal horn of the spinal cord and synapse in laminae I, II, and V. Secondary neurons then ascend in the spinal cord and project to the thalamus and then the somatosensory cortex, limbic, and frontal lobes. It is here at the level of the spinal cord that the phenomenon of *referred pain* can be explained. In deeper levels of the dorsal horn, there is convergence of the afferent nerve fibers from nociceptors from divergent areas of the body. Therefore, nociception from the thigh musculature may converge on the same projection neuron as sensory input from the knee joint, and after transmission and processing of these messages, the message may be interpreted as "knee pain."

Prolonged pain can lead to dorsal horn plasticity, with accompanying increased peripheral sensitivity and lowered pain threshold. About 80 percent of articular fibers are group IV (unmyelinated C) fibers, including both nociceptive and sympathetic efferents. Low-threshold afferents are activated by movement within normal range; second group (high threshold) affrents are activated by movement outside the normal range; third group, or "silent nociceptors," do not respond to movement at all. Several hours after the induction of experimental arthritis, the high-threshold and silent afferents become sensitized and respond to movements in the normal range or are activated without any movement at all. Prostaglandins sensitize fibers to mechanical stimuli, as does mechanical stress on the capsule, ligament, and periarticular tissues. Pain-sensitive structures include the capsule, ligaments, enthesis insertion, periosteum, synovium, subchondral bone, blood vessels, and periarticular structures, but *not* the cartilage.

In a normal joint, pain occurs only with intense pressure or extremes of motion. When the joint is diseased, pain occurs at rest and during movements within the normal range. When joint inflammation is experimentally induced in cats, normally high-threshold afferent sensory fibers are sensitized to movements in the innocuous range, and the normally insensitive units are now mechanosensitive (4). Both develop ongoing activity in the absence of continued stimulation. Afferent fibers, once sensitized, also respond to pressure in adjacent areas, remote areas, and even contralateral limbs. Previously subthreshold afferent inputs from remote regions are now able to excite spinal neurons because of increased sensitivity.

The first detailed descriptions of descending central nervous system (CNS) control of nociceptive input were by Melzack and Wall in 1965 (5). We are now aware of the inhibitory effects of supraspinal input. The midbrain periaqueductal gray matter, the medullary nucleus raphe magnus and reticular formation, and the pontine tegmentum contribute to the production of various neurochemicals such as serotonin, endogenous opioids, and norepinephrine that modulate nociceptive input from the periphery. The modulation of these neurochemicals has shown the most promise in recent pharmacologic developments for the treatment of chronic painful conditions.

PAIN PERCEPTION AND ASSESSMENT

Pain is a subjective experience, and it can not be directly measured or observed. Moreover, not only is the severity of disease not a reliable marker for pain severity, but that pain severity is influenced by much more than the physical process of disease. As the descending cortical influences on pain perception were outlined above, it is imperative to point out that thoughts and emotions contribute to that central descending control of peripheral nociception. An individual's level of stress, anxiety, depression, and the coping skills he has to adapt to life circumstances have great impact on his pain perception. Treating those factors directly improves outcomes in chronic pain syndromes. The treatment of depression and mood disturbances is an important strategy in managing chronic pain from a variety of conditions. Patients with osteoarthritis, similar to most chronic diseases, exhibit higher rates of depression than the general population. Nearly 14 percent of osteoarthritics report levels on the Arthritis Impact Measurement Scale (AIMS) analogous to probable depression, and this rate climbs to 17 percent in those with hip or knee disease and 23 percent in persons with neck involvement (6). The importance of a broader understanding of and approach to pain in persons with OA is underlined by numerous investigators (7–9).

Rating Scales

The measurement of pain is a complex task, given the multidimensional aspects of the pain experience as outlined above. However imperfect different rating scales may be, they are essential for comparing an individual's response to various treatments. In addition to measuring the intensity or quality of pain, rating scales have been developed that attempt to measure the impact of an individual's pain on her function.

Lorig and others described a scale to measure a person's perceived self-efficacy, defined as "one's belief that he can perform a specific behavior or task in the future" (10). It asks about a person's certainty that he can perform a number of tasks in a certain time frame, such as walking one-hundred feet, buttoning three buttons, or turning an outside faucet off and on. Two other subscales measure self-efficacy for reducing pain and for managing mood, pacing, and frustration. This can be used in people with arthritis of any etiology.

The Stanford Health Assessment Questionnaire (HAQ) was also developed for people with both OA and RA (11). It measures disability in nine different activities of daily living.

Other examples of measurement tools that seek to evaluate pain and function are the Lequesne Index and the Western Ontario-McMaster University Arthritic Scale (WOMAC), which were both developed for use in osteoarthritis. The Lequesne index assign points for various levels of pain and function in OA of the hip or knee (12). The WOMAC, developed by Bellamy et al., measures pain, stiffness, and physical function in OA of the hip and knee (13).

Pain in the Elderly

Special consideration should be given to the assessment of pain in the elderly, because the incidence of arthritis increases with age. Crook et al. estimated a rate of persistent pain in those over 81 years old to be 400 per 1,000, whereas the rate for those 10 to 30 was 76 per 1,000 (14). Some patients, however, may feel that pain is a "normal" part of daily life once one reaches the age of 65 and this may cause them to delay seeking the advice of a physician. Although there seems to be a diminution of sense of smell, vision, taste, and some somatic sensation with aging, there is no compelling evidence of altered nociception in the elderly. However, because pain perception includes physical, emotional, and cognitive input, it is possible but not proved that the latter two factors are different in the elderly and thus make the pain experience more or less intense. Comorbid medical conditions, especially with regard to conditions causing cognitive impairment and social isolation, may be relatively unique to the elderly and impact on the experience of pain. Altered pharmacokinetics in the elderly (drug absorption, distribution, metabolism, and elimination) necessitate care in the prescription of drugs.

OSTEOARTHRITIS

Osteoarthritis is a disorder of synovial joints that results in the destruction of articular cartilage, increased formation of subchondral bone, and the formation of new bone at joint margins. Because abnormalities are not restricted to one type of tissue in OA, it has been suggested that "joint failure" can be used to describe the pathogenesis, similar to the kidney failure or heart failure that may result from many different primary tissue disorders. Although a common synonym for OA is *degenerative joint disease*, this term is not entirely correct. It is now known that, at least in the initial stages of the disorder, a misguided effort by the chondrocytes to regenerate cartilage is responsible for many of the clinical features of this condition.

Anatomy and Pathophysiology of Pain in OA

A remarkable feature of OA is its lack of a strict relationship between symptoms and radiographic or clinical exam findings. Less than half of those with radiographic findings consistent with OA have corresponding symptoms. The specific factors that lead to *painful* OA are not clearly understood. In a large, prospective study of individuals with or without radiographic knee OA, psychologic well-being and health status were important predictors of knee pain, independent of radiographic severity (7).

The synovial tissue and subchondral bone are thought to be less sensitive to pain than the other named structures. The development of osteophytes can cause pain through periosteal elevation. Bone cysts have the potential for causing pain, but there does not yet seem to be a radiologic correlation between the presence of bone cysts and pain (15). The increase in growth in the subchondral cancellous bone can cause intraosseous venous engorgement and medullary hypertension, which have been shown to correlate with complaints of pain (16).

Extra-articular pain is a common phenomenon in OA. Bursa, tendons, enthese, and muscle are all supplied with nociceptors. Pain in or surrounding an arthritic joint may be only partially related, or even completely unrelated, to the articular pathology. Tendonitis, bursitis, and muscle strains and sprains are common impairments in persons with arthritic joints (see Table 11.1 for common sources of pain in the OA shoulder). Treatment of these conditions frequently ameliorates pain and functional limitations; the radiographic abnormality of arthritis may have simply been an incidental finding. Similarly, new biomechanical abnormalities around an arthritic joint, such as a knee flexion contracture, may convert a previously nonpainful arthritic joint into a painful one. Reversing these impairments frequently alleviates pain, irrespective of the degree of radiographic joint abnormality. Treatment of pain in arthritis is always based on history and physical examination, not radiographic abnormalities.

Clinical Presentation

OA is a gradual disorder involving one or more joints. The weight-bearing joints (hip, knees, and spine) are most commonly symptomatic, although radiographic evidence of OA of the hand is most common, present in over three-fourths of people over age 65. Pain is usually described as an aching, throbbing discomfort, and its occurrence with motion is the earliest symptom. It is worsened by prolonged weight-bearing activity or immobilization and alleviated with periods of rest. Morning stiffness, lasting less than 30 minutes and relieved by activity, is extremely common.

Patients with advanced disease experience pain at rest and may also report a grinding or grating sensation with joint motion. Their joints may feel unstable or lax, "giving way" during high-performance tasks. Functional limitations are specific to the joint affected. For example, limitations in stair climbing, kneeling and lower body dressing are common with hip or knee arthritis. Signs of the disorder on physical examination include localized tenderness, joint enlargement from proliferation of bone (such as Heberden nodes), and flexion contractures. Joint inflammation and effusions may be present. Periarticular muscle atrophy is common. As a consequence of the primary abnormal joint, secondary joint abnormalities are often present above and below the joint.

Table 11.1. Common Causes of Shoulder Pain in Shoulder Osteoarthritis

Glenohumeral Synovitis
- swelling, warmth and tenderness
- restricted active and passive ROM
- arm held in adduction and internal rotation

Glenohumeral Degeneration
- muscle atrophy
- restricted ROM, particularly flexion, extension, abduction and minimal-to-no rotation
- radiographic evidence of cartilage and bone destruction

AC and SC Joint Degeneration
- shoulder arc painful, limited painful abduction
- tender joint, painful adduction with joint compression

Rotator Cuff Atrophy/Tear/Tendinitis
- impaired active abduction with better or full passive ROM
- painful active or restricted abduction, if acute
- night pain
- radiographs may reveal cephalad migration of humeral head
- arthrography reveals dye passed into bursae if cuff is torn

Impingement Syndrome
- "catch" reported between 60-70 degrees is maximum at 100 to 120 degrees abduction
- pain with compression of subacromial tissue occurs at 90 to 100 degrees flexion
- radiographic abnormalities are evident such as osteophytes and acrominal abnormalities

Subacromial/Subdeltoid Bursitis
- impaired and painful abduction and external rotation
- tenderness over superior lateral shoulder
- swelling, warmth, and erythema
- radiographs usually normal

Adhesive Capsulitis
- diffuse pain and stiffness
- glenohumeral tenderness
- reduced passive and active ROM in all planes arthrogram may be abnormal with reduced joint volume

The diagnosis of OA usually can be determined from the history and physical examination. Characteristic changes on radiographs include osteophytes, cysts, and sclerosis in the subchondral marrow and asymmetric joint space narrowing (Figure 11.1). Whereas more than 90 percent of patients over 40 have radiographic evidence of OA in the weight-bearing joints, only 30 percent have clinical symptoms (17). No laboratory studies are diagnostic, yet those listed in Table 11.2 may be useful in excluding the underlying causes of secondary OA. Similarly, synovial fluid analysis may be useful to exclude other causes of joint pain and

Stage I: Mild Osteoarthritis

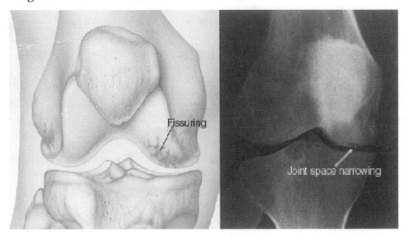

Stage II: Moderate Osteoarthritis

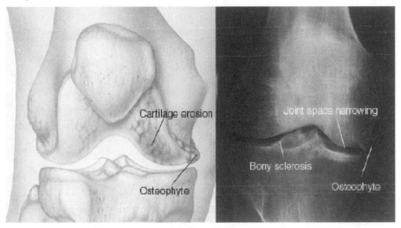

Stage III: Moderately Severe Osteoarthritis

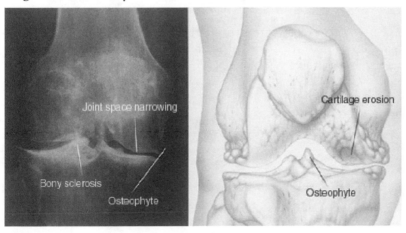

Figure 11.1. Radiographic progression of osteoarthritis of the knee.

Table 11.2. Secondary Osteoarthritis

Causes	Mechanisms
Intraarticular fractures	Damage to articular cartilage or joint incongruity
Ligament and joint capsule	Joint instability
Meniscectomy or meniscal injury	Joint instability and altered joint loading
Joint dysplasias (developmental and hereditary joint and cartilage dysplasias)	Abnormal joint shape and/or abnormal articular cartilage
Aseptic necrosis	Bone necrosis leading to collapse of articular surface and joint incongruity
Hemophilia	Multiple joint hemorrhages
Stickler syndrome (progressive hereditary arthro-ophthalmopathy)	Abnormal joint and/or articular cartilage development
Gaucher disease (hereditary deficiency of enzyme glucocerebrosidase leading to accumulation of glucocerebroside)	Bone necrosis or pathologic bone fracture leading to joint incongruity
Hemochromatosis (excess iron deposition in multiple tissues)	Unknown
Ochronosis (hereditary deficiency of enzyme homogentisic acid oxide leads to accumulation of homogentisic acid)	Deposition of homogenic acid polymers in articular cartilage
Acromegaly	Overgrowth of articular cartilage producing joint incongruity and/or abnormal cartilage
Ehlers-Danlos syndrome	Joint instability
Calcium pyrophosphate deposition disease	Accumulation of calcium pyrophosphate crystals in articular cartilage
Neuropathic arthropathy (Charcot joints, syphilis, diabetes mellitus, syringomyelia, meningomyelocele, leprosy, congenital insensitivity to pain)	Loss of proprioception and joint sensation and eventual joint instability
Paget disease	Distortion of incongruity of joints due to bone remodeling

inflammation in unusual cases. Bone scans, computed tomography (CT), and magnetic resonance imaging (MRI) are rarely necessary; interpretation of the clinically significant abnormalities seen on these films is extraordinarily difficult in light of their poor specificity in this disorder.

Treatment

Pharmacologic Agents. No pharmacologic agents have been shown to alter the course of OA. Pharmacotherapy is aimed at reducing pain and eliminating inflammation.

Analgesics. The American College of Rheumatology guidelines recommend acetaminophen as a first-line pharmaceutical agent in the treatment of OA (18). This is based on studies showing comparable efficacy to naproxen (19) and ibuprofen (20) and its more favorable risk–benefit profile compared to NSAIDs. However, there is still potential for renal or hepatic toxicity in long-term use of acetaminophen, especially in the elderly and when combined with other potentially hepato- and nephrotoxic drugs such as nonsteroidal antiinflammatory drugs (NSAIDs).

Nonsteroidal Antiinflammatory Drugs (NSAIDs). Because of the possible role of local antiinflammatory mediators in OA, some clinicians and researchers contend that NSAIDs are more effective than analgesics for osteoarthritic pain. All NSAIDs are about equally effective in controlling the pain associated with OA. Because it is not well established that an inflammatory component is significant in the pathophysiology of OA, these drugs are thought to act as analgesics via additional pathways to the peripheral cyclo-oxygenase pathway. There is evidence that some NSAIDs may also work centrally, interacting with receptors for endogenous opioids, serotonin, glutamate, and gamma amino butyric acid (GABA) (21).

The high incidence of side effects, particularly gastrointestinal bleeding and hepatic and renal toxicity, has compromised NSAIDs use from the onset. In December 1998, the Food and Drug Administration approved celecoxib, the first of a group of cyclooxygenase-2 (COX-2) inhibitors for use in OA and rheumatoid arthritis. Premarketing studies showed a similar efficacy to naproxen with a lower incidence of gastrointestinal side effects (22). Celecoxib avoids interference with platelet function, but may impart the same risk for hepatic and renal insufficiency as that of NSAIDs. A second COX-2 inhibitor, rofecoxib, was also recently approved for OA.

Opioids. Medications such as codeine, hydrocodone, and oxycodone, and their combinations with NSAIDs and acetaminophen, are common choices for management of acute pain. Elderly patients, those with significant comorbidities, or on numerous medications, are at high risk for side effects from nonsteroidal antiinflammatories. These patients might preferentially benefit from chronic low-dose opioids. However, the chronic use of opioids in any nonmalignant pain condition, including arthritis, is controversial (23). In a retrospective study of 644 rheumatic disease patients, chronic codeine and oxycodone use appeared effective in reducing pain, was associated with mild toxicity, and was not associated with significant dose escalations (24). The retrospective design and risk of recall bias limits generalization of the findings. Whereas opioids may indeed be safe and effective for long-term use in select patients, the American College of Rheumatology guidelines for the management of OA advise against their chronic use, recommending them mainly for acute exacerbations (25). Because there are only a few well-designed, randomized, controlled trials of sufficient length regarding opioid use in arthritis, their use should be closely monitored for the development of dependence, tolerance, and even possible sensitization of the CNS through their long-term use (26).

Tramadol (Ultram®) was FDA-approved in 1995 for the management of moderate and moderately severe pain. Although it selectively binds to m-opioid receptors in the CNS, it is not chemically related to the opioids. Tramadol also offers weak serotonin and norepinephrine re-uptake inhibition (27). It appears to have less potential for tolerance and dependence than other opioid medications and to have fewer drug interactions. In one study in OA, the addition of tramadol was associated with reductions in the daily use of naproxen, although the merits of the trial design are debated (28). However, published data regarding tramadol use for OA are limited and indicate difficulty with side effects such as nausea, vomiting, and dizziness (29).

Tricyclic Antidepressants (TCAs) and Other Antidepressants. TCAs such as amitriptyline, nortriptyline, or doxepin are widely used for their analgesic properties in chronic pain conditions. Contrary to popular belief, their effectiveness as analgesics is unrelated to their mood-elevating properties. Their mechanism of action is thought to be via increasing levels of certain neurotransmitters such as serotonin and norepinephrine in the neuronal synaptic cleft. However, the relative ineffectiveness of the more serotonin-selective agents such as fluoxetine (Prozac®), paroxetine (Paxil®), and others, intimates a more complicated story (30). Studies have shown efficacy in both OA and RA. Low-dose TCAs (such as 10–50 mg nightly) are known to be effective agents in reducing pain and ameliorating the associated sleep disturbances in fibrocytis patients (31).

Topical Agents. Topical capsaicin, a derivative of the common red pepper plant, can be used as an adjuvant treatment to oral analgesics or alone in patients who either may not take or do not wish to take oral medications. Its mechanism of action is thought to be a depletion of substance P stores from the sensory neuron, as well as causing a decrease in its manufacture and transport. It has been shown to be more effective than placebo in four-week randomized controlled trials (32,33). On the other hand, topical trolamine salicylate (Aspercreme® and others) is no more effective than placebo (34).

Complementary Therapies

Acupuncture. Acupuncture involves the insertion of thin needles into the skin at specific points of the body. The goal is to restore *qi*, or vital energy, which when out of balance (according to its practitioners) leads to illness and pain. Acupuncture involves stimulating anatomic skin locations through a variety of techniques, including the use of needles, pressure, and heat. Acupuncture elicits varied biological responses, including the release of opioid peptides, stimulation of the hypothalamus and pituitary, and alterations in immune functions. There are many studies describing the effects of needle acupuncture, but few well-designed clinical trials. It appears efficacious in reducing nausea and pain, including that caused by OA. (35).

Vitamin D. Recent epidemiologic data from the Framingham Osteoarthritis Study suggest that vitamin D might reduce the radiographic progression of arthritis (36). Subjects with low serum 25-hydroxyvitamin D levels had three times the risk of radiographic disease prevention. Although there is no accepted dose recommendation of vitamin D for OA, the current dose recommendation for osteoporosis prevention is 400 to 800 I.U. per day.

Antioxidants. The role of antioxidants in delaying cartilage degeneration has been proposed. Vitamin C, through its effect on the vitamin C-dependent enzyme lysyl-hydroxylase, is required for the stabilization of mature collagen. Animal data has shown a higher risk of experimentally induced arthritis in those with lower serum levels of vitamin C (37). In the Framingham study, individuals with low oral vitamin C intake had a threefold increase in radiographic progression of knee OA. (37).

Chondroitin Sulfate. Chondroitin sulfate (CS), in oral preparation, is a widely popular alternative therapy for OA. It has been proposed that CS may stimulate synthesis of proteoglycan and collagens, while partially inhibiting enzymatic degradation (38). It is not clear how much oral chondroitin is actually absorbed or concentrated in articular cartilage. Several European clinical trials have assessed the efficacy of oral CS in subjects with OA. Morreale performed a randomized, double-blind placebo-controlled trial of CS and diclofenac sodium in 146 subjects with knee OA (39). The NSAID-treated groups showed better early relief of pain and symptoms, which reversed after discontinuation of the drug. The CS groups showed a later therapeutic response that lasted 3 months after the treatment was discontinued. Leeb reported an open, multicenter phase IV clinical trial of sixty-one subjects with hip, knee, or finger OA (40). CS therapy prompted a reduction in total NSAID use and pain reports. Most published trials used doses of 1,200 mg of CS per day.

Glucosamine. Glucosamine is the salt of D-glucosamine, an amino sugar with sulfuric acid. Some investigators believe that oral glucosamine preferentially concentrates in articular cartilage (41). Major side effects are rare and appear to be primarily gastrointestinal. In short-term trials glucosamine has been shown to be effective at reducing pain and stiffness in OA. In four- or eight-week trials, several European studies have compared glucosamine to placebo or nonsteroidal antiinflammatory drugs (42–44). Glucosamine is consistently equal or superior to the comparison drug. These studies are all significantly limited by small sample size. Most published trials used doses of 1,500 mg of glucosamine a day.

Chondroitin and glucosamine are frequently used in combination. There is a wide variation in the concentration of these chemicals in the multitude of marketed products. Most of these preparations, like the widely popular "arthritis cure," combine 1,500 mg of glucosamine with 1,200 mg of CS daily. These products typically cost $40 to $80 per month.

Table 11.3. Intraarticular Steroid Preparations (from Alpiner et. al)

Steroid	Solubility	Duration of Action (T1/2) hours	Hip Dose	Knee Shoulder Dose	Wrist/ Elbow Dose	Small Joints Dose
Betamethasone (Celestone®)	High	36–72	6–12	6–9	3–6	3
Triamcinolone hexacetonide (Aristospan®)	Low	12–72	15–20	10–20	5–10	1–5
Triamcinolone diacetate	Low-intermediate	12–36	30–40	20–40	10–25	5–15
Dexamethasone (Decadron®)	Intermediate	36–72	4–6	2–4	1–2	0.5–1.5
Hydrocortisone (Hydrocortone®)	Low	8–12	30–40	25–40	12.5–37.5	10–25
Methylprednisolone (Depo-Medrol®)	Intermediate	12–36	40-100	20–80	10–40	4–10

Intraarticular Medications

Steroid Injections. There are few well-designed trials of intraarticular steroid use and those mainly report findings from one joint (the knee). In general, the effects appear to be short-lived and nearly indistinguishable from placebo response (45). Glucocorticoids act at the cellular level to control the rate of synthesis of various proteins and inhibit the production of inflammatory mediators. The pharmacokinetic properties of the different steroid preparations should be considered when selecting them for use (see Table 11.3 for a list of intraarticular steroid preparations). The addition of short-acting anesthetics (such as lidocaine) has been associated with the development of reactive effusions from insoluble crystals in the joint, likely from a steroid-preservative reaction. Contraindications to intraarticular steroids include systemic or local infection and intraarticular fracture. Complications, although rare, include increased pain for 24 to 72 hours, infection, systemic steroid absorption, subcutaneous tissue atrophy, and bone or tissue damage.

Viscosupplementation. Hyaluronic acid (hyaluronan and hylan GF-20) injections were recently approved for use in painful knee OA. These compounds, used for years in Europe, Canada, and Japan, are believed to reduce pain, inflammation, and stiffness in knee OA (46–48). Their mechanism of action is unknown. It is proposed that injections of hyaluronic acid temporarily restore elastoviscosity to arthritic synovial fluid, thus reducing stiffness. Through a purely local mechanical effect, hyaluronic acid may reduce inflammation and pain. Research into the disease-modifying capacities of this compound is limited and contradictory. In vitro, hyaluronic acid is proposed to alter the multiple enzymes involved in cartilage degradation (49,50). In an animal model, its use has been reported to delay or reduce posttraumatic cartilage degeneration (51). In contrast, in a canine model of OA, hyaluronic acid–injected knees exhibited more pathologic evidence of degeneration upon sacrifice than those that received saline injections (52).

Clinical research published in peer-reviewed U.S. journals is limited. In a double-blind, placebo-controlled randomized trial, Wobig compared hylan GF-20 to saline in subjects with long-standing knee OA (53). Hylan was superior to saline in the reduction of pain in weight-bearing. The maximum effect of treatment was seen at 8 to 12 weeks. Adams performed a multicenter, randomized double-blind controlled trial of hylan versus continuous NSAID therapy in ninety subjects with knee OA (46). Pain was the primary outcome. The results of the group receiving hylan GF-20 was superior to those receiving NSAID only at the telephone follow-up interview. Although most clinical investigators report modest improvement in pain and function, either comparable or slightly superior to antiinflammatory drugs, research into the disease modifying effect in humans is lacking (54,55).

Hyaluronic acid injections are well tolerated. The most common adverse affects are transient pain or swelling in the knee that lasts for a few days and resolves completely. Up to 10 percent of patients may develop a small, well-circumscribed rash. There have been rare reports of a dramatic synovitis occurring after hyaluronic acid injection. This synovitis responds to intraarticular corticosteroid injection. Hyaluronic acid injection is currently a recommended alternative therapy for knee arthritis. It is best utilized only after standard therapy (weight loss, exercise, analgesics, NSAIDs) fails to provide satisfactory relief of pain in patients who are not candidates for knee replacement surgery. The injections are expensive but are covered by Medicare, Medicaid, and managed care plans with pre-approval.

Exercise

Patients commonly respond to their OA symptoms by limiting activity. The result is restricted joint motion and disuse atrophy. This, in turn, promotes atrophy of cartilage and thinning of bone. Joint integrity is then further compromised, and pain ensues. Quadriceps weakness, specifically, correlates with pain severity in OA. (56). Exercise is an extraordinarily promising avenue to reverse these physical impairments and functional limitations present in persons in OA (57). Exercise has been shown in numerous studies to substantially reduce pain in degenerative and inflammatory arthritis (58) and exercise may impart both protective and remittive actions on the diseased knee joint.

Regular dynamic exercise is associated with increased blood flow and improved cartilage health as well as increased ROM, strength, and periarticular muscle capacity. Exercise programs have been shown to improve flexibility, strength, endurance, function, cardiovascular fitness, and general health status without aggravation of arthritis (59–61). Gentle flexibility exercises performed in the evening can reduce morning stiffness for persons with RA (62). Dance-based aerobic exercise programs reduce pain and disability in persons with RA and OA (63). In contrast to older recommendations against such exercise, aggressive muscle strengthening and endurance exercises improve strength, endurance, and function and reduce pain without exacerbation of disease (64,65). Although isometric strengthening and avoidance of aggressive stretching is appropriate when joints are acutely swollen, either in OA or RA, isometric (or dynamic) exercise, preferably of the closed-kinetic-chain variety, is safe and effective at most other times.

Through the amelioration of biomechanical and other periarticular soft tissue abnormalities, such as reversing a knee flexion contracture, exercise can substantially reduce pain. Tight, inflexible, and weak soft tissues are prone to injury and pain. Flexible, fatigue-resistant muscles function as more efficient shock absorbers, dampening the impact of force through the joint. Strengthening exercise improves quadriceps strength, reduces pain, and improves function in persons with significant knee OA. (66,67).

Orthoses

The use of a cane can decrease the vertical load placed through a weight-bearing joint when used in the contralateral hand. Patients with arthritic spines, hips, and knees frequently report that cushioned heel pads help reduce joint pain while walking. Foot orthotics, such as a total contact arch support with a medial wedge, can reduce knee pain in a patient with genu valgus and a pes planus deformity. An elastic knee sleeve used around an arthritic knee commonly reduces knee pain, despite the absence of biomechanical reasons for this effect. More constrained knee orthotics (such as the knee unloader braces) are effective at reducing pain, particularly in OA that is primarily unicompartmental; however, these rigid orthoses are expensive, cumbersome, and often not well tolerated in patients with significant angular deformities.

Cognitive-Behavioral Therapies (CBT)

These psychologic interventions aim to help patients understand how their thoughts, beliefs, expectations, and behaviors can impact their experience of pain (for details see Chapter 3). CBT then gives patients specific tools such as distraction, imagery, pacing skills, and goal setting to give them some control over their own pain experience. Although there are clear benefits of CBT training for improving pain and physical and psychologic disability, these may tend to lessen over time without reinforcement. Involving a patient's family strengthens the social support system, which may help patients maintain gains for longer periods of time.

There is a need for clarification through clinical research regarding which components of a CBT program are the most helpful and how to match the timing of CBT with an individual patient's readiness to change (68).

Coping skills training has been shown to reduce a patient's ratings of pain and psychological disability in knee OA (69). The Arthritis Self-Management Program

(ASMP), designed to improve coping skills through self-efficacy training, appears to reduce pain and the number of arthritis-related physician visits (70). Telephone-based interventions that involve reviewing educational information, medications, and problem-solving techniques, also reduce pain and improve function without substantially increasing costs (71).

Modalities

Heat. The efficacy of heat modalities in OA has not been proven. Heat is proposed to reduce pain and muscle spasm, as well as facilitate soft tissue stretching (72). Ultrasound, for example, offered no additional benefits when used to facilitate standard physical therapy in the treatment of arthritic knee flexion contractures (73). Contraindications to the use of deep heat include reduced sensation, bleeding, severe inflammation, tumors, or pregnancy.

Electrical Stimulation. Transcutaneous electrical nerve stimulation (TENS) is a widely used electrical modality. TENS is presumed to work by stimulating large-diameter fibers to block propagation of painful stimuli by small fibers. This helps to modulate pain perception at the spinal cord and CNS level. Its use in OA is controversial (73).

Cold. Cold therapy is very useful in the initial treatment of painful acute musculoskeletal syndromes, such as spasm, soft tissue injury, and postoperative conditions. Its effect on joint temperature in OA has been debated (73).

Surgery

When severe pain and functional limitations exist despite maximal nonoperative intervention, joint reconstruction may be indicated. Osteotomy or fusion may provide temporary relief of pain in young patients with OA of the hip or knee who are not yet candidates for joint replacement because of their age. Fusion may be used in persons with severely arthritic knees associated with previous infection or profound weakness. Osteotomy is of greatest benefit when the disease is only moderately advanced. Arthroscopic removal of loose bodies and joint lavage is useful when focal acute pathology, such as a meniscal tear, has caused an acute change in pain in an otherwise minimally involved knee (74).

Total joint replacement (TJR) is an extraordinarily good procedure, relieving pain and substantially improving function in about 90 percent of hip or knee patients (75). Hip replacement is shown to be a cost-savings intervention, even in the very elderly (76). The indication for TJR is articular pain from advanced cartilage loss, refractory to conservative management strategies (including exercise, weight loss, and medications) and associated with a progressive functional decline. Young age is a relative contraindication for surgery. Because the lifespan of hip or knee implants is about 15 to 20 years, young osteoarthritic patients are discouraged from undergoing this surgery until their fourth decade. However, patients with inflammatory arthritis, congenital hip dysplasias, or avascular necrosis are candidates for the procedure at any age. Old age is not a contraindication to TJR. In general, patients over 80 years of age appear to do as well as younger individuals (77). Other surgical procedures, such as cartilage transplant, are not yet indicated or successful in patients with OA.

The rehabilitation of joint replacement patients focuses on regaining functional independence, increasing range of motion in the operated joint, increasing periarticular strength, improving gait and the use of assistive devices, preventing complications such as deep venous thrombosis and infection, and controlling postoperative pain.

RHEUMATOID ARTHRITIS (RA)

Rheumatoid arthritis (RA) is a systemic autoimmune disorder with joint pathology as its main feature. The worldwide prevalence of RA is estimated to be between 1 and 2 percent. This figure may be closer to 10 percent in persons over 65 (78). Other organ systems are affected, and include the cardiovascular system (vasculitis and pericarditis), the pulmonary system (nodules, interstitial fibrosis), and the nervous system (mononeuritis multiplex).

Anatomy and Pathophysiology of Pain in RA

The involvement of the synovium and joint capsule in RA provides more obvious sources of nociception than do the pathological abnormalities in OA. However, the same potential sources of nociception presumably apply in RA as in OA, including a sensitized CNS and its afferent nerves.

Clinical Presentation

RA is a clinical diagnosis, present when a patient has symmetrical polyarthritis and morning stiffness for more than 60 days. There is no simple diagnostic test to establish the diagnosis of RA. The diagnosis is based on a thorough clinical evaluation, referring to the revised American Rheumatism Association criteria (see Table 11-4) (18). RA can involve multiple organ systems and is associated with significant systemic disease. There may be three subtypes of RA, each with its own natural history. Type I RA is a self-limited process, usually postviral, rarely rheumatoid factor (RF) positive. Type II disease is persistent but minimally aggressive. Type III disease is severe, progressive, and associated with rapid radiographic abnormalities and disability. RA is associated with premature mortality (79,80).

Treatment

As a consequence of the intermingled physical and functional impairments present in this disease, successful treatment of pain in RA requires a multifaceted approach. RA is managed using medications, splinting, and rest to suppress pain

Table 11.4. 1988 Revised American Rheumatism Association Criteria for the Diagnosis of RA

Criteria	Definition
Morning stiffness	Morning stiffness in and around the joints lasting at least 1 hour before maximal improvement
Arthritis of three or more joint areas	At least three joint areas have simultaneously had soft tissue swelling or fluid (not bony overgrowth alone) observed by a physician. The 14 possible joint areas are (right or left) PIP, MCP, wrist, elbow, knee, ankle, and MTP joints
Arthritis of hand joints	At least one joint area swollen as above in wrist, MCP, or PIP joint
Symmetric arthritis	Simultaneous involvement of the same joint (as in 2) on both sides of the body (bilateral involvement of PIP, MCP, or MTP joints is acceptable without absolute symmetry)
Rheumatoid nodules	Subcutaneous nodules, over bony prominences, or extensor surfaces, or in juxta-articular regions, observed by a physician
Serum rheumatoid factor	Demonstration of abnormal amounts of serum rheumatoid factor by any method that has been positive in less than 5 percent of control subjects
Radiographic changes	Radiographic changes typical of RA on posteroanterior hand wrist radiographs, which must include erosions or unequivocal bony decalcification localized to or most marked adjacent to the involved joints (osteoarthritis changes along do not qualify)

Abbreviations: PIP, proximal interphalangeal: MCP, metacarpophalangeal; MTP, metatarsophalangeal. For classification purposes, a patient is said to have RA if he or she has satisfied at least four of the seven criteria. Criteria 1 through 4 must be present for at last 6 weeks.

and inflammation; exercise to maintain joint motion, strength, and cardiovascular endurance; functional training including the use of adaptive and assistive devices; education in joint protection, energy conservation, and disease self-management; orthotics; environment modification; and psychosocial, vocational, and avocational interventions. First and primarily inflammation must be suppressed, because this is the cause of joint pain and deterioration. Then, rehabilitative measures are useful. These concepts are described in the following sections.

Pharmacotherapy

Traditionally, the pharmacotherapy of RA has been based on a pyramidal approach to treatment (81). Patients with milder disease and most patients when first diagnosed are treated with the drugs shown on the low end of the pyramid. However, patients whose disease is considered progressive Type III (such as those who present with radiographic erosions) should immediately begin second-line therapy with the drugs identified higher on the pyramid, including disease-modifying antirheumatic drugs (DMARDs). The decision as to whether a patient has self-limited or progressive RA usually can be made within 1 to 3 months, and aggressive treatment begun as soon as possible. Methotrexate is the most widely used DMARD, because of its fairly low toxicity and strong antiinflammatory properties. The dosage is generally 7.5 mg to 15 mg per week, either orally or by injection. Early combination chemotherapy, using two or more DMARDs, has come into favor for patients who present with advanced disease (81). Steroids and surgery, on the lateral aspects of the pyramid, may be useful at many stages of intervention. Low dose prednisone (7.5 mg a day or less) is an effective alternative to DMARD therapy for patients with refractory disease. This dose may be associated with much fewer steroid-induced side effects (diabetes, osteopenia, hypertension, etc.). Newer biologic therapies (such as tumor necrosis factor [TNF] and interleukin inhibitors) offer promising alternatives in the treatment of refractory disease (82,83). These agents specifically target the cells and cell products responsible for the pathophysiologic mechanisms of RA. For example, TNF helps regulate cell proliferation and cell death, stimulates the release of proinflammatory cytokines, stimulates the production of proteases (such as collagenase), and enhances cell movement through the joint (82). It is yet unclear when in the course of RA to use biologic therapies, and whether to use them in combination or in place of traditional DMARDs. These drugs are usually introduced in DMARD-refractory patients; however, despite this lack of clear evidence, the trend is to use these agents earlier in the course of treatment in patients who have aggressive, erosive disease. These agents are associated with side effects, particularly those related to immune suppression, such as infection. This aggressive approach is an alternative to more traditional pharmacotherapy, which has not clearly been shown to reverse the onset of inevitable erosive disease (80).

Topical Agents. Capsaicin has shown similar effectiveness in RA as in OA (see topical agents section under Osteoarthritis).

TCAs and Antidepressant Therapy. Clinical depression appears very commonly in RA. In a sample of 6,153 consecutive rheumatic patients (1,152 with RA), 25 percent of the RA patients self-reported depressive symptoms consistent with possible depression and 20 percent had probable depression (84). RA patients with depression have poorer function, are more likely to spend days in bed, and report greater pain (85). Depression and anxiety predict pain and functional limitations (86). Several investigators have reported the analgesic effect of low-dose antidepressants in RA. Low-dose therapy with TCAs appears to reduce joint pain, particularly in the patient who also shows signs of depression (87).

Narcotic Analgesics. The controversial issues regarding chronic opioid use in persons with rheumatic diseases is covered in the corresponding osteoarthritis section of this chapter.

Intraarticular Medications

Corticosteroids. Single-joint inflammations occur regularly in RA, despite acceptable systemic management of inflammation. Rapid resolution of inflammation is essential to protect cartilage and soft tissues from damage. Single-joint injections of corticosteroid are effective at achieving a rapid, local response with relatively few side effects. The principles regarding injectable solutions, contraindications, and technique apply equally in rheumatoid and osteoarthritis (see previous section Intraarticular Medications).

Hyaluronic Acid. The use of injectable hyaluronic acid derivatives has not been studied in RA.

Exercise

Exercise is one of the few available interventional strategies having proven efficacy. Exercise reverses many of the deteriorating effects of RA and increases aerobic capacity, muscle strength, and force generation. Exercise significantly reduces pain. Additional benefits that occur are decreased depression, reduced fatigue, resolution of sleep disturbances, increased activities of daily living, and and increased level of independence (60,63,88–91).

Traditionally, physicians and other health care professionals have discouraged patients with RA from exercising because of concern about accelerated joint damage. In the acute phases of inflammation, range-of-motion and isotonic strengthening are believed to increase joint temperature and swelling and potentially accelerate joint deterioration. There is also concern about the deleterious effects of particular strengthening exercises on unstable joints. Unfortunately the overemphasis on these *theoretical* negatives by health care providers has greatly overshadowed the important benefits of exercise in arthritis. It is well known that those with RA have poorer muscle strength and endurance than the general population (63,92,93). Recent studies strongly indicate that aerobic and resistance exercises are significantly beneficial to RA patients, improving flexibility, strength, endurance, function, and cardiovascular fitness without aggravating symptoms (60,63,88,94). For example, one study included RA subjects with symptomatic weight-bearing joints in a 12-week graded aerobic exercise program. Significant gains in aerobic capacity, overall physical activity, 50-foot walk time, grip strength, and flexibility were demonstrated and maintained after 1 year (63); there was a corresponding decrease in anxiety and depression. A combined dance-based aerobic exercise program and educational problem-solving and skills-building program showed increases in quality of life measures and 50-foot walk time (60,88). Yet another study of RA subjects indicated that a program of muscle strengthening exercises raised scores on physical fitness tests (94).

Physicians should offer a specific exercise prescription that includes duration, intensity, and frequency for each RA patient. Beforehand, assessment of joint instability and inflammation is critical so that potentially harmful exercises may be excluded. During acute joint inflammation it is important not to overstretch periarticular tissues, because their reduced tensile strength may lead to tears. Isometric exercise is recommended during inflammation; it is used in conjunction with dynamic resistive and aerobic exercise programs once inflammation subsides. Adequate warm-up and cool-down, using gentle stretching and light aerobics, ensures safety and comfort.

Aquatic exercise is highly recommended for RA patients. The warmth and buoyancy of a heated pool provides an almost pain-free environment in which to exercise. Regular pool therapy has been demonstrated to improve strength and conditioning. Other aerobic exercise, such as low-impact aerobics, bicycling, and walking, are recommended to improve cardiovascular conditioning without increasing pain or inflammation.

Patients with RA who have not exercised in a structured program before or those with identified physical impairments (such as joint contractures) should be referred to a physical therapist. This will best enable them to learn specifically which exercises are best for them and precisely how to perform them for the greatest benefit.

Psychologic Therapies

Biofeedback. Relative to placebo or no treatment groups, a biofeedback-assisted group therapy program has been shown to reduce pain behavior and active joint count in persons with RA. These gains were maintained at follow-up (20).

Cognitive and Behavioral Therapies (CBT). (Refer to the CBT section under osteoarthritis for general principles.) One of the goals of psychologic interventions in general, and CBT in specific, is to increase a patient's perception of self-efficacy. Self-efficacy is defined as a person's belief in his or her own power to successfully manage a challenging situation. Even after controlling for disease severity, patient reports of high self-efficacy are significantly correlated with decreased pain and improved mood (95). Stress management training, as one component of CBT, reduces self-reported pain and improves coping strategies in persons with RA (96).

Modalities

Heat. Superficial heat (hot packs, paraffin, wax baths, fluidotherapy, infrared radiation, and hydrotherapy) is used primarily to reduce pain and improve flexibility. Heat may reduce muscle guarding, increase blood flow, and increase pain threshold. Heat increases extensibility of connective tissues, theoretically facilitating range-of-motion therapies. The efficacy of superficial heat has not been proven. However, many patients report improvement following heat treatments (97) despite the absence of substantiating literature (98). The daily use of heat does not appear to affect disease progression (99). However, because joint and skin temperatures elevate following superficial heat application, heat should be avoided during acute inflammatory flares. Deep heat (short wave diathermy and ultrasound) elevates joint, muscle, and connective tissue temperatures. Again, current literature does not support its use (73,100).

Cold. Cold treatments (cold packs, ice massage, cold baths, and vapocoolant sprays) are used to reduce pain, swelling, and inflammation by slowing nerve conduction, decreasing muscle activity, releasing endorphins, or promoting vasoconstriction. Cold is believed to reduce joint temperature by reducing skin temperature (101). Literature substantiating these effects is limited.

Transcutaneous Electrical Nerve Stimulation (TENS). Based on the gate theory of pain by Melzack and Wall, TENS application theoretically reduces pain through stimulating large sensory fibers, which then overwhelm sensory receptors and block small pain fiber transmission to the spinal cord (5). TENS is reported to reduce pain in RA (102). The most common modes of TENS are high-frequency, low-frequency, and burst mode. High-frequency TENS uses a continuous train of 100-microsecond pulses in a frequency range of 70 to 100 Hz. Electrodes are placed around the painful joint. Low-frequency TENS uses wide 250-microsecond pulses at a frequency range of 1 to 3 Hz. Electrodes are placed over motor points in the myotomes of muscles around the painful joint. In burst-mode TENS, current frequency is 70 Hz, delivered in small bursts at a rate of 3 per second. There is little evidence to support the use of one mode of TENS over another in rheumatoid arthritis (103).

Local and Systemic Rest

Local Joint Rest. In RA, splints are used to reduce pain and inflammation through local rest, and to correct deformity and improve function. Splints are believed to reduce pain and inflammation through strict immobilization of the joint (104,105). Numerous investigators document the efficacy of splints in reducing pain (72). Although the duration of wear to achieve pain reduction is not clear, most clinicians prescribe splint use throughout the day and night when inflammation is present and at night for several weeks once the inflammation has resolved. Patients are taught to self-manage splint use. Resting splints are used to reduce inflammation and pain. Custom fabricated splints are expensive, but are often better tolerated than prefabricated splints.

Joint Protection Techniques. Repetitive joint loading and motion can increase pain in abnormal joints. Joint loading can be reduced through the modification of daily activities. For example, when carrying heavy items, an individual with an impaired hip should carry those items in the ipsilateral hand or split the weight and carry half in each hand. Recreational activities should be low-impact, such as swimming or bicycling. When standing at the sink, persons with back impairments should use a stool to elevate one leg. The Arthritis Foundation provides outstanding practical literature on energy conservation and joint protection techniques for individuals with RA (Arthritis Foundation, Atlanta, Georgia 1-800-741-4008).

Systemic Rest. Adequate general rest, including restorative sleep, is necessary for general health and is imperative in the presence of chronic disease. General body rest is a known strategy to reduce systemic inflammation in RA. However, the known adverse effects of rest, including rapid reductions in strength and endurance, limit its use as a systemic therapy. During periods of acute inflammation, daily periods of prolonged rest (30 to 60 minutes in duration) are typically recommended.

Surgery

Total joint replacement has revolutionized the quality of life for patients with RA. Although nonprosthetic interventions, such as arthrodesis, tendon repair, and synovectomy, still play an important role, patients with RA are candidates for joint replacement at any age.

Cervical Spine. The cervical spine is frequently involved in RA, in as many as 70 percent of patients. The three most common radiographic instabilities in the rheumatoid cervical spine are atlantoaxial subluxation (AAS), subaxial subluxation, and basilar invagination of the odontoid. Cervical fusion is a common procedure in RA when pain and functional loss from cervical instability is refractory to other interventions. AAS is the most common type of instability and is a result of the destruction and laxity of the transverse and apical ligaments. The indications for surgery are refractory pain, progressive neurologic deficit in the presence of an anterior or posterior atlantodental interval of 14 mm or less, basilar invagination of at least 5mm, and subaxial subluxation with a sagittal diameter of the canal less than 14 mm (106). The surgical indications include decompression or fusion of the cervical spine or a combination of the two. Surgery is more likely to provide symptomatic relief in patients with neck and radicular pain than in those with neurologic deficit.

Shoulder. Most rheumatoid shoulder surgery involves the glenohumeral joint. Synovectomy can relieve pain and improve range of motion when the articular surfaces are smooth. Surgical rotator cuff tear repair is frequently unsuccessful in RA patients and is rarely indicated. Glenohumeral arthroplasty provides predictable pain relief, but is more successful at restoring range of motion if the rotator cuff is still intact at the time of surgery. When conservative therapies fail, painful acromioclavicular disease is sometimes amenable to excision of the distal end of the clavicle, acromioplasty, and subacromial decompression.

Elbow, Wrist, and Hand. Synovectomy and total elbow arthroplasty are the most common surgical procedures at the elbow. Elbow arthroplasty is successful in about 50 to 75 percent of patients in most reported studies (107). A number of surgical procedures have been designed to reduce pain and improve function at the wrist and hand, and prosthetics exist for the wrist and metacarpal (MCP) joints. Pain relief is the primary goal. In view of the poor published results from wrist arthroplasty, this surgery is not recommended (108). Wrist arthrodesis is a more predictable choice.

Hip. Hip replacement is a common, extraordinarily successful surgery to reduce pain and improve function in RA. Most studies report near complete relief of pain in over 95 percent of cases. Infection is more common in patients with RA than OA, but occurs in less than 1 percent of cases. Aseptic loosening is the principal cause of revision surgery. Revision rates are about 15 percent at 10 to 15 year follow-up in RA patients.

Knee. Arthroscopic synovectomy is occasionally warranted for short-term pain relief in RA patients. Radiation ablative synovectomy is emerging as an alternative to surgical synovectomy. Like THA surgery in the hip, total knee arthroplasty (TKA) is the surgical standard for the treatment of the painful rheumatoid knee. TKA surgery is successful in providing dramatic pain relief in about 85 percent of RA patients. The longevity of these implants is approximately 15 to 18 years.

Foot and Ankle. Arthrodesis of the first metatarsal (MTP), arthroplasty of the first MTP, metatarsal head resection, and osteotomies are well-described procedures in the treatment of metatarsalgia and painful hallux valgus. Talonavicular fusion reduces hindfoot pain in about 80 percent of patients with refractory, painful talonavicular arthritis. Ankle arthrodesis is the most predictable surgery in reducing ankle pain, but is often associated with complications. Ankle arthroplasty is not yet a procedure with consistent results and is therefore very rarely indicated.

CONCLUSIONS

Arthritis is one of the most common underlying conditions in patients complaining of pain. Research continues at a rapid pace into the chemical and biomechanical etiologies of joint disease and more specific treatments will likely follow. Regardless of the pathophysiology of the particular arthritis, the general principles of physiatric pain management still apply. These include maximization of the anatomic substrate through correcting faulty postures and strengthening surrounding musculature, pacing, optimizing the psychosocial milieu, and the judicious use of medication and surgical techniques. Like any chronic painful condition, successful treatment of OA and RA involves the artful application of these principles in a program individualized to each patient.

REFERENCES

1. Lawrence RC, Helmick CG, Arnett FC et al. Estimates of the prevalence of arthritis and selected musculoskeletal disorders in the United States. *Arthritis Rheum* 1998; 41:778–99.

2. Yelin E and Callahan LF. The economic cost and social and psychological impact of musculoskeletal conditions. *Arthritis Rheum* 1995; 38:1351–1362.

3. Wyke B. The neurology of joints: a review of general prinicples. *Clin Rheum Dis* 1981; 7:223–239.

4. Schaible HG and Grubb BD. Afferent and spinal mechanisms of joint pain. *Pain* 1993; 55:5–54.

5. Melzack R, Wall PD: Pain mechanisms: A new theory. *Science*. 150:971–979, 1965.

6. Dexter D, Brandt K. Distribution and predictors of depressive symptoms in osteoarthritis. *J Rheumatol* 1993; 21:279–286.

7. Davis MA, Ettinger WH, Neuhaus JM, Barclay JD, Segal MR. Correlates of knee pain among U.S. adults with and without radiographic knee osteoarthritis. *J Rheumatol* 1992; 19(12): 1943–1948.

8. Wegener ST. Psychosocial aspects of rheumatic disease: The developing biopsychosocial framework. *Curr Opin Rheumatol* 1991; 3:300–304.

9. Summers MN, Haley WE, Reveille JD, Alarcon GS. Radiographic assessment and psychologic variables as predictors of pain and functional impairment in osteoarthritis of the knee or hip. *Arthritis Rheum* 1988; 31:204–209.

10. Lorig K, Chastain, RL, Ung E, et al. Development and evaluation of a scale to measure perceived self-efficacy in people with arthritis. *Arthritis Rheum* 1989; 32:37–44.

11. Fries JF, Spitz P, Kraines RG et al. Measurement of patient outcome in arthritis. *Arthritis Rheum* 1980; 23:137–145.

12. Lequesne MG, Mery C, Samson M et al. Indexes of severity for osteoarthritis of the hip and knee. *Scand J Rheumatol* 1987; 65S:85–89.

13. Bellamy N, Buchanan WW, Goldsmith H et al. Validation study of WOMAC: A health status instrument for measuring clinically important patient relevant outcomes to antirheumatic drug therapy in patients with osteoarthritis of the hip or knee. *J Rheumatol* 19; 15:1833–1840.

14. Crook J, Rideout E , Browne G. The prevalence of pain complaints in a general population. *Pain* 1984; 18:299–314.

15. McCarthy C, Cushnaghan J, Dieppe P. Osteoarthritis. In: Wall PD, Melzack R (eds.), *Textbook of Pain*, 3rd edition. Edinburgh: Churchill Livingstone, 1994.

16. Arnoldi CC, Djurhuus JC, Heerfordt J et al. Intraosseous phlebography, intraosseous pressure measurements and 99mTc polyphosphate scintigraphy in patients with various painful conditions in the hip and knee. *Acta Orthopaedica Scandinavica* 1980; 51:19–28.

17. Brandt KD and Slemenda CW. In: Schumacher HR, Klippel JH, Koopman WJ (eds.), *Primer on the Rheumatic Diseases,* 10th edition. Atlanta: The Arthritis Foundation, 1993.

18. American College of Rheumatology Ad Hoc Committee on Clinical Guidelines. Guidelines for the initial evaluation of the adult patient with acute musculoskeletal symptoms. *Arthritis Rheum* 1996; 39:1–8

19. Williams HJ, Ward JR, Egger MJ et al. Comparison of naproxen and acetaminophen in a two-year study of treatment of osteoarthitis of the knee. *Arthritis Rheum* 1993; 36:1196–1206.

20. Bradley JD, Brandt KD, Katz BP et al. Comparison of an antiinflammatory dose of ibuprofen, an analgesic dose of ibuprofen, and acetaminophen in the treatment of patients with osteoarthritis of the knee. *N Eng J Med* 1991; 325:87–91.

21. McCormack K. Nonsteroidal antiinflammatory drugs and spinal nociceptive processing. *Pain* 1994; 59:9–43.

22. Fort J. Celecoxib, a COX–2–specific inhibitor: The clinical data. *Am J Orthopedics* 1999; 28(3Supp):13–18.

23. Harden RN, Bruehl SP, Backonja MM. The use of opioids in treatment of chronic pain: An examination of the ongoing controversy. *J Back Musculoskel Rehab* 1997; 9:155–180.

24. Ytterberg SR, Maren ML, Woods SR. Codeine and oxycodone use in patients with chronic rheumatic disease pain. *Arthritis Rheum* 1998; 41(9):1603–1612

25. Hochberg MC, Altman RD, Brandt KD et al. Guidelines for the medical management of osteoarthritis. *Arthritis Rheum* 1995; 38:1535–1546.

26. Mao J, Price DD, Mayer DJ. Experimental mononeuropathy reduces the antinociceptive effects of morphine: Implications for common intracellular mechanisms involved in morphine tolerance and neuropathic pain. *Pain* 1995; 61:353–364.

27. Katz WA. The role of tramadol in the management of musculoskeletal pain. *Today's Therapeutic Trends* 1995; 13:177–186.

28. Scnitzer TJ, Kamin M, Olson WH. Tramadol allows reduction of naproxen dose among patients with naproxen-responsive osteoarthritis pain. A randomized, double-blind, placebo controlled study. *Arthritis Rheum* 1999:42(7):1370–1377.

29. Wollheim FA. Current pharmacologic treatment of osteoarthritis. *Drugs* 1996; 52Suppl3:27–38.

30. Monks R. Psychotropic drugs. In:Wall PD, Melzack R (eds.), *Textbook of Pain,* 3rd edition. Edinburgh: Churchill Livingtone, 1994.

31. Carette S, McCain GA, Bell DA, Fam AG. Evaluation of amitriptyline in primary fibrositis : A double-blind, placebo-controlled study. *Arthritis Rheum* 1986; 29:655–659.

32. Deal CL, Schnitzer TJ, Lipstein E et al. Treatment of arthritis with topical capsaicin: A double blind trial. *Clin Ther* 1991; 13:383–395.

33. McCarthy GM and McCarty DJ. Effect of topical capsaicin in the therapy of painful ostcoarthritis of the hands. *J Rheumatol* 1992; 19:604–607.

34. Algozzine et al. Trolamine salicylate cream in osteoarthritis of the knee. *JAMA* 1982; 247:1311–1313.

35. Acupuncture. NIH Consensus Statement. 1997 Nov 3–4; 15(5):1–34.

36. McAlindon TE, Felson DT, Zhang Y et al. Relation of dietary intake and scrum levels of vitamin D to progression of osteoarthritis of the knee among participants of the Framingham study. *Ann Int Med* 1996; 125:353–359.

37. McAlindon TE, Jacques P, Zhang Y et al. Do antioxidant micronutrients protect against the development and progression on knee osteoarthritis? *Arth Rheum* 1996:39(4); 648–656.

38. Pipitone VR. Chondroprotection with chondroitin sulfate. *Drugs Exp Clin Res* 1991; 17:3.

39. Morreale P. Comparison of the antiinflammatory efficacy of chondroitin sulfate and diclofenac sodium in patients with knee osteoarthritis. *J Rheumatol* 1996; 23:1385.

40. Leeb BF, Petera P, Neumann K. [Results of a multicenter study of chondroitin sulfate (Condrosulf) use in arthroses of the finger, knee and hip joints] {German}. *Wiener Medizinische Wochenschrift* 1996; 146:604–614.

41. Barclay TS, Tsourounis C, McCart GM. Glucosamine. *Ann Pharmacother* 1998; 32:574–579.

42. Drovanti A. Therapeutic activity of oral glucosamine sulfate in osteoarthritis: A placebo-controlled double-blind investigation. *Clin Ther* 1980; 3:260.

43. Qi GX, Gao SN, Giacovelli G et al. Efficacy and safety of glucosamine sulfate versus ibuprofen in patients with knee osteoarthritis. *Arzneimittelforschung* 1998; 48:469–474.

44. Vas AL. Doubleblind clinical evaluation of the relative efficacy of ibuprofen and glucosamine sulfate in the management of osteoarthritis of the knee in outpatients. *Curr Med Res Opin* 1982; 8:145–149.

45. Creamer P. Intra-articular corticosteroid injections in osteoarthritis: do they work and if so, how? *Ann Rheum Dis* 1997; 56:634–36.

46. Adams ME, Atkinson MH, Lussier AJ et al. The role of viscosupplementation with hylan G–F 20 (Synvisc) in the treatment of osteoarthritis of the knee: A Canadian multicenter trial comparing hylan G–F 20 alone, hylan G–F 20 with nonsteroidal antiin-

flammatory drugs (NSAIDs) and NSAIDs alone. *Osteoarthritis and Cartilage* 1995; 3:213–225.

47. Balazs EA and Denlinger JL. Viscosupplementation: A new concept in the treatment of osteoarthritis. *J Rheumatol* 1993; supp 39; 20:3–9.

48. Scale D, Wobig M, Wolpert W. Viscosupplementation of osteoarthritic knees with hylan: A treatment schedule study. *Current Therapeutic Research* 1994; 55:220–232.

49. Yasui T, Akatsuka M, Tobetto K. Effects of hyaluronan on the production of stromelysin and tissue inhibitor of mettaloproteinase–1 in bovine articular chondrocytes. *Biomedical Research*. 1992; 13:343–348.

50. Tobetto K, Nakai K, Akatsuka M, et al: Inhibitory effects of hyaluronan on neutrophil mediated cartilage degredation. *Connect Tissue Res* 1993; 29:181–190.

51. Armstrong S, Read R, Ghosh P. The effects of intraarticular hyaluronan on cartilage and subchondral bone changes in an ovine model of early osteoarthritis. *J Rhematol.* 21:680–688, 199.

52. Brandt KD. Osteoarthritis. In: *Harrison's Principles of Internal Medicine*. New York: McGraw-Hill, 1994; 13:1692–1698.

53. Wobig M, Dickhut A, Maier R et al. Viscosupplementation with hylan G–F 20: A 26–week controlled trial of efficacy and safety in the osteoarthritic knee. *Clin Ther* 1998; 20:410–423.

54. Creamer P, Sharif M, George E, et al. Intraarticular hyaluronic acid in osteoarthritis of the knee: An investigation into mechanisms of action. *Osteoarthritis and Cartilage,* 2; 133–140, 1994.

55. Listrat V, Ayral X, Patarnello F et al. evaluation of the potential structure modifying activity of hyaluronan (hyalgan) in osteoarthritis of the knee. *Osteoarthritis and Cartilage.* 1997; 5:153–160.

56. Felson DT, Zhang Y, Anthony JM, Naimark A, Anderson JJ. Weight loss reduces the risk for symptomatic osteoarthritis in women. The Framingham Study. *Ann Intern Med* 1992, 116(7):535–539.

57. Alpiner NM, Oh TN, Brander VA. Rehabilitation in joint and connective tissue diseases. *SAE Study Guide* 1995, 76(55) 532.

58. VanBaar ME, Assendelft WJ, Dekker J et al. Effectiveness of exercise therapy in patients with osteoarthritis of the hip or knee: a systematic review of randomized clinical trials. *J Rheumatol* 1998; 25(12); 2432–2439.

59. Kovar PA, Allegrante JP, MacKenzie CR, et al. Supervised fitness walking in patients with osteoarthritis of the knee. *Ann Intern Med* 1992; 116:529–534.

60. Perlman SG, Connell KJ, Clark A et al. Dance-based aerobic exercise for rheumatoid arthritis. *Arthritis Care Res* 1990; 3:29–35.

61. Semble EL, Loeser RF, Wise CM. Therapeutic exercise for rheumatoid arthritis and osteoarthritis. *Semin Arthritis Rheum* 1990; 20:32–40.

62. Byers PH. Effect of exercise on morning stiffness and mobility in patients with rheumatoid arthritis. *Res Nurs Health* 1985; 8:275–281.

63. Minor MA, Hewitt JE, Webel RR et al. Efficacy of physical conditioning exercise on inpatients with RA and OA. *Arthritis Rheum* 1989; 32:1396–1405.

64. Fisher NM, Pendergast DR, Gresham GE, Calkins E. Muscle rehabilitation: Its effect on muscular and functional performance of patients with knee OA. *Arch Phys Med Rehabil* 1991; 72:367–374.

65. Ekdahl C, Andersson SI, Moritz V, Svensson B. dynamic v. static training in patients with RA. *Scand J Rheumatol* 1990; 19: 17–26.

66. Chamberlain MA, Care G, Harfield B. Physiotherapy in osteoarthritis of the knees. A controlled trial of hospital versus home exercises. *Int Rehabil Med* 1982, 4:101–106.

67. Feinberg J, Marzouk D, Sokolek C, Katz B, Bradley J, Brandt K. Effects of isometric versus range of motion exercises on joint pain and function in patients with knee osteoarthritis (abstract). *Arth Rheum* 1992, 35 (Suppl 5): R28.

68. Keefe FJ and Caldwell DS. Cognitive behavioral control of arthritis pain. *Med Clinics N Am* 1997; 81:277–290.

69. Keefe FJ, Caldwell DS, Williams DA et al. Pain coping skills training in the management of osteoarthritic knee pain: A comparative study. *Behav Ther* 1990; 21:49–62.

70. Lorig KR, Mazonson PD, Holman HR. Evidence suggesting that health education for self-management in patients with chronic arthritis sustained health benefits while reducing health care costs. *Arthritis Rheum* 1993; 36: 439–446.

71. Weinberger M, Tierney WM, Cowpar PA et al. Cost-effectiveness of increased telephone contact for patients with osteoarthritis: A randomized controlled trial. *Arthritis Rheum* 1993; 36:243–246.

72. Nicholas JJ, Gruen H et al. Splinting in rheumatoid arthritis. I. Factors affecting patient compliance. *Arch Phys Med Rehab* 63:92–94, 1982.

73. Falconer J, Hayes, KW, Chang, RW. Effect of ultrasound on mobility in osteoarthritis of the knee. A radomized clinical trial. *Arth Care Res* 5:29–35, 1992.

74. Chang RW, Falconer J, Stulberg SD et al. A randomized controlled trial of arthroscopic surgery versus closed needle lavage for patients with osteoarthritis of the knee. *Arth Rheum* 1993; 36:289–296.

75. Harris WH and Sledge CB. Total hip and total knee replacement, parts 1 and 2. *N Eng J Med* 1990; 323:725–31, 801–807.

76. Chang RW, Pellissier JM, Hazen GB. A cost-effectiveness analysis of total hip arthroplasty for osteoarthritis of the hip. *JAMA* 1996; 275:858–865.

77. Brander VA, Malhotra S, Jet J et al. Outcome of hip and knee arthroplasty in persons aged 80 years and older. *Clin Ortho Rel Res* 1997; 345:67–78.

78. Wilder RL. Rheumatoid arthritis: epidemiology, pathology and pathogenesis. In: Schumacher HR, Klippel JH, Koopman WJ (eds.), *Primer on the Rheumatic Diseases,* 10th edition. Atlanta: Arthritis Foundation, 1993, 86–89.

79. Pincus T, Callahan LF. Reassessment of twelve traditional paradigms concerning the diagnosis, prevalence, morbidity, and mortality of rheumatoid arthritis. *Scan J Rheum* 1989, Suppl.79:67.

80. Pincus T, Callahan LF. Early mortality in rheumatoid arthritis predicted by poor clinical status. *Bull Rheum Dis* 1992; 41:4.

81. Wilske KR, Healy LA. Remodeling the pyramid: A concept whose time has come. *J Rheumatol* 1989; 16(5):565–567.

82. Elliot MJ, Maini RN, Feldmann M. Repeated therapy with monoclonal antibody to TNFa (cA2) in patients with RA. *Lancet* 1994; 344:1125–1127.

83. Group GLS. Double-blind controlled Phase III multicenter clinical trial with interferon gamma in rheumatoid arthritis. *Rheumatol Int* 1992:12:175–185.

84. Hawley DJ, Wolfe F. Anxiety and depression in patients with rheumatoid arthritis: A prospective study of 400 patients. *J Rheumatol* 1988; 15:932–941.

85. Katz PP, Yelin EH. The development of depressive symptoms among women with RA: The role of function. *Arthritis Rheum* 1995; 38: 49–56.

86. Hagglund HJ, Haley WE, Reveille JD, Alarcon GS. Predicting individual differences in pain and functional impairment among patients with RA. *Arthritis Rheum* 1989; 32:851–858.

87. Frank RG, Hagglund KJ. Mood Disorders. In: Wegener ST, Belza BL, Gall EP (eds.), *Clinical Care in the Rheumatic Diseases.* Atlanta: American College of Rheumatology, 1996:125–130.

88. Gerber LH. Exercise and arthritis. *Bull Rheum Dis* 1990; 39:1–9.

89. Nordemar R. Physical training in rheumatoid arthritis: a controlled long-term study. II. Functional capacity and general attitudes. *Scand J Rheum* 1981; 10:25–30.

90. Nordemar R, Ekblom B, Zachrisson L et al. Physical training in rheumatoid arthritis: A controlled long-term study. I. Functional capacity and general attitudes. *Scand J Rheum* 1981; 10:17–23.

91. Hicks SE. Exercise in patients with inflammatory arthritis and connective tissue disease. *Rheum Dis Clinics NA* 1990; 16(4):845.

92. Clark SR, Burckhardt CS, Bennett RM. Exercise for prevention and treatment of illness. In *Exercise for prevention and treatment of illness.*

93. Basmajian JV and Wolf SL. In: Gerber LH, Hicks JE (eds.), *Therapeutic Exercise*, 5th edition. Baltimore: Williams and Wilkins, 1990; 340.

94. Herbison GJ, Ditunno Jr, Jaweed MM. Muscle atrophy in rheumatoid arthritis. *J Rheumatol* 1987; S15(14):78–81.

95. Lefebvre JC, KeefeFJ, Affleck G et al. The relationship of arthritis self-efficacy to daily pain, daily mood, and daily pain coping in rheumatoid arthritis patients. *Pain* 1999; 80:425–435.

96. Parker JC, Smarr KL, Buckelew SP et al. Effects of stress management on clinical outcomes in rheumatoid arthritis. *Arthritis Rheum* 1995; 38:1807–1818.

97. Williams J, Harvey J, Tannenbaum H. Use of superficial heat versus ice for the rheumatoid arthritic shoulder: A pilot study. *Physiotherapy Canada* 38:8–13, 1986.

98. Green J, McKenna F, Redfern EJ, Chamberlain MA: Home exercises are as effective as outpatient hydrotherapy for osteoarthritis of the hip. *Br J Rheumatol* 32:812–815, 1993.

99. Mainardi CL, Walter JM, Spiegel PK, et al. Rheumatoid arthritis: Failure of daily heat therapy to affect its progression. *Arch Phys Med Rehabil* 1979:60(9); 390–393.

100. Hashish I, Harvey W, Harris M. Antiinflammatory effects of ultrasound therapy: evidence for major placebo effect. *Br J Rheumatol* 25:77–81, 1986.

101. Oosterveld FGJ, Rasker JJ< Jacobs JWG, Overmars HJA. The effect of local heat and cold therapy on the intraarticular and skin surface temperature of the knee. *Arthritis Rheum* 1992; 35:146–151.

102. Kumar VN, Redford JB. Transcutaneous nerve stimulation in rheumatoid arthritis. *Arch Phys Med Rehabil* 63:75–78, 1987.

103. Hayes KW. Physical Modalities. In: Wegener ST, Belza BL, Gall EP (eds.), *Clinical Care in the Rheumatic Diseases*. Atlanta: American College of Rheumatology, 1996: 79–82.

104. Partridge REH, Duthie JJR. Controlled trial of the effect of complete immobilization of the joints in rheumatoid arthritis. *Ann Rheum Dis* 22:91–99, 1963.

105. Gault SJ, Spyker JM: Beneficial effects of immobilization of joints in rheumatoid arthritis and related arthritidities: A splint study using sequential analysis. *Arthritis Rheum* 12:34–44, 1969.

106. Boden SD. Rheumatoid arthritis of the cervical spine. Surgical decision making based on predictors of paralysis and recovery. *Spine* 1994; 19(20):2275–2280.

107. Goldberg, VM, Figgie HE, Inglis AE, Figgie MP. Current concepts review: Total elbow arthroplasty. *J Bone Joint Surg* 1988; 70–A:778–783.

108. Jolly SL, Ferlic DC, Clayton ML, Dennis DA, Stringer EA. Swanson silicone arthroplasty of wrist in rheumatoid arthritis: A long-term follow-up. *J Hand Surg* 1992:17:142–149.

12 | Pain Management and Cancer

Helene Henson, M.D.
Uma Monga, M.D.

The focus of this chapter is to review common cancer pain syndromes, outline assessment of these syndromes, and review the progress made in cancer pain management, emphasizing the need for interdisciplinary treatment approaches to various painful cancer conditions.

Cancer pain is common and extremely heterogeneous. Although the exact prevalence is not known, pain is reported by nearly 50 percent of patients at all stages of the disease and by more than 70 percent of patients with advanced neoplasms (1). The prevalence of pain varies depending on the cancer site, stage of the disease, and the population studied. For example, Greenwald et al. (1987) reported that moderate to severe pain occurred in more than 50 percent of patients with lung cancer, in about 38 percent of patients with prostate and uterine cancer, and in 60 percent of patients with pancreatic cancer (2). Portenoy et al. (1992) reported a pain prevalence rate of 33 percent in patients attending an outpatient ambulatory clinic, but the prevalence of pain was 74 percent in advanced cancer patients reported by a hospital team (3,4). According to Daut et al. (1982), 40 to 50 percent of patients with advanced cancer experience moderate to severe pain, and in 25 to 30 percent the pain is severe or excruciating (5). In another study, 84 percent of the patients receiving hospice care for advanced cancer reported pain (6).

Pain leads to various psychosocial problems. According to Storm et al. (1992), the high risk of suicide during the first two years after diagnosis is in part caused by severe pain and the failure of physicians to meet the somatic and psychosocial needs of the patient (7).

In response to the need for pain management, several practice guidelines and algorithms have been developed (8–11). In 2000, the National Comprehensive Cancer Network (NCCN) published practice guidelines (version 2000) for treating cancer pain (see Figures 12.1 through 12.5) (12). Despite these guidelines, unrelieved cancer pain remains a problem not only for the patient and family but for the treating physician as well.

There are several barriers to the implementation of cancer pain management (see Figure 12.6). Pain control has been a low priority in the healthcare industry. Healthcare providers are reluctant to accept pain relief as one of their responsibil-

233

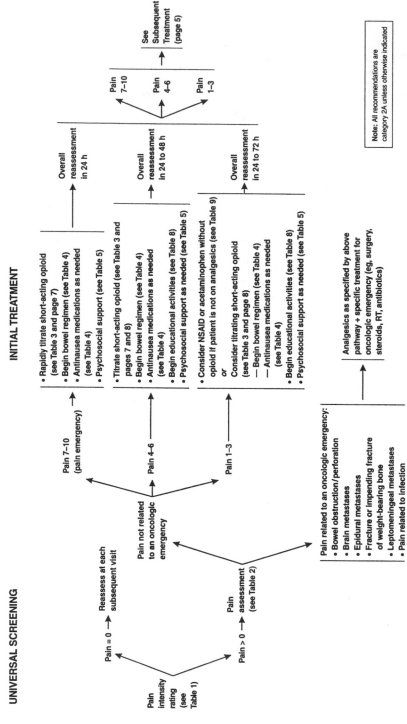

Figure 12.1. NCCN cancer pain guidelines. (Reproduced with permission from *Oncology* 2000; 14:135–150; Natural Comprehensive Cancer Network, Rockledge, PA.)

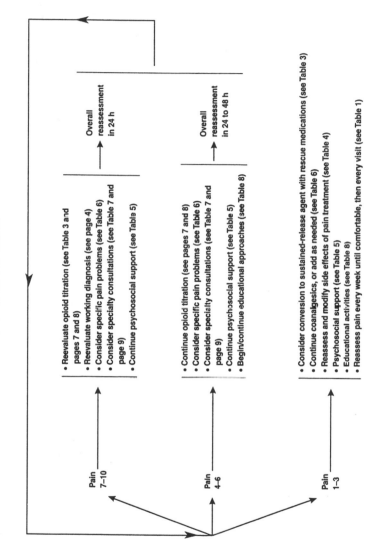

SUBSEQUENT TREATMENT

Pain 7–10
- Reevaluate opioid titration (see Table 3 and pages 7 and 8)
- Reevaluate working diagnosis (see page 4)
- Consider specific pain problems (see Table 6)
- Consider specialty consultations (see Table 7 and page 9)
- Continue psychosocial support (see Table 5)

Overall reassessment in 24 h

Pain 4–6
- Continue opioid titration (see pages 7 and 8)
- Consider specific pain problems (see Table 6)
- Consider specialty consultations (see Table 7 and page 9)
- Continue psychosocial support (see Table 5)
- Begin/continue educational approaches (see Table 8)

Overall reassessment in 24 to 48 h

Pain 1–3
- Consider conversion to sustained-release agent with rescue medications (see Table 3)
- Continue coanalgesics, or add as needed (see Table 6)
- Reassess and modify side effects of pain treatment (see Table 4)
- Psychosocial support (see Table 5)
- Educational activities (see Table 8)
- Reassess pain every week until comfortable, then every visit (see Table 1)

Figure 12.2. NCCN cancer pain guidelines (cont.).

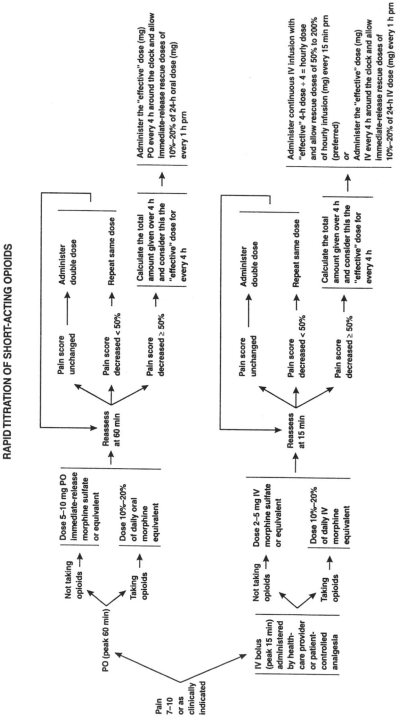

Figure 12.3. NCCN cancer pain guidelines (cont.).

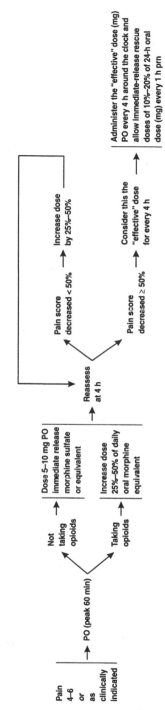

SLOWER TITRATION OF SHORT-ACTING OPIOIDS

Pain 4–6 or as clinically indicated → PO (peak 60 min)

Not taking opioids → Dose 5–10 mg PO immediate release morphine sulfate or equivalent

Taking opioids → Increase dose 25%–50% of daily oral morphine equivalent

→ Reassess at 4 h

Pain score decreased < 50% → Increase dose by 25%–50%

Pain score decreased ≥ 50% → Consider this the "effective" dose for every 4 h → Administer the "effective" dose (mg) PO every 4 h around the clock and allow immediate-release rescue doses of 10%–20% of 24-h oral dose (mg) every 1 h prn

Figure 12.4. NCCN cancer pain guidelines (cont.).

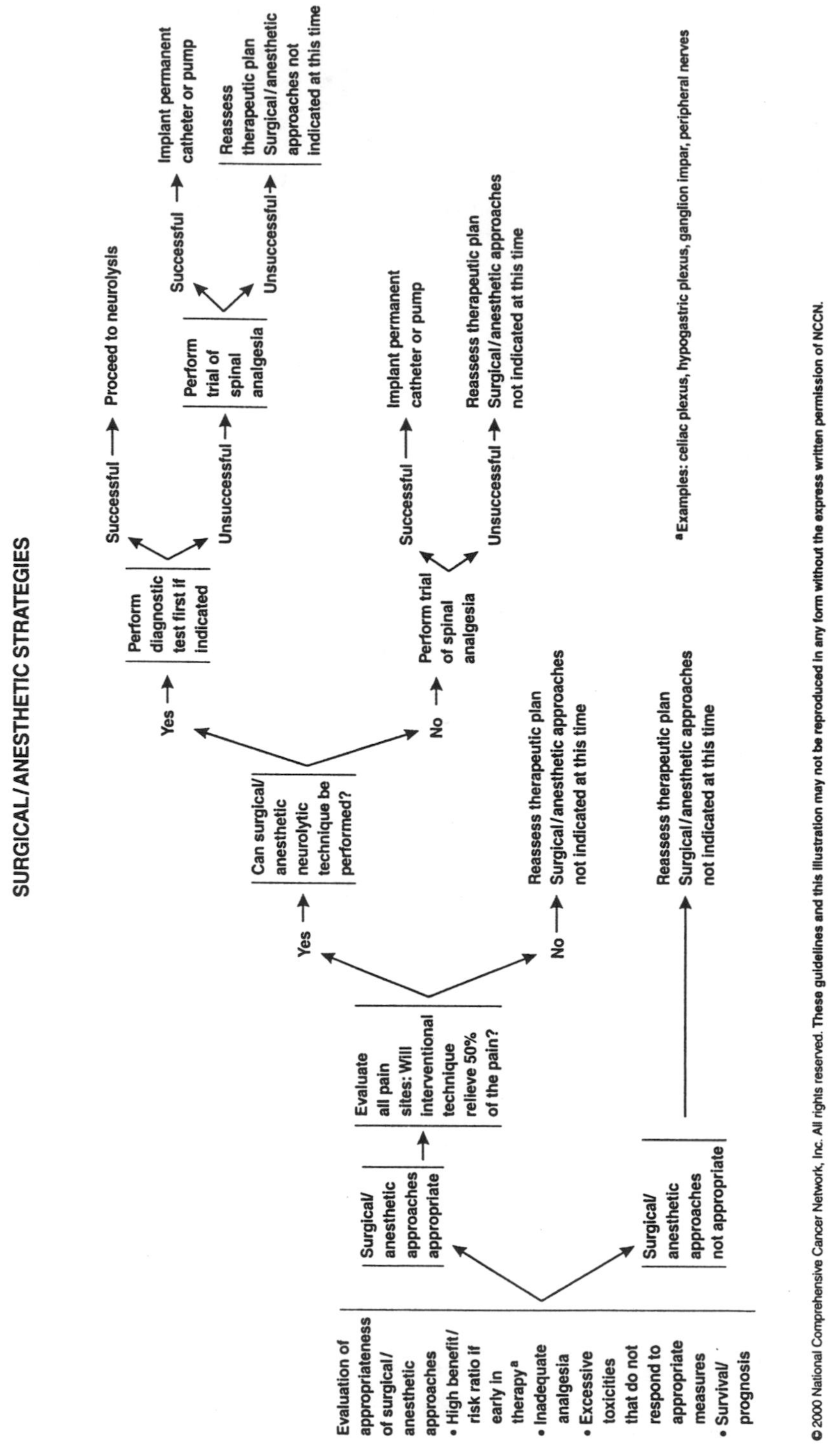

SURGICAL/ANESTHETIC STRATEGIES

Evaluation of appropriateness of surgical/anesthetic approaches
- High benefit/risk ratio if early in therapy[a]
- Inadequate analgesia
- Excessive toxicities that do not respond to appropriate measures
- Survival/prognosis

→ Surgical/anesthetic approaches appropriate → Evaluate all pain sites: Will interventional technique relieve 50% of the pain?

→ Surgical/anesthetic approaches not appropriate → Reassess therapeutic plan Surgical/anesthetic approaches not indicated at this time

Evaluate all pain sites: Will interventional technique relieve 50% of the pain?
- Yes → Can surgical/anesthetic neurolytic technique be performed?
- No → Reassess therapeutic plan Surgical/anesthetic approaches not indicated at this time

Can surgical/anesthetic neurolytic technique be performed?
- Yes → Perform diagnostic test first if indicated
- No → Perform trial of spinal analgesia

Perform diagnostic test first if indicated
- Successful → Proceed to neurolysis
- Unsuccessful → Perform trial of spinal analgesia
  - Successful → Implant permanent catheter or pump
  - Unsuccessful → Reassess therapeutic plan Surgical/anesthetic approaches not indicated at this time

Perform trial of spinal analgesia
- Successful → Implant permanent catheter or pump
- Unsuccessful → Reassess therapeutic plan Surgical/anesthetic approaches not indicated at this time

[a] Examples: celiac plexus, hypogastric plexus, ganglion impar, peripheral nerves

Figure 12.5. NCCN cancer pain guidelines (cont.).

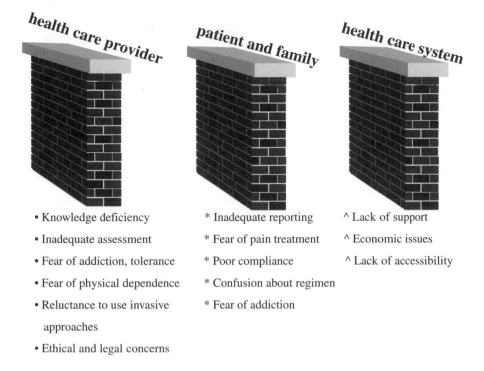

health care provider

- Knowledge deficiency
- Inadequate assessment
- Fear of addiction, tolerance
- Fear of physical dependence
- Reluctance to use invasive
  approaches
- Ethical and legal concerns

patient and family

* Inadequate reporting
* Fear of pain treatment
* Poor compliance
* Confusion about regimen
* Fear of addiction

health care system

^ Lack of support
^ Economic issues
^ Lack of accessibility

Figure 12.6. Barriers to cancer pain management.

ities, often because they lack the clinical knowledge or resources needed to alleviate pain (13). Healthcare providers may fail to recognize and treat cancer pain (14). Several authors report that one of the major barriers to treating cancer pain is the insufficient education of doctors worldwide in cancer pain management (15–17). Furthermore, pain caused by cancer and its treatment is often considered inevitable.

Patients, too, may be reluctant to discuss pain problems with their physicians and other care providers. They may have many concerns regarding addiction, tolerance, and physical dependence. These concerns may not surface until strong therapeutic relationships have developed. In a recent study of physicians, patient reluctance to report pain and take opioids was considered among the top four barriers to effective treatment (18).

CANCER PAIN SYNDROMES

Cancer pain may be classified according to its temporal patterns (acute, chronic, breakthrough); neurophysiologic mechanisms (visceral, neuropathic, and somatic); and specific cancer-related causes. Pain in cancer patients may be the result of the tumor itself and anticancer treatments, or it may be unrelated to the cancer and its treatment (see Table 12.1) (19).

Table 12.1. Etiology of Pain in Cancer Patients

Direct tumor involvement (70%)
    Invasion of bone
    Invasion or compression of neural structures
    Obstruction of hollow viscus or ductal systems of solid viscus
    Vascular obstruction or invasion
    Mucous membrane ulceration or involvement

Diagnostic or therapeutic procedures (20%)
    Procedure related pain
        bone marrow aspiration
        biopsy
        lumbar puncture
    Acute postoperative pain or postoperative syndromes
        postthoracotomy
        postmastectomy
        postamputation
    Postradiation
        injury to plexus
        injury to spinal cord
        mucositis
        enteritis
    Postchemotherapy
        mucositis
        peripheral neuropathy
        aseptic necrosis

Cancer-induced Syndromes (<10%)
    Paraneoplastic syndromes
    Pain associated with debility
        bedsores
        constipation
        bladder spasm
        postherpetic neuralgia

Pain unrelated to the malignancy or its treatment (<10%)

Reprinted with permission from Grossman SA, Saats PS, *Oncology*, volume 8, number 3, 1994 p. 94.

    Direct tumor involvement of bone, nerve, or viscera is the most common cause of cancer-related pain and is responsible for pain in approximately two-thirds of patients with metastatic cancer (20). Most painful metastases (50 percent) are caused by tumor invasion of bone; the remaining patients experience pain as a result of gastrointestinal tract, nerve, or soft tissue invasion.

    Pain resulting from cancer treatments such as surgery, chemotherapy, and radiation therapy accounts for 19 to 28 percent of painful conditions (21). Postsurgery pain is usually acute and severe. It is commonly seen in patients undergoing thoracotomy, mastectomy, radical neck dissection, amputation, and nephrectomy. Postsurgical pain may be caused by wound infection, nerve injury, or injury to other soft tissues. Chemotherapy may cause painful polyneuropathy, mucositis, cranial neuralgia, and phlebitis. Postradiation pain syndromes are secondary to fibrosis of the brachial or lumbosacral plexus, myelopathy, mucositis, esophagitis, and bone necrosis.

In some patients the pain is not related to the cancer or the cancer therapy. About 3 to 10 percent of patients have this etiology (22). Accurate diagnosis in this group can alter both therapy and prognosis. It is important to understand that physical, emotional, social, spiritual, and cultural facets affect the perception, experience, and severity of pain.

PAIN MANAGEMENT

Although there have always been efforts to palliate cancer pain, the idea that pain relief can and should be a part of the standard of care for the cancer patient is relatively new (13). Pain is a multidimensional problem (see Figure 12.7). A conceptual framework of cancer pain management has been provided by Ahlers et al. (23) and McGuire (1995) (24). This framework identifies six dimensions of cancer pain: physiologic (organic etiology); sensory (intensity, quality, location); affective (depression, anxiety); cognitive (influence of pain on thought processes, meaning of pain); behavioral (involvement in treatment plan); and sociocultural (demographic, social, and cultural influences). This multidimensional framework encompasses the basic concepts of impairment, disability, and handicap. It is recommended that all patients with cancer should be screened for pain using this model every time they are seen.

A full assessment of pain in cancer patients therefore includes a comprehensive history and physical examination with specific reference to pain quality, intensity, and location. The history should also include the duration and course of pain. Note should be made of any aggravating and alleviating factors. Associated symptoms, such as sleep deprivation, fatigue, nausea, and vomiting should be documented. Assessment of functional limitations secondary to pain should be carried out. A history of previous interventions for pain relief, including drug therapy, should be documented. In addition, the pain should be evaluated in terms of the role it plays in the overall suffering of the patient and his care providers. Psychosocial functioning and provision of family support must be considered. The physician must be aware that patient attitudes and fears may make it difficult to perform a comprehensive assessment. Finally, a review of laboratory and imaging studies must be included in this assessment, and other appropriate investigations should be performed to elucidate pain mechanisms.

Undertreatment of cancer pain may be caused by an inadequate assessment of the problem. It is important to determine the underlying cause of pain before deciding on possible methods of pain control. This also helps to determine what other specific therapy is required along with analgesics.

General Management

Pain in cancer is not just a medical issue, and pain management should not be seen in isolation, but as part of a continuum of care provided by a group of professionals (25). The impact of pain on many of the aspects of the quality of life also must be considered (see Figure 12.7) (26). The Agency for Health Care Practice and Research (AHCPR) guidelines stress the need for a collaborative multidisciplinary approach to the management of cancer pain, with the patient acting as the central member of this multidisciplinary team (8). Furthermore, pain management should be tailored to the individual patient so that the need for crisis intervention is minimized.

The goals of pain management are to decrease pain and improve the quality of life. These goals should be achieved by effective utilization of resources. Some of the critical elements of such a management program are: (*a*) to allow a patient to make choices, so that her own values and preferences are taken into account in decision making; (*b*) to recognize the patient's needs; (*c*) to provide timely interventions; and (*d*) to do no further harm. Disease modification should always be considered in each patient and, therefore, surgery, radiation therapy, or chemotherapy may be appropriate in some circumstances (27).

To achieve optimum results, patient and family education is very important. Patients need instruction regarding the importance of a balanced diet and a regular exercise program. An explanation about the side effects of drugs and other

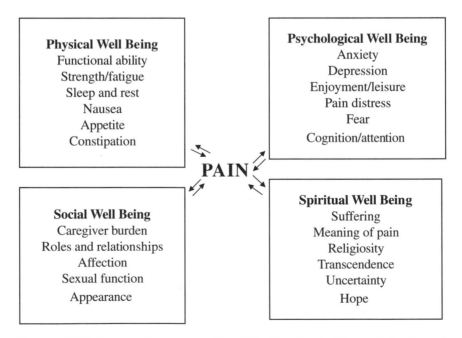

Figure 12.7. Impact of pain on quality of life. Reprinted with permission from Ferrell, BR, *Oncology*, volume 13, supplement 2, May 1999, p. 16.

treatment interventions should be provided, as well as information on coping with those side effects. Patients should be asked to keep a record of pain severity, intensity, frequency, and duration. Patients should also keep note of activity level and other symptoms. Patients and their families should be reassured that pain control is possible. It is important to allow adequate time for the patient and his family to discuss their concerns.

Pharmacotherapy

There are several specific issues that must be considered with the use of pain medications in cancer patients. Many of these patients are elderly or may be taking several medications, thus increasing the potential for drug interaction. The occurrence of malnutrition and the increased incidence of liver and kidney damage by concomitant disease processes affects the choice of medications and the dosages that can be prescribed. Malnourished patients have lower levels of serum proteins and therefore have fewer binding sites, which may increase the risk for adverse effects or toxicity.

In 1986, the World Health Organization (WHO) developed a three-step analgesic ladder for cancer pain management (9). The essential element in the WHO guidelines is the sequential use of drugs by mouth and by the clock. The feasibility and efficacy of the analgesic ladder has been reported in various studies (28–31).

The first step in the analgesic ladder includes the use of nonsteroidal antiinflammatory drugs (NSAIDs) and other nonopioid drugs for mild to moderate pain. An opioid should be added to the NSAID if pain persists or increases in intensity. Opioids conventionally used for moderate pain constitute the second ladder analgesic ladder. The opioids of higher concentration are recommended if the pain continues unrelieved or is severe at the outset. Adjuvant drugs are regularly prescribed according to the patient's needs.

WHO Step I: Nonopioid Analgesics. Nonopioid analgesics, including nonsteroidal antiinflammatory drugs (NSAIDs), are the first line medications for mild to moderate pain. They are most useful in patients with bone pain, and have limited efficacy in patient with neuropathic pain. The safe administration of nonopioid analgesics requires familiarity with their potential adverse effects (32).

Aspirin is one of the most commonly used drugs in clinical practice. It binds with protein and is metabolized through the liver. It is excreted through the kidneys. Side effects include gastrointestinal irritation, gastric ulceration, and tinnitus. Caution should be taken in prescribing aspirin to malnourished patients or patients with liver and end-stage renal disease.

Acetaminophen is an analgesic with a good safety profile. The hepatotoxicity of acetaminophen is dose-dependent and increases in patients with a history of previous liver disease or alcohol abuse.

Both short- and long-term administration of NSAIDs has been reported in cancer pain management (29,33–35). NSAIDs may delay the need for escalating opioid doses or may allow the use of lower doses, thus resulting in fewer central nervous system (CNS) side effects. Risk factors for increased side effects include age, previous renal or gastrointestinal diseases, hypovolemia, and concomitant use of drugs such as anticoagulants. There is a great variability in drug response; failure in using one NSAID can be followed by success with another NSAID. Furthermore, NSAID analgesia is characterized by a *ceiling effect*, meaning that there exists a dose above which additional increments do not provide additional analgesia (36).

The antiinflammatory and subsequent analgesic effects of NSAIDs are believed to be achieved through a peripheral mechanism, related to the inhibition of the enzyme cyclooxygenase, and a consequent reduction of inflammatory mediators (37). Concomitant prophylactic treatment with antacids or H2 receptor antagonists may be indicated to reduce the risk of gastric and duodenal ulcerations. It is reported that newer selective cyclooxygenase-2 (COX-2) inhibitors, such as rofecoxib (Vioxx®) and celecoxib (Celebrex®), do not interfere with the synthesis of protective prostaglandins in gastric mucosa, thus decreasing the gastrointestinal side effects. The COX-2 inhibitors may be of benefit in treating pain in cancer patients (38).

WHO Step II: Weak Opioid Analgesics.

Opiate medications, or derivatives of morphine, produce analgesia by binding to specific receptor sites in the CNS. They are recommended for moderate to severe pain, or pain that has not responded to the first line of medications.

It is common to initiate therapy either with codeine, oxycodone, or hydrocodone, combined with aspirin or acetaminophen. To avoid adverse effects or overdosage, therapy is begun with the lowest possible dose and titrated upward as needed. The patient should always be placed on a scheduled dosing routine to provide the most optimal pain control possible. To decrease the risk of addictive behavior, the patient should be placed on long-acting agents with rescue doses of immediate-release medication for breakthrough pain. Individualization of therapy is emphasized to minimize side effects and to improve the response (39). The physician must be aware of the potential development of physical tolerance after prolonged use of a specific opiate medication and the great variability in response to different opioid drugs.

The WHO step II opioids include hydrocodone (10 mg every 3 to 4 hours), oxycodone (10 mg every 3 to 4 hours), with APAP or ASA, and tramadol. Tramadol (Ultram®) is an opioid agonist that binds to the opioid receptors in the CNS, but has a lower incidence side effects and allegedly lower abuse potential than other opioids. The usual dose for tramadol is 50 mg QID. Relatively low protein binding occurs using tramadol, but dosages may need to be lowered in patients with liver or kidney damage. Similar to the NSAIDs, there is a great variability in the response of a patient to different opioid drugs (39).

WHO Step III: Strong Opioids.

A change from step II to step III is usually implemented when analgesia for increasing pain from cancer progression is inadequate or when the side effects of the drugs administered become intolerable. For moderate to severe pain, strong opioids plus nonopioids are prescribed. Examples of stronger opioids include morphine (in both an immediate release formulation administered at 10 mg every 3 to 4 hours, and a sustained-release form administered at 30 mg q 12 hour), hydromorphone (4 to 6 mg every 3 to 4 hour), oxycodone (20 mg q 12 hour), methadone, and fentanyl. Fentanyl is available for transdermal administration; however many patients require oral rescue doses (8).

In step III, oral opioid analgesics remain the preferred method of delivery primarily because of convenience and cost. If oral dosing is not possible, other routes of opioid administration are available, including transdermal, intrathecal (IT), intramuscular (IM), subcutaneous (SQ), intravenous (IV), rectal (PR), and via a nebulizer.

Transdermal application of fentanyl (Duragesic®), may be helpful in patients who have difficulty of taking oral medications. It may provide 48 to 72 hours of pain relief. Because it takes from 12 to 24 hours for the serum concentration from transdermal patches to stabilize, a shorter acting form of opioid should be prescribed during this period to achieve pain relief.

Morphine can be administered intrathecally or via an epidural route. This approach allows the use of lower doses of the medications with a comcomitant decreased risk of side effects and a more consistent level of pain control. There is a risk of infection, and proper care for surgical sites is recommended. Morphine can also be delivered through intramuscular, subcutaneous, and intravenous injections. Patient-controlled analgesia (PCA) may be prescribed in certain circumstances, such as during the late stages of the disease.

Common side effects of opioid analgesics include gastrointestinal symptoms such as nausea, vomiting, and constipation, and neurologic manifestations such as delirium, attention deficits, and disorientation. Respiratory depression may occur.

The role of weak opioids in the treatment of moderate pain has been questioned in a meta-analysis by Eisenberg et al. (40). The authors examined twenty-five randomized control trials of the use of NSAIDs in cancer patients. The conclusions drawn from their study were that (a) the efficacy of single-dose NSAIDs is greater than placebo and is approximately equivalent to 5 to 10 mg of parenteral morphine; (b) the analgesic efficacy achieved with single and multiple doses of weak opioids is no greater than that achieved with NSAIDs alone; and (c) neither single or multiple doses of weak opioid and NSAID combinations produce greater analgesia than NSAIDs alone. However, others do not share this conclusion (31,41). A note of caution is necessary in the interpretation of this meta-analysis, because the studies available for inclusion in the meta-analysis formed a heterogeneous group (42).

Adjuvant Analgesics

Numerous adjuvant analgesics from diverse drug classes are commonly used in the management of cancer pain (43). It is generally accepted that the adjuvant analgesics should be used to complement an optimal opioid regimen in patients with cancer pain (43). Furthermore, the existence of large interindividual and intraindividual response variability to these drugs must be recognized. Adjuvant analgesics may be utilized at any stage in the analgesic ladder for treatment of pain in cancer patients. Examples of adjuvant drugs include antidepressants, anticonvulsants, local anesthetics, neuroleptics, and topical agents.

Antidepressant Medications. The efficacy of tricyclic antidepressants (TCAs) has been established for the management of chronic pain, especially for neuropathic or musculoskeletal pain. The indication for use of an antidepressant in cancer patients is persistent neuropathic pain that has failed to respond satisfactorily with opioids. Relative contraindications for the use of TCAs include significant cardiac arrhythmias or the presence of conduction block, symptomatic prostate hypertrophy, or narrow-angle glaucoma. A commonly used TCA is amitriptyline, which is dosed at 10 to 25 mg at night, with the dose gradually increased every few days to 150 mg per day. Another common TCA is nortriptyline, dosed at 25 mg at night, and increased to 150 mg per day. Although antidepressant actions may well contribute to the benefits produced by these drugs in patients with pain, the drugs also have clear primary analgesic effects (43). Pain relief usually occurs earlier than mood changes in chronic pain patients.

Anticonvulsant Medications. Anticonvulsant drugs are widely accepted in the management of chronic neuropathic pain, particularly for intense shooting pain or pain that has a paroxysmal onset (44). The response of the individual patient to the drugs in this category can vary remarkably. Furthermore, there have been no studies to determine the relationship between plasma level and pain relief with these drugs (43). Carbamazepine (Tegretol®, at 200 to 800 mg per day orally) is demonstrated to be helpful in the treatment of neuropathic and other types of pain with dysesthetic and paroxysmal qualities. The presence of leukopenia is a relative contraindication for the use of carbamazepine. Carbamazepine should not be used if the patient is scheduled to receive cytotoxic chemotherapy. Other drugs in this group include phenytoin, clonazepam, and valproic acid.

Gabapentin (Neurontin®) is another adjuvant analgesic. Serum levels of gabapentin are not effected in malnourished patients, because the drug is not highly bound with protein. It is recommended to start at a low dose, such as 100 to 300 mg taken orally at nighttime, and to gradually titrate up to a TID dosage. Divided dosages of up to 300 to 400 mg three times a day may be required (45). Monitoring of liver and renal function is recommended every month for 6 months after starting the medication. Weaning the patient off the drug is recommended because of the risk for rebound seizure activity.

Antiarrhythmics. Dejgard et al. described the use of mexiletine, an oral antiarrhythmic, for the treatment of chronic painful diabetic neuropathy (46). When other medications fail to produce adequate pain relief, mexiletine can be tried; however, a significant side effect profile limits its usage, including palpitations, tremor, and dizziness. Lidocaine may also be used for refractory neuropathic pain via intravenous continuous infusion over 30 minutes at a dosing schedule of 5 mg/kg (8).

Steroidal Agents. In patients with a significant inflammatory response, corticosteroids are often prescribed in combination with opioids to control pain. The prescription of these drugs is essential in the emergency treatment of elevated intracranial pressure and epidural spinal cord compression (8,47). Steroids are part of the standard therapy for tumor-induced spinal cord compression (48). They are also useful in metastatic bone disease and in neuropathic pain. However, these drugs should be used cautiously in cancer patients with suppressed immunity and in those with a history of gastric ulcers or gastrointestinal bleeding (49). Prophylaxis with an H2 blocker may be needed to prevent gastric ulcerations. Other undesirable effects such as myopathy, hyperglycemia, weight gain, and dysphoria may occur during prolonged steroid therapy (8).

Dexamethasone (16 to 24 mg/day) or prednisone (40 to 100 mg/day) may be added to opioids for the management of pain in brachial or lumbosacral plexopathy (8). In acute cases, 50 to 100 mg of dexamethasone in 50 mL of dextrose and water is given via intravenous drip. After the intravenous dose, 4 mg of the drug is given orally every 6 hours. If the patient is going to be treated with radiotherapy, dexamethasone is continued until completion of radiotherapy. Thereafter, corticosteroid use should be gradually tapered.

Other Drugs

Clonidine, an alpha-adrenergic agonist, is shown to produce analgesia and can be administered by transdermal, intravenous, oral, and epidural routes to suppress CNS noradrenergic activity and peripheral sympathetic tone (50–54). Clonidine is a nonspecific analgesic that may be considered for refractory neuropathic pain. Sedation is the major side effect, and hypotension and bradycardia may occur. Max et al. reported the beneficial effects of clonidine in the management of pain in patients with postherpetic neuralgia (55). Eisenach et al. used epidural clonidine for intractable cancer pain (56). Baclofen, an antispasticity medication available both in oral and intrathecal forms, has also been used in patients with neuropathic pain (57).

Topical compounds such as capsaicin and local anesthetics may be considered for neuropathic pain secondary to peripheral nerve injury (58). Watson et al. reported beneficial effects from the local application of topical capsaicin in patients with postmastectomy pain syndrome (59). It was concluded that a cream containing 0.025 percent capsaicin can be an effective analgesic in at least some types of neuropathic pain. Patients may experience a burning sensation with capsaicin application. This feeling may disappear over time. The use of a local anesthetic may also be of benefit in refractory neuropathic pain (60).

Endocrine Therapy

Endocrine therapy has few side effects, making it the preferable palliative treatment modality in hormone-responsive tumors. In metastatic breast cancer, about 33 percent of all patients obtain pain relief after hormone manipulation, and about 50 percent of estrogen receptor–positive prostate cancer patients experience pain relief (61) from endocrine therapy. Tamoxifen dosed at 10 to 20 mg orally twice a day is quite useful for pain control in both pre- and postmenopausal women, although exacerbation is common and may require adjuvant analgesics for a short time (62). Side effects are minimal, and the drug usually is well tolerated. Pannuti and associates (1997) used medroxyprogesterone (MAP), given at a dose of 1500 mg intramuscularly daily, in breast, prostate, and renal cancers (63). Thirty-seven of forty patients (92 percent) with breast cancer pain reported pain relief with MAP. This study showed that tumor hormone responsiveness was not necessary to obtain pain relief (63). Leuprolide, a leuteinizing hormone releasing hormone (LHRH) analog, is highly effective as an initial agent for bone pain (62). Flutamide, an antiandrogen, given orally at 250 mg per day, is also effective and well tolerated (64). Patients who relapse after responding to one type of endocrine therapy may benefit from another type.

REHABILITATION APPROACHES

The basic principles of rehabilitation include prevention of complications resulting from inactivity or immobilization and restoration of function. Inactivity results in deconditioning, both physical and psychological, with a decline in cardiovascular function, loss of bone mass, and muscle weakness and atrophy. Inactive patients are at a higher risk of developing pressure ulcers and infections. The goal of rehabilitation is to identify functional limitations and to train or educate patients on how to regain as much independent function as possible.

The physiatric modalities such as electrical stimulation (TENS, functional electrical stimulation, electrical massage), heating modalities, and cryotherapy may provide direct pain relief. Other approaches include prescribing assistive devices, braces, therapeutic exercises, biofeedback, trigger point injections, acupuncture, and behavioral modification techniques.

Physical Modalities to Control Pain

Modalities are beneficial as primary interventions in a variety of nonmalignant pain syndromes and have been used for soft tissue, orthopedic, and some neuropathic pain syndromes. However, their role in the management of cancer pain has not been clearly identified. Recent reviewers of rehabilitation medicine limit their comments on the management of pain in cancer patients to the use of narcotics, adjuvant medications, anesthetics, and neurosurgical procedures (65,66). Yet, physical modalities may decrease the need for analgesic medication.

Heat. Cutaneous stimulation includes the application of superficial heat or cold. Superficial heat is applied by hot packs, hot water bottles, hot compresses, electric heating pads, or immersion in whirlpool baths. Although some authors report beneficial effects from superficial heat in reducing cancer pain (67–69), other authors caution against the use of heat over tumor sites out of concern that it may increase tumor growth and the metastatic spread of the disease (70–71).

The use of ultrasound, a deep heating modality, is also controversial. Hayashi (1940) showed that tumor growth may be accelerated both by ultrasound and by short-wave exposure (72). Local ultrasound in mice is reported to enhance the subcutaneous growth of malignancy (73). Lehmann and De Lateur (1990) recommend avoiding the application of ultrasound over areas where a malignant tumor could be reached by an unknown quantity of ultrasound energy (74).

AHCPR clinical practice guidelines for the management of cancer pain conclude that in view of the lack of research findings that clearly contraindicate the use of superficial heat, it can be used as a method of pain control in patients with cancer (8). Furthermore, it is recommended that modalities to deliver deep heat (such as ultrasound, diathermy, and microwave) be used with caution in patients with active cancer and not be applied directly over a cancer site or on sites having received recent radiation therapy (75). To minimize the risk of burns, the temperature of applied heat must be carefully monitored, especially in patients who are cognitively impaired or who have impaired sensation in the area of application (69).

Cryotherapy. Ice packs, cold towels, or commercially prepared chemical gel packs are another form of cutaneous stimulation. Sealed cold packs should be applied to produce a comfortable level of intensity. The usual duration for application is about 15 minutes. Care should be taken over insensate areas, and cold should not be applied over radiated skin or limbs with poor circulation (75,76).

Massage. Massage is another modality that may be used to aid relaxation and help ease general aches and pains in a variety of conditions. However, the role of massage in the management of pain in cancer patients has not been studied except for the pain resulting from postmastectomy lymphedema. Massage may decrease pain in specific areas by increasing superficial circulation (69,77) and improving venous and lymphatic return. Care should be taken that techniques are gentle and used with caution, to avoid damage to the devitalized tissues. Ferrell-Torry and Glick (1993) reported that massage in cancer patients reduced their perceptions of pain and anxiety and enhanced relaxation (78). However, according to Knapp (1990), massage is contraindicated in malignancies because tumor tissues may be spread beyond confined limits to promote metastases or an extension of the malignancy (79).

Pneumatic massage and compression garments may be particularly helpful for lymphedema-related pain. The exact prevalence of postmastectomy pain in women undergoing surgical procedures on the breast is unknown. The incidence of lymphedema has been reported to occur in between 6 and 67 percent of patients, and prevalence of postmastectomy pain has been placed at 4 to 50 percent (80–85). Many patients experience worsening of pain with the increasing size of the limb. Compression garments are either prefabricated or custom-made, with a sequential gradient of pressure that passes from the distal aspect of the extremity to the more proximal segment. A number of sequential electronic pumping devices are also available, having variable cost and complexity. However, no one pumping device works best for all patients. Pumping should be avoided in the presence of active infection in the involved extremity, bleeding diatheses, and in those receiving chemotherapy.

Transcutaneous Electrical Nerve Stimulation (TENS). TENS is reported to be effective in musculoskeletal pain problems. Few studies have found TENS to have beneficial effects in the management of cancer pain (86,87). In one study, thirty-six of thirty-seven patients reported good or complete pain relief at 1 to 10 days of treatment. However, only in four of these subjects was the benefit maintained at 30 days (86). Specific syndromes that may respond to TENS include those caused by nerve injuries, back pain associated with metastatic lesions, and post-surgical pain. TENS is not effective for pain related to chemotherapy-induced peripheral neuropathy, disease of hollow viscus, or chronic cancer-related pain (88). Complications from TENS are rare. Most problems are caused by skin irritation, burn, or allergy to the jelly, tape, or electrodes used. It is recommended by manufacturers that the TENS stimulator should not be used in the presence of a cardiac pacemaker or over the cardiac sinus, or in patients suffering from dysrhythmias.

Exercise. Pain often leads to lengthy periods of immobility that may result in joint stiffness and muscle weakness, which may lead to further pain and a reluctance to remain active. Appropriate exercise may help to break this cycle. Exercise should be prescribed to strengthen muscles, mobilize stiff joints, and restore balance and coordination. Exercise enhances a patient's comfort and provides cardiovascular conditioning. In one study, patients used position change or exercise as a self-initiated strategy for pain relief. Eighty-six percent reported pain relief with a change of position, and 25 percent reported pain relief after exercise. Therefore, cancer patients should be encouraged to remain active and participate in self-care activities as long as possible (89,90).

However, caution should be practiced in exercising weak and paralyzed muscles. Overstretching should be avoided. Exercises should not be carried out if they increase pain. Exercise that involves weight bearing should be avoided when pathological fracture is likely. During acute pain, passive range-of-motion and isometric exercises should be advised.

Orthoses and Assistive Devices. At times, immobilization or restriction of movement is recommended during acute episodes of pain or to stabilize fractures. Braces may provide support and stabilization and thus relieve stress and pain. Braces can either be prefabricated or custom molded depending on the patient's needs. Those with pain as a result of metastatic disease of the long bones and spine benefit most from bracing.

The Sarmiento brace provides shoulder stabilization in patients who have disease or a pathologic fracture involving the shoulder joint (91). It is prescribed to prevent further fracture or soft-tissue damage to the joint by limiting shoulder range of motion while permitting hand and finger function to continue.

Painful lower extremity bone lesions may be treated with bypass orthoses that help to redistribute weight bearing to more stable and less painful tissues. Examples include the patella tendon weight-bearing orthosis and the ischial weight-bearing brace for lesions around the foot, lower leg, and knee respectively.

Weakness and poor positioning of the limbs may result in contracture and pain that impacts functional independence. A patient with weakness in dorsiflexion of the foot may benefit from an ankle–foot orthosis (AFO). The use of the AFO, along with proper physical therapy, may help to relieve pain and enable patients to ambulate with greater ease.

The most frequently prescribed orthoses are for patients with back pain secondary to metastatic involvement of the vertebral column. The brace prescription depends on the spinal level of pain and the degree of stabilization required (92). The braces range from corsets to custom body jackets. According to Brennan, bracing is more beneficial in those patients in whom the back pain worsens when strain is applied to the spine (88). Pain does not need to radiate, nor must it be of a neuropathic quality, to be relieved. In patients with a stable spine, soft, prefabricated devices such as neck collars, corsets, and sacroiliac belts may be adequate in controlling pain. These braces are easy to don and are tolerated well, and they do not restrict range of motion. If the pain relief is not adequate, more rigid braces should be prescribed.

Patients with compromised spinal integrity secondary to surgery or extensive vertebral lesions need greater stabilization. The Knight spinal orthosis is prescribed to provide control of the lumbosacral spinal segment in flexion, extension, and lateral bending. The Taylor brace provides flexion and extension control of the thoracolumbosacral segment. The Knight–Taylor orthosis adds lateral control to the Taylor brace. In patients with an unstable fracture, a custom body jacket provides maximum control and immobilization.

It must be recognized that the prolonged use of these devices may be detrimental, because their use may lead to muscular atrophy. Caution should be taken in prescribing any brace for patients who have desensate or hyperpathic tissue, especially if the device is going to be in direct contact with the skin. Care should likewise be taken if the patient's mental status is compromised. It is important to provide appropriate training in use of the orthosis. Follow-up evaluation should be carried out to see that the right kind of orthosis has been delivered and whether it is solving the problem for which it has been prescribed.

Crutches and Canes. Crutches, canes, and a variety of walkers are assistive devices that also aid in limiting pain and improving patient function. These assistive devices typically lessen weight bearing by altering the distribution of mass while ambulating. If total relief from weight bearing is required on the affected side, double-supported ambulation using either canes or crutches is recommended. When prescribing gait aides, it is important to evaluate upper extremity strength and to be certain of the integrity of the bones. Weight transfer from the lower extremities to the arm may predispose the patient to bony injury if a metastatic lesion is present in the upper extremity (88).

Patients with severe pain and limited mobility may benefit from using a wheelchair. In extreme cases, lifts may be advisable for transferring patients from the bed to the chair. A variety of wheelchair and bed cushions are available that can be prescribed when pain is increased by weight bearing. During immobilization, optimum body alignment and the proper positioning of various joints is important to promote comfort, prevent contracture, and provide pain relief. For example, the immobilized wrist should be placed in 30 degrees of dorsiflexion with the thumb opposed to fingers. Ankles should be at 90 degrees of flexion, with 5 to 10 degrees of flexion at the knee. This positioning, whether provided through custom-molded polypropylene splints, plaster casts, or off-the-shelf padded metallic boots, allows for maximal function after an immobilization period (70). Bedridden patients require frequent change of whole body position to prevent pressure ulcers. Ultimately, both patients and families should be provided with instructions regarding positioning and orthotic devices so that prolonged immobilization can be avoided. Proper training in the use of these assistive devices and braces is of paramount importance to prevent falls from improper use, which can have devastating consequences that include fractures and traumatic brain injury.

Psychosocial Approaches to Cancer Pain

There is an increased frequency of psychiatric disorders in cancer patients with pain, including primary adjustment disorder with depressed or anxious mood and major depression (23,93,94). These mental status changes may be endogenous or associated with cancer treatments, including the use of narcotics and steroids (95). Uncontrolled pain is, in fact, a major factor in cancer suicide (96), and the incidence of pain, depression, and delirium increases with greater debilitation and in advanced stages of illness (97). Studies show that cancer patients who receive active, structured psychological support report less pain and live longer (98,99).

Although most physicians rely on traditional approaches to treat cancer pain, there are alternative specialized treatments for chronic pain, including biofeedback, relaxation, and hypnosis, which can be combined with traditional methods for the treatment of both pain and depressive symptoms (100).

Supportive psychotherapy is useful in treating depression in cancer pain patients. The goals of psychotherapy with these patients are to provide emotional support, continuity, information, and to assist in adaptation to the crisis. It is important to emphasize past strengths and teach new coping strategies such as relaxation, cognitive coping, self-observation, assertiveness, and communication skills. Spiegel and Bloom demonstrated the beneficial effects of supportive group therapy and hypnosis in patients with breast cancer (101,102).

Psychosocial approaches are an important component of any comprehensive pain management plan. Psychosocial interventions may include both cognitive and behavioral techniques. Cognitive techniques focus on perception and thought, and are designed to influence how one interprets events. Behavioral techniques are directed toward helping a patient develop skills to cope with pain and to modify his reactions to pain. These approaches recognize that how a patient thinks affects how he feels, and changing how a patient thinks about pain can change his sensitivity, feelings, and reactions to it (103). Psychosocial interventions thus help the patient achieve a sense of control over his pain, which in turn may decrease his perception of pain (104). These strategies should be introduced early in the course of illness so that patients can learn and practice while they have sufficient strength and energy (8).

In chronic cancer pain, cognitive behavioral techniques are most effective when they are employed as part of a multimodal, multidisciplinary approach used in conjunction with appropriate analgesics and physical modalities (105).

Specific cognitive-behavioral techniques useful in treating cancer pain include passive relaxation with mental imagery, cognitive distraction or focusing, music therapy, and biofeedback (106–110). *Distraction* is the strategy of focusing attention on stimuli other than pain (111,112). Distractions may be internal, such as counting, praying, or singing to oneself, or external, such as listening to music and talking to family members and friends. It appears that distraction works best for pain that is acute and relatively mild, but that it is not very effective for controlling chronic or high levels of pain (112).

Hypnosis has been used in the management of pain resulting from a variety of disorders, including burns and rheumatoid arthritis (101,113–117) The evidence supporting the effectiveness of hypnosis in alleviating the chronic pain associated with cancer seems strong. Hypnosis is a state of heightened awareness and focused concentration that can be used to manipulate the perception of pain and thus alter the subjective experience of pain. The techniques most often used include physical relaxation and imagery that provide a substitute focus of attention for the painful sensation. Using self-hypnosis, a patient can learn to control and transform the pain signal into one that is less uncomfortable. Some patients prefer to move a pain to another part of their body. A patient can also be taught to not fight pain, because pain is only enhanced by focusing attention to it. In a randomized prospective study, a combination of hypnosis and group psychotherapy resulted in a 50 percent reduction in pain among patients with metastatic breast cancer (101).

Biofeedback is used to provide comfort and minimize pain in adults and children undergoing bone marrow aspirations, spinal taps, and other painful procedures (118). The basis of biofeedback is the utilization of augmentative techniques to make the patient cognitively aware of normally autonomous physiological function (119). The underlying goal is to teach a patient to consciously control systemic functions that are usually only nominally affected by volitional thoughts. Various amplification systems are available that interface with the patient via surface-contact devices such as thermal sensors and electromyography and pulse-rate monitors. Feedback is provided by auditory or visual cues. The effectiveness of electrocardiomyography (EMG) biofeedback has been reported in tension headaches and chronic low back pain (120,121). EMG biofeedback may be most helpful in cancer patients who have pain resulting from musculoskeletal problems. This modality, however, has not been tested in cancer patients.

SPECIFIC PAIN SYNDROME

Bone Pain

Bone metastases can cause pain and compromise the quality of life (122). Although more than 25 percent of patients with bone metastases have no symptoms, the remaining 75 percent have pain as the dominant complaint (123). Pain characteristics are variable, depending on the site of involvement. Patients may describe a generalized aching pain or a severe, sharp, and stabbing pain.

Bone metastases are often the first sign of disseminated disease. Certain primary tumors, including those of prostate, breast, and lung, routinely metastasize to bone (124,125). These metastases commonly cause increased bone destruction, although increased bone formation (osteolysis) is seen in prostate cancer (osteosclerosis), or a combination of both processes can occur (126–129).

More than 80 percent of bone metastases are found in the axial skeleton (124,130), thus leading to morbidities that impair the quality of life (22). The spine, pelvis, and ribs are often the earliest sites of metastases. Skull, femora, humeri, scapulae, and sternum are involved later. Cancers of prostate, bladder, uterine cervix, and rectum tend to involve the bones of the pelvis (131,132).

The relationship between bone invasion and pain is unclear (122). Patients may have multiple bone lesions without associated bone pain. Conversely, patients may have considerable pain without radiologic evidence of bone metastases (20,133). Furthermore, the exact mechanism of pain resulting from bone metastases is not known.

Osteolytic lesions are associated with the greatest structural weakening and are most likely to cause pathologic fractures. Pathologic fractures have been reported to occur in 8 to 30 percent of all patients with bone metastases (129,134–136), with most (80 percent) of the fractures occurring in patients with breast, kidney, lung, and thyroid primaries (137–138). The proximal portion of the long bones in both the upper and lower extremity are commonly at risk, leading to significant disability in ambulation even with assistive devices such as crutches and walkers.

Epidural spinal cord compression is one of the most serious complications of bone metastasis and is an oncologic emergency. Early diagnosis and intervention is critical to preserving neurologic function and preventing disability. Spinal cord compression occurs in about 5 percent of patients and is usually associated with tumors of the breast, lung, prostate, or unknown primary (139,140). Any patient who has a bone-seeking cancer and who presents with back and neck pain should be considered at high risk.

Spinal cord compression may not always produce clear neurologic deficits. More than 90 percent of patients have a history of back pain, with or without radicular distribution (139,141). Fifty percent of patients have bladder and bowel incontinence, and less than 50 percent of these patients are able to walk at the time of initial evaluation. Early diagnosis and intervention is important, because a majority of patients who are ambulatory at the time of presentation can retain that ability with appropriate intervention.

The diagnosis of bone metastases, even in patients with an unknown primary, can usually be established from the clinical history, serum alkaline phosphatase, plain radiography, and bone scintigraphy (137). Although an increased level of alkaline phosphatase is not pathognomonic for the presence of bone metastases, total serum alkaline phosphatase is elevated in about 80 percent of prostate cancer patients and in about 40 percent of breast cancer patients (124). Plain x-rays can be used as a simple screening tool, with the understanding that 30 to 50 percent of the cortical bone must be destroyed before metastases are visible on plain films. Bone scan is more sensitive in identifying abnormalities, but the findings are less specific. Trauma, infection, and inflammation can also produce abnormal bone scans. Computed tomography (CT) or magnetic resonance imaging (MRI) scans may give additional information, especially for lesions in the spine or when early detection is required. These may also be essential in determining the extent of involvement of the neural structures.

In the management of bone pain, although the ultimate prognosis is poor, patients with bony metastases may survive for several months or years and will require the treatment of symptoms related to their disease. Apart from pain, bone metastases may lead to pathologic fracture, hypercalcemia, neurologic deficits, and immobility. The management of metastatic bone disease requires the efforts of a multidisciplinary team including orthopedic surgeons, radiation oncologists, neurologists, diagnostic and nuclear medicine consultants, physiatrists, and therapists. The goals of treatment are to relieve pain, prevent development of pathological fractures, and to improve function and mobility with an ultimate objective of improving the quality of life. An algorithm for bone pain management secondary to metastatic disease has been published by Kori et al. (142) (see Figure 12.8).

The liberal and carefully titrated use of opioids is the mainstay of treatment for bone pain (75). Dosage requirements for opioids are quite variable and require frequent assessment of the patient's response. During the acute stage of pathologic fracture or epidural spinal cord compression, intravenous morphine or hydromorphone is prescribed to control pain. PCA pumps allow the flexibility to control pain both at rest and with activity. In movement-related pain, the oral route may not adequately control pain, and a PCA pump may be more effective in providing comfortable weight bearing and walking. Once the pain is stabilized, an equianalgesic oral dose of a controlled-release preparation such as morphine or oxycodone can be prescribed (142). Transdermal fentanyl may also provide adequate pain relief.

Fractures of the arm are usually managed conservatively with radiotherapy or immobilization with a sling (124). In patients with multiple metastases involving both upper and lower extremities, arm fractures should be treated surgically with internal fixation by use of either intramedullary rods or a prosthetic replacement (138) so that the patient may ambulate with crutches or a walker.

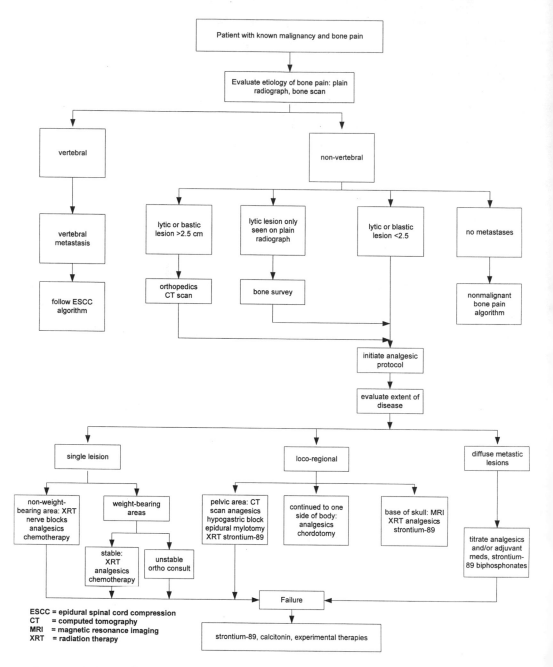

Figure 12.8. Summary Algorithm for Bone Pain Management. Reproduced by permission from Kori SH, et al., *Cancer Control:* Journal of the Moffitt Cancer Center Volume 4, 1997 p. 157.

The femur is the most common site of pathologic fractures. Although Cheng and colleagues (1980) reported good results with radiotherapy alone (143), fractures of the femur are usually managed surgically (144). The surgical procedure used depends on the site of fracture. For femoral neck fractures, total hip replacement is indicated, whereas inter- and subtrochanteric fracture requires plate-and-screw fixation. Fractures of the femoral shaft are best treated with intramedullary rod fixation.

The management of impending hip fractures remains controversial. It is unlikely for pathologic fracture to occur in cases having less than 50 percent of cortical bone destruction. However, the probability of fracture increases considerably, to about 70 percent, when more than 50 percent of the bone cortex is destroyed (135). Cheng and colleagues (1980) believe that these patients could be managed without early surgical intervention (143). In their study of 59 cases of osteolytic metastases involving weight-bearing bones, having lesions causing less than 59 percent bone destruction, none of the patients developed pathological fractures after treatment with 30 Gy XRT as an initial dose (143).

The optimum treatment of spinal cord compression is controversial. Spinal cord lesions can be managed conservatively in patients who do not have neurologic deficits or evidence of bony instability. Conservative options include radiotherapy, bed rest, and external immobilization. The management of pain in patients with evidence of neurologic cord compression incorporates radiotherapy alone or surgery with postoperative radiotherapy.

Surgery. Traditionally, decompression of the spinal cord is carried out by a posterior laminectomy with or without internal stabilization, though some investigators recommend an anterior approach (92). Internal fixation is indicated in patients with possible bony instability. Surgical stabilization allows early mobilization. Common indications for surgical intervention include (*a*) lytic lesions with a diameter of >2 to 3 cm; (*b*) cortical destruction of >50 percent; or (*c*) impending fractures because of metastasis in weight bearing bones. Patients should have an anticipated survival of longer than six months, be in stable enough condition to permit operation, and have sufficient strength and cognition to allow for increased postoperative mobility. The details of surgical procedures and guidelines for various types of fractures have been discussed in a number of review articles (124,129,136,138,144).

Radiotherapy. In patients with bone metastases, radiotherapy is used for pain control rather than for curative purposes. The mechanism of pain relief through radiotherapy is believed to be associated with tumor shrinkage and the subsequent relief of pressure from the sensitive neural structures. It may also aid in healing and stabilizing the bone.

Several retrospective studies have reported that local radiotherapy is an effective palliative intervention for painful metastases (124,133,145,146). However, pain relief varies from patient to patient. Some patients may experience pain relief during the treatment regimen, whereas many others actually have increased pain caused by inflammation and positioning. Patients and families should be informed that it might take 10 to 14 days for pain relief to occur following radiotherapy.

A number of prospective studies have examined the role of radiation therapy for relief of bone pain (147–151). It appears that at doses of 8 Gy and higher, there is no strong evidence for a dose–response relationship and no consistent advantage of multiple fractions over one or two large fractions (149). It can be concluded that in most patients local radiotherapy for painful localized bone metastases can be given as a single treatment of 8 Gy (122).

In patients with multiple bone metastatic lesions, multiple separate fields or half-body radiation is given. The onset of pain relief occurs within 1 to 14 days of treatment, with about 50 percent of the patients noting pain relief within 48 hours (145). However, there may be appreciable side effects.

Although its role is unproven, a number of retrospective studies have emphasized that postoperative radiotherapy may be beneficial (122), and it is the current standard treatment in most centers. Radiotherapy is usually given in 10 fractionated treatments at a dose of 25 to 30 Gy to inhibit local regrowth of the tumor and to induce recalcification. It has been suggested that doses exceeding 30 Gy should be avoided because of impaired healing (122). Daily travel and lying on the treatment table may increase the patient's discomfort (152). The use of single-fraction and short-course radiotherapy is being studied to improve the quality of life (153).

Radiopharmaceuticals. The U.S. FDA has approved ^{32}P (sodium phosphate), ^{89}Sr (strontium chloride), and ^{153}Sm lexidronam for the treatment of bone pain of osteoblastic metastases. Patients with diffuse metastases and multiple sites of pain are good candidates for radiopharmaceuticals such as strontium-89 (152,154). One advantage is that strontium can be given to treat pain in previously irradiated sites. Only in a patient with an abnormal bone scan (increased osteoblastic activity) will the radiotracer accumulate in a site of osseous metastases to a sufficient extent to have a therapeutic effect (155). As with radiotherapy, patients may initially experience an increase in their pain, and it may take an average of 7 to 14 days for adequate pain control to occur. The principal toxic effect of strontium-89 is bone marrow suppression, with the nadir occurring at 2 to 8 weeks posttreatment.

Bisphosphonates. Bisphosphonates are new agents that have been shown to reduce the bony complications associated with breast cancer (156–160). In one study, 382 women receiving chemotherapy with at least one lytic lesion were randomized to either 90 mg pamidronate or placebo intravenously over 2 hours on a monthly basis for 12 months. Pamidronate was superior to placebo in terms of time to occurrence of the first skeletal complication, proportion of women with any skeletal complication, and change in pain severity (157). The American Society of Clinical Oncology expert panel suggests that the highest priority be given to women with multiple lytic bone metastases or disease in weight-bearing bones or vertebrae. The optimum duration of treatment with bisphosphonate use is unknown. It is suggested that once initiated, treatment should be continued until there is evidence of substantial decline in a patient's general performance status.

Visceral Pain

Tumor infiltration of the viscera causes nociceptor activation from stretching, distension, or inflammation. The result is a poorly localized pain. Patients may describe gnawing or cramping pain, suggesting the obstruction of a hollow viscus, or the pain may be deep, aching, and throbbing, because of the involvement of the organ capsule or mesentery.

Pain resulting from visceral infiltration may be referred in the distribution of a dermatome, sclerotome, or a myotome. Dermatomal referred pain is usually superficial, whereas sclerotomal and myotomal referred pain is deep in a single spinal segment. The exact pathophysiology of referred pain is not known but it might be related to the dual innervation of multiple structures, or chemical irritation by tumor-mediated substances (161).

Visceral pain is the presenting symptom in 75 percent of pancreatic cancer patients (162). The pain is usually described as deep and aching. Localization varies depending on the underlying site of obstruction. The pain is reported in the periumbilical area in patients with pancreatic duct obstruction, whereas patients with biliary tract obstruction experience pain localized to the right upper abdominal quadrant. Forward flexion of the abdomen may provide some relief.

Patients with liver metastases present with malaise, weight loss, and right upper quadrant pain. The pain is often described as aching and dull, or sharp and colicky. Physical examination may reveal an enlarged liver and there may be tenderness on palpation. At times, the pain is referred to the right suprascapular area or the back.

In the management of visceral pain, nonsteroidal antiinflammatory drugs and opioids in appropriate dosage are effective in controlling pain of visceral origin. At times, patients are unable to tolerate oral medications, and may develop dose-limiting side effects. Neurolytic blockade of the celiac axis may be required in patients who do not respond or who become refractory to pharmacotherapy.

The celiac plexus innervates the gastrointestinal tract, adrenals, ureters, liver, and abdominal vessels. A celiac plexus block interrupts the abdominal nociceptive transmission without interfering with normal somatic peripheral nerve endings. Celiac plexus blocks are most frequently indicated in pancreatic and intra-abdominal cancer, with significant pain relief occurring in 70 to 94 percent of patients (163,164). Apart from procedure-related pain, which usually subsides within 20 to 30 minutes, other complications include hypotension, diarrhea, subarachnoid and epidural inflammation, pneumothorax, and lower chest pain. The diarrhea is self-limiting, and attempts should be made to prevent dehydration. It is recommended that a close follow-up after discharge be carried out to evaluate the efficacy of the intervention and to adjust medications.

Neuropathic Pain

Neuropathic pain in cancer patients is caused either by direct tumor infiltration of the nerve or by cancer treatment. Direct infiltration or compression of a peripheral nerve is most common. Tumor infiltration may involve a single peripheral nerve or several peripheral nerves, including the brachial and lumbosacral plexus. Pain is described initially as dull and aching, and is unilateral in the distribution of the involved nerve. There may be tenderness on percussion over the nerve route. Later, the pain becomes constant and burning in character. Numbness, allodynia, and hyperesthesias are often present. The patient may also present with nerve root impingement, which causes a radicular type of pain.

Metastatic infiltration of a nerve plexus by tumor often results in severe pain and neuromuscular weakness. Plexus involvement can have a significant impact on the functional status and quality of life of cancer patients. The true incidence and prevalence of plexus metastases is not known.

Cervical Plexopathy. Involvement of the cervical plexus most commonly is caused by the extension of squamous cell carcinoma of the head and neck, lymphomas, or metastases from systemic tumors, such as lung and breast tumors, to cervical lymph nodes and vertebrae. The major clinical presentation is pain that usually radiates to the neck, shoulder, and throat. Neck movement and swallowing may make the pain worse. Sensory deficits in the distribution of the plexus may be present. Involvement of the sympathetic trunk may result in a unilateral Horner's syndrome. Involvement of the cervical plexus implies a close proximity of the tumor to the spine, and epidural cord compression at this level may result in life-threatening respiratory paralysis.

MRI or CT scan of the cervical plexus can confirm the diagnosis of metastatic cervical plexopathy. MRI is the preferred procedure, because it provides the best anatomical detail. When neck stability is in question, standard cervical spine radiograph or CT scan is recommended.

The treatment of cervical plexopathy is primarily directed at relieving the pain. Severe impending epidural involvement may respond to focal radiotherapy to the involved area or chemotherapy for the primary tumor. In some patients, cervical nerve blocks or selective rhizotomy may be necessary to improve the quality of life (165).

Brachial Plexopathy. Brachial plexopathy may result from tumor infiltration and radiotherapy. Traction injury related to upper extremity positioning during a prolonged procedure might also cause plexopathy. Pain is the most common presenting symptom in patients with metastatic tumor infiltration of the brachial plexus (166–168). The pain is severe and constant, and may be associated with marked muscle weakness and wasting in the distribution of the nerves involved. In contrast, pain is not a common symptom in radiation-induced plexopathy (166–168). However, Thomas et al. (1972), while attempting to define differentiating characteristics of radiation-induced brachial plexopathy and metastatic brachial plexopathy, concluded that no single clinical symptom or sign permitted distinction between the two groups (166).

However, Kori and colleagues (1981) believe that a distinction between tumor infiltration and radiation-induced plexopathy can be made on clinical grounds (168). In a review of 100 patients with brachial plexopathy, 78 patients were considered to have tumor-infiltrated plexopathy and 22 had radiation-induced injury. The major difference between the two groups was anatomic involvement of the plexus and the severity of pain. Brachial plexus lesions secondary to tumor infiltration usually affect the lower plexus and involve the lower trunk or medial cord, producing weakness in intrinsic hand and wrist flexors muscles. Sensory symptoms are in the C8–T1 distribution (168). Radiation-induced plexopathy typically involves the upper trunk, thus resulting in weakness of shoulder elevation, external rotation of the arm, and weakness of supination and flexion of the forearm. In these cases the sensory symptoms and signs are most prominent over the deltoid muscle. It was further noted that weakness develops later in the course of tumor plexopathy (168).

Severe pain was the presenting complaint in 75 to 89 percent of the metastatic plexopathy group, compared to only 18 percent of the radiation group. In metastatic plexopathy, the pain was routinely localized to the shoulder and axilla with radiation down the medial arm, forearm, and into the fourth and fifth fingers. Distressing paresthesias, hypesthesia, heaviness, and weakness were the major complaints in the radiation group, and lymphedema of the arm was significantly more common, probably because of intense fibrosis of the plexus and lymphatic tissues (168). It was concluded that early and severe pain, hand weakness (C8–TI), and Horner syndrome suggest metastatic plexopathy. By contrast, painless weakness of shoulder abduction and arm flexors with progressive lymphedema suggests radiation-induced plexopathy. Furthermore, if more than 6,000 R is given and if neurologic symptoms appear within a year, the diagnosis is probably radiation damage.

Helpful diagnostic studies for plexopathy include electromyography and nerve conduction studies as well as diagnostic imaging. EMG/NCS may help to localize the site of the lesion electrophysiologically, whereas MRI helps to visualize tumor infiltration and radiation fibrosis. MRI can also help to evaluate the adjacent spinal cord. It is of particular importance to evaluate the epidural space as well, because patients with malignant brachial plexopathy are at high risk for epidural extension of the disease (169,170). CT provides an excellent alternative and has the advantage of providing an improved definition of the vertebral bony involvement and stability.

Lumbosacral Plexopathy. Lumbosacral plexopathy is not common. Thomas and colleagues (1985) described a retrospective study of radiation-induced and neoplastic lumbosacral plexopathy (171). Twenty cases of radiation-induced plexopathy and thirty cases of neoplastic involvement of the plexus were identified. In radiation-induced plexopathy, the predominant initial symptom was weakness of the legs in twelve of the twenty patients, followed by numbness or paresthesias in six and pain in two patients. Symptoms were predominantly bilateral. Although pain was uncommon as the initial symptom in radiation cases, it was eventually present in 50 percent of the cases, located mostly in legs and described as aching, burning, pulling, and cramping. Muscle weakness occurred in all radiation patients (171). In the tumor group, pain was the first and most unrelenting symptom in all but two patients. Proximal regions such as low back, buttock, hip, and thigh were commonly involved. The onset was typically unilateral and in 90 percent of cases remained confined to one side. Pain was often worse at night. Progression in this group was much faster, with severe deficit occurring within weeks or months. Muscle weakness was also common (171).

To differentiate the etiology of lumbar plexopathy, CT scan of the abdomen and pelvis was found to be most valuable in neoplastic disease, disclosing a tumor mass, lymphadenopathy, or bone erosion in 78 percent of cases. EMG on the other hand, was most useful in diagnosing radiation-induced plexopathy, with 57 percent of these patients showed "myokymic" discharges (171).

Treatment

Antitumor therapies such as radiotherapy to the involved field and chemotherapy for the underlying neoplasm represent the primary treatment for metastatic plexopathy. However, results have been variable. Radiation therapy of 2,000 to 5,000 R to the plexus relieved pain in only 46 percent of the patients (168). Neurologic improvement was minimal. Nisce and Chu (1968), conversely, reported that 491 patients with breast cancer had complete pain relief for a mean period of 6 months (172).

Stellate ganglion block with local anesthetic or neurolytic agents may relieve plexopathy pain. However, neurolysis of the plexus will result in a nonfunctional extremity.

In patients with radiation-induced plexopathy, distressing paresthesias disappeared spontaneously over time and a lymphedematous paretic limb was the most distressing problem (168). Conservative pain management for plexopathies includes NSAIDs and opioids, and adjuvant medications such as TCAs and anticonvulsants, may be helpful. Hydroxyzine is a mild anxiolytic with sedating and analgesic properties that is useful in the anxious cancer patient with pain. This drug also has antiemetic activity.

CONCLUSIONS

Pain is commonly associated with cancer. Cancer pain is not of a single distinct quality, but is highly variable in presentation. It is a multidimensional symptom that often requires multispecialty intervention.

Pain in cancer may be associated with direct tumor infiltration, cancer treatment, or may occur as an independent variable separate from the cancer itself. Along with patient and family education, treatment options include pharmaceuticals, surgical intervention, radiation therapy, physical modalities, and psychological/

psychosocial techniques. Yet, with all these options available, cancer pain remains widely undertreated.

As long ago as 1986, the WHO provided a cancer pain relief guidelines. The following year, Ventafridda et al. demonstrated that use of this analgesic ladder could provide relief for more than 75 percent of patients with pain caused by cancer. Unfortunately, at the present, only a small minority of patients have access to this simple analgesic scheme (173).

It follows that pain need not be an inevitable consequence of a cancer diagnosis. Multiple treatment options are available. More healthcare providers, however, must identify pain management as a critical component of cancer treatment protocols and become knowledgeable in the various treatment methods.

REFERENCES

1. Higginson I. Innovations in assessment: Epidemiology and assessment of pain in advanced cancer. In: Jensen TS, Turner JA, Weisenfield-Hallin (eds.) Proceedings of the 8th World Congress on Pain, Progress in Pain Research and Management. Seattle: IASP Press, 1997; pp. 707–716.
2. Greenwald HP, Bonica JJ, Berbner M. The prevalence of pain in four cancers. *Cancer* 1987; 60:2563–2569.
3. Portenoy RK, Miransky J, Tahler T, et al. Pain in ambulatory patients with lung or colon cancer: Prevalence, characterization, and effect. *Cancer* 1992; 70:1616–1624.
4. Ellershaw JE, Peat SJ, Boys LC. Assessing the effectiveness of a hospital palliative care team. *Pall Med* 1995; 9:145–152.
5. Daut RL, Cleeland CS. The prevalence and severity of pain in cancer. *Cancer* 1982; 50:1913–1918.
6. Twycross RG. Clinical experience with diamorphine in advanced malignant disease. *Int J Clin Pharmacol* 1974; 67:184–198.
7. Storm HH, Christensen N, Jensen OM. Suicide among Danish patients with cancer: 1971–1986. *Cancer* 1992; 69:1507–1512.
8. Management of cancer pain. Clinical Practice Guidelines No. 9. Agency for Health Care Policy and Research; Jacox A, Carr. DB, Payne R, Co–Chairs of the Guideline Panel, HCPR Publication no. 94–0592. Rockville, Md.: Agency for Health Care Policy and Research, U.S. Department of Health and Human Services, Public Health Service, March, 1994.
9. World Health Organization. *Cancer Pain Relief and Palliative Care*. Technical Reports Series 804, Geneva, Switzerland: World Health Organization,1992.
10. World Health Organization. *Cancer Pain Relief*, 2nd ed. Geneva: World Health Organization, 1996.
11. Health and Welfare Canada. *Cancer Pain*. A Monograph on management of cancer pain. Publication no. H42–2/5 1984e. Ottawa: Minister of Supply and Services, 1984.
12. National Comprehensive Cancer Network Cancer Pain Guidelines. *Oncology* 2001; 14:138–139, 141–143.
13. Cleeland CS, Nakamura Y, Mendoza TR, et al. Dimensions of the impact of cancer in a four-country sample: New information from multidimensional scaling. *Pain* 1996; 67: 267–273.
14. Von Roenn JH, Cleeland CS, Gonin R, Hatfield A, Pondaya KJ. Physicians' attitudes and practice in cancer pain management. A survey for the Eastern Cooperative Oncology group. *Ann Int Med* 1993; 119:121–126.
15. Elliott TE, Elliott BA. Physician acquisition of cancer pain management knowledge. *J Pain and Symptom Management* 1991; 6:224–229.

16. Weissman DE. Cancer pain education for physicians in practice: Establishing a new paradigm. *J Pain and Symptom Management* 1996; 12:364–371.

17. Billings JA, Block S. Palliative care in undergraduate medical education, status report and future directions. *JAMA* 1997; 278:733–738.

18. Cleeland CS, Jajan NQA, Scott CB, et al. Cancer pain management by radiotherapist: A survey of radiation therapy oncology group physicians. *Int Radiat Oncol Biol Phys* 2000; 47:203–208.

19. Grossman SA, Staats PS. Current management of pain in patients with cancer. *Oncology* 1994; 8:93–107.

20. Foley KM. The treatment of cancer pain. *N Eng J Med* 1985; 313:84–95.

21. Foley KM. Clinical assessment of cancer patient. *Acta Anaesthesiol Scand Suppl* 1982; 74:91–96.

22. Foley KM. Pain syndromes in patients with cancer. In: Portenoy R, Kanner R (eds.), *Pain Management: Theory and Practice*. Philadelphia: FA Davis, 1996; pp. 191–216.

23. Ahlers TA, Blanchard EB, Ruckdeschel JC. The multidimensional nature of cancer-related pain. *Pain* 1983; 17:277–288.

24. McGuire D. The multiple dimensions of cancer pain: A framework for assessment and management. In: McGuire D, Yarbro C, Ferrel B (eds.), *Cancer Pain Management*, 2nd ed. Boston: Jones & Bartlett, 1995; pp. 1–17.

25. Levy MH. Effective integration of pain management into comprehensive cancer care. *Postgraduate Med J* 1991; 67: 35–43.

26. Ferrell BR. Patient and family caregiver perspectives. *Oncology* (suppl 2) 1999; 13:15–19.

27. Simpson KH. Philosophy of cancer pain management. In: Simpson KH, Budd K (eds.), *Cancer Pain Management: A Comprehensive Approach*. Oxford: University Press, 2000; pp.1–6.

28. Ventafridda V, Tamburini M, Sbanotto A, et al. A validation of the WHO method for cancer pain relief. *Cancer* 1987; 59:850–856.

29. Zech DF, Grond S, Lynch J, et al. Validation of World Health Organization Guidelines for cancer pain relief: A 10 year prospective study. *Pain* 1995; 63: 65–76.

30. Jadad AR, Browman GP. WHO analgesic ladder for cancer pain management: Stepping up the quality of its evaluation. *JAMA* 1995; 274: 1870–1873.

31. Mercadante S. World Health Organization Guidelines: Problem areas in cancer pain management. *Cancer Control* 1999; 6: 191–197.

32. Cherny NI. The management of cancer pain. *CA* 2000; 50:70–116.

33. Ventafridda V, De Conno E, Pancrai AE et al. Nonsteroidal antiinflammatory drugs as the first step in cancer pain therapy: Double-blind within patient study comparing nine drugs. *J Int Med Res* 1990; 18:21–29.

34. Mercadante S, Sapio M, Caligara M, et al. Opioid-sparing effect of diclofenac in cancer pain. *J Pain Symptom Manage* 1997; 14: 15–20.

35. Portenoy RK. Pharmacologic management: Non-opioid and adjuvant analgesics. *Hem Onc Ann* 1994; 2:423–431.

36. Stein WM. Cancer pain in the elderly. In: Ferrell BR and Ferrell BA (eds.), *Pain in the Elderly*. Seattle: IASP Press, 1996; pp. 69–80.

37. Vane JR. Inhibition of prostaglandin synthesis as a mechanism for aspirinlike drugs. *Nat New Biol* 1971; 231:232 235.

38. Simon LS. Nonsteroidal antiinflammatory drugs and their effects: The importance of COX "selectivity." *J Clin Rheumatol* 1996; 2:135–140.

39. Cherny NJ, Chang V, Frager G, et al. Opioid pharmacotherapy in the management of cancer pain: A survey of strategies used by pain physicians for the selection of analgesic drugs and routes of administration. *Cancer* 1995; 76:1283–1293.

40. Eisenberg E, Berkey CS, Carr DB, et al. Efficacy and safety of nonsteroidal antiinflammatory drugs for cancer pain: A meta-analysis. *J Clin Oncol* 1994; 12: 2756–2765.

41. Schug SA, Zech D, Grond S., et al. A long-term study of morphine in cancer pain patients. *J Pain Symptom Manage* 1992; 7: 259–266.

42. Ballantyne Jane. Nonnarcotic analgesic use in acute and cancer pain: Results of selected Meta-analyses. *Cancer Control* 1999; 6:26–30.

43. Portenoy RK, Tahler HT, Kornblith AB, et al. Symptom prevalence, characteristics and distress in a cancer population. *Quality Life Res* 1994; 3:183–189.

44. Swerdlow M. Anticonvulsant drugs and chronic pain. *Clin Neuropharmacol* 1984; 7:51–82.

45. Janjan NA. Introduction. *Seminars Radiation Oncology* 2000; 10:169–174.

46. Dejgard A, Petersen P, Kastrup J. Mexiletine for treatment of chronic painful diabetic neuropathy. *Lancet* 1988; 1:9–11.

47. Vecht CJ, Verbiest HBC. Use of glucocorticoids in neuro-oncology. In: Wiley RG (ed.), *Neurologic Complication of Cancer*. New York: Marcel Dekker, 1995; p. 199.

48. Byrne TN. Spinal cord compression from epidural metastases. *N Eng J Med* 1992; 327:614–619.

49. Carson JL, Willett LR. Toxicity of nonsteroidal antiinflammatory drugs. An overview of the epidemiological evidence. *Drugs* 1993; 46:243–248.

50. Zeigler D, Lynch SA, Muir J, Benjamin J, Max MB. Transdermal clonidine versus placebo in painful diabetic neuropathy. *Pain* 1992; 48: 403–408.

51. Ono H, Mishima A, Ono S, Fukuda H, Vasko MR. Inhibitory effects of clonidine and tizanidine on release of substance P from slices of rat spinal cord and antagonism by alpha adrenergic receptor antagonists. *Neuropharmacology* 1991; 30:585–589.

52. Kawamata T, Omote K, Kawamata M, Iwasaki H, Namiki A. Antinociceptive interaction of intrathecal alpha2 adrenergic agonists, tizanidine and clonidine, with lidocaine in rats. *Anesthesiology* 1997; 87:436–448.

53. Kroin JS, McCarthy RJ, Penn RD, Lubenow TR, Ivankovich AD. Intrathecal clonidine and tizanidine in conscious dogs: Comparison of analgesic and hemodynamic effects. *Anesth Analg* 1996; 82:627–635, 1996.

54. Semenchuk MR, Sherman S. Effectiveness of tizanidine in neuropathic pain: An open label study. *J Pain* 2000; 1:285–292.

55. Max MB, Schafer SC, Culnane M, Dubner R, Gracely RH. Association of pain relief with drug side effects in postherpetic neuralgia: A single-dose study of clonidine, codeine, ibuprofen, and placebo. *Clin Pharmacol Ther* 1988; 43:363–371.

56. Eisenach J, DuPen S, Dubois M, et al. Epidural clonidine analgesia for intractable cancer pain: The Epidural Clonidine Study group. *Pain* 1995; 61:391–399.

57. Fromm G, Terence C, Chatta A. Baclofen in the treatment of trigeminal neuralgia. *Ann Neurol* 1984; 15:240–247.

58. Watson CP, Evans RJ, Watt VR. Postherpetic neurologia and topical capsaicin. *Pain* 1988; 33: 333–340.

59. Watson CP, Evans RJ, Watt VR. The post mastectomy pain syndrome and the effect of topical capsaicin. *Pain* 1989; 38: 177–186.

60. Rowbotham MC. Topical analgesic agents. In: Fields HJL, Liebeskind JC (eds.), *Pharmacological Approaches to the Treatment of Chronic Pain: New Concepts and Critical Issues*. Seattle: IASP Press; 1994; 211–227.

61. Rose C, Mouridsen HT. Endocrine therapy of advanced breast cancer. *Acta Oncol* 1988; 27:721–728.

62. Nelson KA, Walsh TD. The use of chemotherapy in cancer pain treatment. In: Arbit E (ed.), Management of Cancer-related Pain. New York: Futura, 1993; pp. 143–149.

63. Pannuti F, Martoni A, Rossi AP, et al. The role of endocrine therapy for relief of pain due to advanced cancer. In: Bonica JJ, Ventafridda V (eds.), *Advances in Pain Research and Therapy*. 1979.

64. Sogani PC, Ray B, Whitmore WF. Advanced prostate carcinoma: Flutamide therapy after conventional endocrine treatment. *Urology* 1975; 6:164–166.

65. Walsh NE. Cancer pain. *Phys Med State Art Rev* 1991; 5:133–153.

66. King JC, Kelleher WJ. The chronic pain syndrome: The interdisciplinary rehabilitative behavioral modification approach. *Phys Med State Art Rev* 1991; 5:165–186.

67. Barbour LA, McGuire DB, Kirchhoff KT. Nonanalgesic methods of pain control used by cancer outpatients. *Oncol Nurs Forum* 1986; 13:56–60.

68. Rhiner M, Ferrell BR, Ferrell BA, Grant MM. A structured non-drug intervention program for cancer pain. *Cancer Practice* 1993; 1:137–143.

69. McCaffery M, Wolff M. Pain relief using cutaneous modalities, positioning, and movement. In: Turk DC, Feldman CS (eds.). Special issue: noninvasive approaches to pain management in the terminally ill. *Hospice J* 1992; 8:121–153.

70. Lee MHM, Itoh M, Yang GW, Eason AL. Physical therapy and rehabilitation medicine. In: Bonica JJ (ed.), *The Management of Pain*, 2nd ed. Vol 2. Philadelphia: Lea & Febiger 1990; p. 1769–1788.

71. Pfalzer L. Physical agents and the patient with cancer. *Clin Manage Phys Ther* 1992; 12:83–86.

72. Hayashi S. Der einfluss del ultraschallwellen und utrakurtzwellen auf den maligen tumor. *Jpn J Med Sci Biophy* 1940; 6:138.

73. Sicard-Rosenbaum L, Lord D, Danoff JV, et al. Effects of continuous therapeutic ultrasound on growth and metastasis of subcutaneous murine tumors. *Phys Ther* 1995; 75:3–13.

74. Lehmann JF, de Lateur BJ. Therapeutic heat. In: Lehmann JF (ed.) *Therapeutic Heat and Cold*, 4th ed. Baltimore, Md.: Williams & Williams; 1990, p. 417–581.

75. Jacox A, Carr DB, Payne R. New clinical-practice guidelines for the management of pain in patients with cancer. *N Eng J Med* 1994; 330:651–655.

76. Whitney SL. Physical agents: Heat and cold modalities. In: Scully R, Barnes M (eds.), *Physical Therapy*. Philadelphia: JB Lippincott Co., 1989; pp. 844–875.

77. Fairchild VM, Salerno LM, Wedding SL, Weinberg E. Physical therapy. In: Raj PP (ed.), *Practical Management of Pain: With Special Emphasis on Physiology of Pain Syndromes and Techniques of Management*. Chicago: Yearbook Medical Publishers, 1986; pp. 839–852.

78. Ferrell-Torry AT, Glick OJ. The use of therapeutic massage as a nursing intervention to modify anxiety and the perception of cancer pain. *Cancer Nurs* 1993; 16:93–101.

79. Knapp ME. Massage. In: Kottke FJ and Lehmann JF (eds.), *Krusen Hand Book of Physical Medicine and Rehabilitation*, 4th ed. Philadelphia: WB Saunders, 1990; pp. 433–435.

80. Markowski J, Wilcox J, Helm P. Lymphedema incidence after specific postmastectomy therapy. *Arch Phys Med Rehabil* 1981; 62: 449–452.

81. Carroll D, Rose K. Treatment leads to significant improvement: Effect of conservative treatment on pain in lymphedema. *Professional Nurse* 1992; 32–36.

82. Stevens PE, Dibble SL, Miaskowski C. Prevalence, characteristics, and impact of postmastectomy pain syndrome: An investigation of women's experiences. *Pain* 1995; 61:61–68.

83. Kisson M, Querci della Rovere G, Easton D, Westbury G. Risk of lymphedema following the treatment of breast cancer. *Br J Surg* 1986; 73:580–584.

84. Aitken D, Minton J. Complications associated with mastectomy. *Surg Clin North Am* 1983; 63: 1331–1352.

85. Brennan M. Lymphedema following the surgical treatment of breast cancer: A review of pathophysiology and treatment. *J Pain Symptom Manage* 1992; 7: 110–116.

86. Ventafridda V. Transcutaneous nerve stimulation in cancer pain. In: Bonica JJ, Ventafridda, VV (eds.), *Advances in Pain Research and Therapy*. New York: Raven Press, 1979; pp. 509–515.

87. Avellanosa AM, West CR. Experience with transcutaneous nerve stimulation for relief of intractable pain in cancer patients. *J Med* 1982; 13:203–213.

88. Brennan M. The role of physiatry. In: Arbit E (ed.), *Management of Cancer-related Pain*. Mount Kisco, N.Y.: Futura Publishing Co., 1993; pp. 179–191.

89. Kohl HW, LaPorte RE, Blair SN. Physical activity and cancer: An epidemiological perspective. *Sports Med* 1988; 6:222–237.

90. Kovar PA, Allegrante JP, MacKenzie R, Peterson MGE, Gutin B, Charlson ME. Supervised fitness walking in patients with osteoarthritis of the knee: A randomized trial. *Ann Intern Med* 1992; 116:529–534.

91. Sarmiento A, Sinclair WF. Fracture orthoses. In: *Atlas of Orthotics: Biomechanical Principles and Applications*. St. Louis: CV Mosby; 1975.

92. Cybulski GR. Methods of surgical stabilization for metastatic disease of the spine. *Neurosurg* 1989; 25:240–252.

93. Woodforde JM, Fielding JR. Pain and cancer. *J Psychosomatic Res* 1970. 14:365–370.

94. Breitbart W. Psychiatric management of cancer pain. *Cancer* 1989; 63:2336–2342.

95. Bruera E, Brenneis C, Paterson AH, et al. Use of methyl-phenidate as an adjuvant to narcotic analgesics in patients with advanced cancer. *J Pain Symptom Manage* 1989; 4:3–6.

96. Breitbart W. Suicide in cancer patients. *Oncology* 1987; 1:49–53.

97. Bukberg J, Penman D, Holland J. Depression in hospitalized cancer patients. *Psychosom Med* 1984; 43:199–202.

98. Fawzy FI, Cousins N, Fawzy NW, Kemeny ME, Elashoff R, Morton DA. Structured psychiatric intervention for cancer patients. I. Changes over time in methods of coping and affective disturbance. *Arch Gen Psychiatry* 1990; 47:720–725.

99. Spiegel D, Bloom JR, Kraemer HC, Gottheil E. Effect of psychological treatment on survival of patients with metastatic breast cancer. *Lancet* 1989; 2:888–891.

100. Nickelson C, Brende JO, Gonzalez J. What if your patient prefers an alternative pain control method? Self hypnosis in the control of pain. *South Med J* 1999; 92:521–523.

101. Spiegel D, Bloom JR. Group therapy and hypnosis reduce metastatic breast cancer pain. *Psychosom Med* 1983; 4:333–339.

102. Speigel D. The use of hypnosis in controlling cancer pain. *CA Cancer J Clin* 1985; 4:221–231.

103. McGrath PA, ed. *Pain in Children: Nature, Assessment, and Treatment*. New York: Guilford Press, 1990.

104. Citron ML, Johnson-Early A, Boyer M, et al. Patient controlled analgesia for severe cancer pain. *Arch Inter Med* 1986; 146:734–736.

105. Breitbart W, Holland J. Psychiatric aspects of cancer pain. In: Foley KM (ed.), *Advances in Pain Research and Therapy*, XVI. New York: Raven Press, 1990; pp. 73–87.

106. Cleeland CS. Nonpharmacologic management of cancer pain. *J Pain Symptom Control* 1987; 2:523–528.

107. Fishman B, M, Jacobsen PB, Przo M. Cognitive-behavioral interventionals in the management of cancer pain: Principles and applications. *Med Clin North Am* 1987; 71:271–287.

108. Beck SL. The therapeutic use of music for cancer-related pain. *Oncol Nurs Forum* 1991; 18:1327–1337.

109. Munro S, Mount B. Music therapy in palliative care. *Can Med Assoc J* 1978; 119:1029–1034.

110. Pfaaf VK, Smith KE, Gowen D. The effects of music assisted relaxation on the distress of pediatric cancer patients undergoing bone aspiration. *Child Health Care* 1989; 18:232–236.

111. McCaffery M, Beebe A. *Pain: Clinical Manual For Nursing Practice*. St. Louis: CV Mosby Co., 1989.

112. McCaul KD, Malott JM. Distraction and coping with pain. *Psychol Bull* 1984; 95:516–533.

113. Hilgard E, LeBaron S. Relief of anxiety and pain in children and adolescents with cancer: Quantitative measures and clinical observations. *Int J Clin Exper Hypnosis* 1982; 30:417–442.

114. Anderson KO, Bradley LA, Young LD, McDaniel LK, Wise CM. Rheumatoid arthritis: Review of psychological factors to etiology, effects, and treatment. *Psychol Bull* 1985; 98: 358–387.

115. Syrjala KL, Cummings C, Donaldson GW. Hypnosis or cognitive behavioral training for the reduction of pain and nausea during cancer treatment: a controlled clinical trial. *Pain* 1992; 48:137–146.

116. Patterson DR, Everett JJ, Burns GL, Matvin JA. Hypnosis for the treatment of burn pain. *J Consult Clin Psychol* 1992; 60:713–717.

117. Genuis ML. The use of hypnosis in helping cancer patients control anxiety, pain, emesis: A review of the literature. *Am J Clin Hypn* 1995; 37:317–325.

118. Jay S, Elliott C, Varni J. Acute and chronic pain in adults and children with cancer. *J Consult Clin Psychol* 1986; 54:601–607.

119. Basmajian JV. Biofeedback in rehabilitation: A review of practices and principles. *Arch Phys Med Rehabil* 1981:62:469–475.

120. Biedermann HJ, Monga TN. Relaxation oriented EMG biofeedback with back pain patients: Evaluation of paraspinal muscles activity. *Clin Biofeedback Health* 1985; 8:119–123.

121. Biedermann HJ, McGhie A, Monga TN, Shanks GL. Perceived and actual control in EMG treatment of back pain. *Behav Res Ther* 1987; 25:137–147.

122. Nielsen OS, Munro AJ, Tannock IF. Bone metastasis: Pathophysiology and management policy. *J Clin Oncol* 1991; 9:509–524.

123. Wagner G. Frequency of pain in patients with cancer. *Recent Results Cancer Res* 1984; 89:64–71.

124. Lote K, Walloe A, Bjersand A. Bone metastasis. Prognosis, diagnosis and treatment. *Acta Radiol Oncol* 1986; 25:227–232.

125. Patanaphan V, Salazar OM, Risco R. Breast cancer: Metastatic patterns and their prognosis. *South Med J* 1988; 81:1109–1112.

126. Carter RL. Patterns and mechanisms of bone metastases. *J Royal Soc Med* 1985; (suppl 9)78:2–6.

127. Carter RL. Patterns and mechanism of localized bone invasion by tumors: Studies with squamous carcinomas of the head and neck. *Crit Rev Clin Lab Sci* 1985; 22:275–315.

128. Mundy GR. Bone resorption and turnover in health and disease. *Bone* 1987; (suppl 1)8: 9–16.

129. Paterson, AGH. Bone metastases in breast cancer, prostate cancer, and myeloma. *Bone* 1987: 8 (suppl 1); 17–22.

130. Miller F, Whitehill R. Carcinoma of the breast metastatic to the skeleton. *Clin Orthop* 1984; 184:121–127.

131. Jacobs SC. Spread of prostate cancer to bone. *Urology* 1983; 21:337–344.

132. Tofe AJ, Francis MD, Harvey WJ. Correlation of neoplasms with incidence and localization of skeletal metastases. *J Nucl Med* 1975; 16:986–989.

133. Poulsen HS, Nielsen OS, Klee M., et al. Palliative radiation of bone metastases. *Cancer Treat Rev* 1989; 16:41–48.

134. Fisher G, Mayer DK, Struthers C. Bone metastasis: Part 1–pathophysiology. *Clin J Oncol Nurs* 1997; 1:29–35.

135. Fidler M. Incidence of fracture through metastases in long bones. *Acta Orthop Scand* 1981; 52:623–627.

136. Albright JA, Gillespie TE, Butaud TR. Treatment of bone metastases. *Semin Oncol* 1980; 7:418–433.

137. Malawer MM, Delaney TF. Treatment of metastatic cancer to bone. In: DeVita VT Jr, Hellman S, Rosenberg SA (eds.), *Cancer, Principles, and Practice of Oncology.* Philadelphia: Lippincott, 1989; pp. 2298–2317.

138. Oda MAS, Schurman DJ. Monitoring of pathological fracture. In: Stoll BA, Parbhoo S (eds.), *Bone Metastases Monitoring and Treatment.* New York: Raven Press, 1983; pp. 271–288.

139. Rodriguez M, Dinapoli RP. Spinal cord compression with special reference to metastatic epidural tumors. *Mayo Clic Proc* 1980; 55:442–448.

140. Sundereson, N, DiGiacinto GV, Hughes JEO. Neurosurgery in the treatment of cancer pain. *Cancer* 1989; 63:2365–2377.

141. Latini P, Maranzano E, Ricci S, et al. Role of radiotherapy in metastatic spinal cord compression: Preliminary results from a prospective trial. *Radiother Oncol* 1989; 15:227–233.

142. Kori SH, LaPerriere JA, Kowalski MB, Rodriguez C, Dinwoodie W. Management of bone pain secondary to metastatic disease. *Cancer Control* 1997; 4:153–157.

143. Cheng DS, Seitz CB, Eyre HJ. Non-operative management of femoral, humeral, and acetabular metastases in patients with breast carcinoma. *Cancer* 1980; 45:1533–1537.

144. Harrington KD. *Orthopedic Management of Metastatic Bone Disease*. St. Louis: Mosby, 1988.

145. Hoskin PJ. Scientific and clinical aspects of radiotherapy in the relief of bone pain. *Cancer Surv* 1988; 7:69–86.

146. Arcangeli G, Micheli A, Arcangeli G, Giannarelli D, La Pasta O, Tollis A, et. al. The responsiveness of bone metastases to radiotherapy: The effect of site, histology and radiation dose on pain relief. *Radiotherapy and Oncology* 1989; 14:95–101.

147. Tong D, Gillick L, Hendrickson FR. The palliation of symptomatic osseous metastases. Final results of the study by the radiation therapy oncology group. *Cancer* 1982; 50:893–899.

148. Madsen EL. Painful bone metastasis: Efficacy of radiotherapy assessed by the patients: A randomised trial comparing 4 Gy x 6 vs. 10 Gy x 2. *Int J Radiat Oncol Biol Phys* 1983; 9:1775–1779.

149. Price P, Hoskin PJ, Easton D, et al. Prospective randomised trial of single- and multi-fraction radiotherapy schedules in the treatment of painful bony metastases. *Radiother Oncol* 1986; 6:247–255.

150. Price P, Hoskin PJ, Easton D, et al. Low-dose single fraction radiotherapy in the treatment of metastatic bone pain: A pilot study. *Radiother Oncol* 1988; 12:297–300.

151. Cole DJ. A randomized trial of a single treatment versus conventional fractionation in the palliative radiotherapy of painful metastases. *Clin Oncol* 1989; 1:59–62.

152. Janjan NA. Radiation for bone metastases: Conventional techniques and the role of systemic radiopharmaceuticals. *Cancer* 1997; 80:1628–1645.

153. Barak F, Werner A, Walach N, et al. The palliative efficacy of a single-dose of radiation in treatment of symptomatic osseous metastases. *Int J Radiat Oncol Biol Phys* 1987; 13:1233–1235.

154. Dickinson CZ, Hendrix NS. Strontium-89 therapy to painful bony metastases. *J Nucl Med Technol* 1993; 21:133–137.

155. Silberstein EB. Systemic radiopharmaceutical therapy of painful osteoblastic metastases. *Sem Radiation Oncol* 2000; 10:240–249.

156. Hortobagyi GN, Theriault RL, Porter, L. et al. Efficacy of pamidronate in reducing skeletal complication in patients with breast cancer and lytic bone metastases. *N Eng J Med* 1996; 335:1785–1791.

157. Hortobagyi GN, Theriault RL, Lipton A, et al. Long- term prevention of skeletal complications of metastatic breast cancer with pamidronate. Protocol 19 Arcdia Breast Cancer Study Group. *J Clin Oncol* 1998; 16:2038–2044.

158. Theriault RL, Lipton A, Hortobagyi GN, et al. Pamidronate reduces skeletal morbidity in women with advanced breast cancer and lytic bone lesions: A randomized, placebo-controlled trial. Protocol 18 Aredia Breast Cancer Study Group. *J Clin Oncol* 1999; 17:846–854.

159. Berenson JR, Lichtenstein A, Porter L. et al. Efficacy of pamidronate in reducing skeletal events in patients with advanced multiple myeloma. *N Eng J Med* 1996; 334:488–493.

160. Hillner BE. The role of Bisphosphonates in metastatic breast cancer. *Sem Radiation Oncol* 2000; 10:250–253.

161. Payne R. Anatomy, physiology and pharmacology of nocioception. In: Arbit E (ed.), *Management of Cancer-Related Pain*. New York: Futura, 1993; pp. 21–36.

162. Elliott K. Cancer pain syndromes and classification. In: Arbit E (ed.), *Management of Cancer-Related Pain*. New York: Futura, 1993; pp. 29–53.

163. Thompson G, Moore D. Abdominal pain and celiac plexus nerve block. *Anesth Analg* 1977; 56:1.

164. Ischia S, Luzzani A, Ischia A, et al. A new approach to the neurolytic block of the celiac plexus: The transaortic technique. *Pain* 1983; 16:333–341.

165. Jaeckle KA. Nerve plexus metastases. *Neurol Clin* 1991; 9:857–866.

166. Thomas JE, Colby MY Jr. Radiation-induced or metastatic brachial plexopathy? Diagnostic dilemma. *JAMA* 1972; 222:1392–1395.

167. Match RM. Radiation-induced brachial plexus paralysis. *Arch Surg* 110:384–386, 1975.

168. Kori SH, Foley KM, Posner JB. Brachial plexus lesions in patients with cancer: 100 cases. *Neurology* 1987; 31:45–50.

169. Portenoy RK. Epidemiology and syndromes of cancer pain. *Cancer* 1989; 63:2289–2307.

170. Jaeckle KA, Young DF, Foley KM. The natural history of lumbosacral lexopathy in cancer. *Neurology* 1985; 35: 8–15.

171. Thomas JE, Cascino TL, Earle JD. Differential diagnosis between radiation and tumor plexopathy of the pelvis. *Neurology* 1985; 35: 1–7.

172. Nisce LZ, Chu FC. Radiation therapy of brachial plexus syndrome from breast cancer. *Radiology* 1968; 91:1022–1025.

173. Stjernsward J, Koroltchouk V, Teoh N. National policies for cancer pain relief and palliative care. *Palliative Med* 1992; 273–276.

13 | Burn Pain—Evaluation and Management

Karen J. Kowalske, M.D.

Burn injury can produce the most excruciating pain that an individual will ever experience. With loss of the epidermis and a portion of the dermal layer, nerve endings are exposed. The nerve endings depolarize spontaneously and are stimulated by the environment, thus producing an overwhelming volume of painful nociceptive input. Opioids are the mainstay of burn pain treatment (1,2). Long-acting opioids or patient-controlled analgesia (PCA) is used to treat constant background pain (3,4). Procedural or acute pain is treated with short-acting opioids, nitrous oxide, or ketamine (5,6,7). General anesthesia is reserved for only the most painful procedures (8). Because of the overwhelming nature of the burn experience, the majority of patients have superimposed affective pain and anxiety (9). This component can be treated with anxiolytics, but also responds to alternative methods such as relaxation techniques, hypnosis, or distraction with videos or music (10). The pediatric and geriatric population often have their pain needs grossly underestimated and are undermedicated despite clear evidence that they experience severe pain and may require medication doses similar to the adult population (11). A full understanding of the nature and extent of burn pain is essential for the rehabilitation professional to facilitate appropriate treatment for this unique population.

Burn injury is quite common. Each year in the United States approximately 1.5 million people suffer a burn injury (12). Of these, 500,000 people are seen in an emergency room and over 50,000 are admitted to the hospital (12). Approximately 5,500 deaths per year are attributed to the complications of burn injury (12). All of these individuals have pain associated with their injuries. This pain is initially related to the magnitude and type of tissue and nerve damage sustained and the resultant inflammatory process.

MECHANISM OF BURN PAIN

With loss of the epidermal and dermal layers, nerve endings are exposed. These nerve endings spontaneously depolarize and produce severe pain. Wound care, including the scrubbing or sharp debridement techniques necessary to remove necrotic eschar, also stimulates the exposed nerve endings, thus producing ongoing painful nociceptive input (13,14). Keeping the wound covered partially relieves this discomfort but by no means takes it away completely. Full thickness burns, which involve the entire dermal layer, are classically described as insensate but most patients experience pain at the wound margins and in the surrounding tissues. Also, the majority of wounds that appear full thickness actually have varying wound depth, with some areas of deep partial thickness, which spares the nerve ending and produces pain (15). In response to the tissue trauma, inflammation occurs and histamine is released. This hypersensitizes the adjacent tissues and produces an associated pain response in the unburned surrounding skin (7,13,14).

EXTENT OF BURN

Burn size combined with burn depth is used to determine overall injury severity. Larger burns have a significantly longer recovery course, requiring approximately one day of hospitalization for each percent of the total body surface area (TBSA) burned (15,16). Mortality and morbidity are also related to the TBSA. In the past, percent TBSA + age, approximated the following burn injury. With the use of good fluid resuscitation and aggressive antibiotic treatment, this is no longer completely accurate, but it still can be used as a gauge of burn severity (16,17). The TBSA can be calculated in many ways. The *Rule of Nines* is an estimation method that is commonly used because it is easy to remember, but is not the most accurate measurement system. The TBSA is divided into 11 major body parts, each of which contain a 9 percent surface area with the remaining 1 percent for the perineum. The head and each arm represent 9 percent. The anterior trunk, back, and each leg represent 18 percent TBSA (16). Another simple method for estimating burn size is using the palm of a patient's hand to represent 1 percent TBSA (16). The Lund and Browder chart is more accurate and is useful for calculating burn size in children (16).

BURN DEPTH AND PROGNOSIS FOR HEALING

Traditionally, burn depth was classified as first, second, and third degree. Today, burn depth has been reclassified as superficial (first degree), partial (second degree), full (third degree), and deep full thickness (fourth degree). All of these burns produce pain; what appears to be a mild burn may produce significant pain.

Superficial burns (first degree) involve only the epithelium and are usually related to sunburn. The skin is red, moist, and may be edematous. Pain levels are mild to moderate. The skin does not blister, but may peel over 3 to 7 days. This depth of burn heals without scarring or pigmentation changes (16).

Partial thickness burns (second degree) are subdivided into three categories: superficial, mid-, and deep. Superficial partial thickness burns involve the epidermis and the superficial layer of the dermis. They are shiny, red, weeping, and are moderately painful. These wounds heal in 7 to 14 days and produce minimal or no scarring. Mid-partial thickness burns are blistered and range in color from pink to red. These wounds are moderately to severely painful, but usually heal in 14 to 21 days. Pigment changes and scarring may occur. Deep partial thickness burns involve the epidermis and most of the dermis with sparing of the base of hair follicles. Because the hair follicle is lined with epithelium, re-epithelization of these wounds can occur. Nerve endings are usually spared and pain is excruciating, especially when exposed to air. These wounds initially have a thick yellow eschar but are deep cherry red when fully debrided. Healing usually occurs over 21 to 28 days, but will produce a significant amount of thick hypertrophic scarring (16). If these wounds are larger than a quarter or in a functionally or cosmetically important area like the face or dorsal hands, skin grafting may be performed to maximize outcome (16).

Full thickness burns (third degree) involve the entire dermis down to subcutaneous tissue. Wounds are usually dull white and leathery appearing. Areas of full thickness burn larger than 2 to 3 cm require skin grafting or will otherwise take months to epthelilize from the wound margin (16). Although classically described as insensate, these wounds may vary in depth with partial sparing of nerve endings that cause pain (7). Also, the wound margins and surrounding skin become hypersensitive and produce pain (7).

Deep full thickness burns (fourth degree) are usually caused by prolonged hot contact or an electrical injury. Prolonged hot contact produces a wound that is charred in appearance. Electrical wounds are pale in appearance and may have a relatively small skin component despite significant underlying muscle necrosis. Fourth-degree burns are truly insensate except for the wound margin and require flap coverage or amputation to achieve wound closure (18). These patients are candidates for neuropathic or phantom-type pain, which will require specific intervention (19).

In general, wound closure decreases pain, but as the nerve endings regrow through scar tissue, scar pain occurs (7). Also, long-term therapy, as outlined below, continues to produce pain for the burn patient.

PAIN ASSESSMENT TOOLS

We can accurately assess the pain associated with burn injuries only through patient self-report. This method is subjective, but can be made quantitative and useful for research by the development and use of statistically validated scales. Visual analog scales, numerical scales, and verbal descriptive scales are widely used to evaluate burn pain (20). The visual analog scale has a slight advantage for research purposes, because it may be more sensitive to treatment changes and it can be analyzed using parametric statistics. In contrast, the ordinal scales require the use of nonparametric statistics. Picture scales may be more useful for those who do not speak or read English, and for young children. The Descriptor Differential Scale of Pain Effect, the Visual Analog Scale of Pain Effect, and the Pain Discomfort Scale may be more useful for evaluating the affective component of pain (20). The Magill Pain Questionnaire is a more categorical tool used to differentiate the sensory and affective components of the pain response in burn patients (21).

Pain in very young children can be assessed by observation of physiologic changes, but this is not a very reliable measure of the actual pain experience. Pain in children is best evaluated by using age-appropriate picture or verbal scales (20).

Unfortunately even with the best of scales, there is still a low correlation of pain assessment between the healthcare provider versus that of the patient. Using the visual analog scale, studies show that only 30 to 55 percent of nurses are able to rate pain within one pain scale level of where patients rate themselves (20). Inaccurate assessment of pain impairs the ability to accurately assess the patient's medical condition and can negatively impact the amount of medication a patient receives and his subsequent quality of life (22).

MANAGEMENT OF BURNS

Initial treatment for all burn wounds is twice-daily dressing changes. Fifty to 85 percent of adult burn patients report severe pain with dressing changes, despite the use of numerous medications (23). When the dressing is removed, the nerve endings are exposed and pain is generated. The wound eschar is then debrided either with scrubbing or sharp excision. This is the most painful aspect of burn care and requires very aggressive medical management (19). With frequent dressing changes over a prolonged period of time, hypersensitivity develops in the burn and surrounding tissues (7). Covering the exposed nerve endings provides some pain relief. Topical agents such as silver sulfadiazine are first line for coverage. This bacteriostatic agent keeps the wound bed moist and protects the nerve endings (24). A wide variety of other dressings are available. Fine mesh gauze, biobrane, xenograft (pig skin), and allograft (cadaver skin) can also be used to cover and protect a wound. These dressings are used on clean wounds, including mid-partial thickness burns or deeper wounds that no longer have eschar (24). Autographing provides definitive coverage for deep partial thickness and full thickness wounds. Skin grafting decreases the pain at the grafted site but produces pain at the new area of partial thickness skin loss at the donor site (7). Besides wound care, many other aspects of acute burn care are also painful. These include escharotomies and fasciotomies, frequent blood draws, intramuscular injections, as well as numerous intravenous and intra-arterial line placements.

Burn rehabilitation treatments are another daily source of pain. Stretching of burned skin produces pain, so that patients have a tendency to rest in a position of skin shortening. This "position of comfort" becomes the "position of contracture" (25). Initial therapy is designed to facilitate sustained stretch across these areas. The patient must also be positioned in the stretch position, which includes using shoulder boards to stretch the axillas, elbow extension splints, volar wrist positioning splints, derotation straps for the thighs, and neutral ankle positioning splints (25,26).

Once a patient is more mobile, splinting or casting is used to keep the wounds and subsequent scar stretched and to facilitate a good functional outcome.

Pressure garments and face masks are used to control scarring (7). Unfortunately, these necessary treatments perpetuate constant background pain. Passive range-of-motion to the point of pain, which is essential for maximizing range of motion, continues throughout the course of burn recovery. Healed scar may be hypersensitive to touch. This is treated by desensitizing deep massage of the scar. This can be quite painful but is the only treatment for this condition. Exercise for reconditioning may cause muscle pain. Reinforcement of the importance of rehabilitation for recovery may help patients cope better with the associated pain.

Although burn patients commonly have neuropathy, significant neuropathic pain is unusual. If neuropathic pain does occur, it can be treated as is neuropathic pain in other populations. It is usually unresponsive to opioid analgesia. Tricyclic antidepressants (TCAs) and antiepileptics are the mainstay of treatment and can be safely used for burn patients. If pain persists despite standard interventions, it may respond to continuous infusion of low dose lidocaine (27).

Permanent pain after burn injury is unusual. Most patients have minimal or no pain once the wounds are healed and the scars are fully mature (18 to 24 months). Some patients can continue to have pain because of prolonged wound healing or recurrent open wounds related to methicillin-resistant *Staphylococcus aureus*. Itching is a common problem following wound healing and may be related to a combination of dry skin, neuropathic changes, and nerve regeneration. Dysesthesias within the scarred areas is seen in as many as 80 percent of patients at 1-year post-burn (28).

Burn pain may be made worse by psychologic factors including fear of pain or disfigurement, anxiety related to loss of control, the distress of losing family members or material possessions at the time of the injury, and the development of depression (28).

Pharmacologic Management of Burn Pain

Opioids. Opioids have been the mainstay of acute burn pain management for over 150 years (1,2). Immediate pain management for a patient with a major burn can include frequent small doses of intravenous morphine (25 to 50 micrograms/kg/hr), using careful titration to avoid respiratory depression (7). Following resuscitation, patients may remain on intravenous morphine either as PCA, nurse controlled analgesia (NCA), or continuous IV infusion (7).

Initially, all analgesics or anesthetics should be titrated to effect. However, when dosing after the first 24 hours, decreased plasma protein levels increase the bioavailability of the free drug. Also, changes in the volume of distribution and clearance of drugs must be taken into account. Other factors to consider are the effects of nephrotoxic or hepatotoxic drugs, malnutrition, parenteral nutrition, and underlying systemic illness (11). As long as significant surface areas remain open, requiring frequent dressing changes and local wound debridement, intravenous opioids should be administered. As the wounds heal spontaneously or after surgical wound closure, patients can be converted to oral opioids for procedural and background pain.

The oral dose for morphine can be calculated by multiplying the IV dose by a factor of 3, allowing for individual variability. Oral medications should be administered 20 to 30 minutes prior to wound care, to allow time for adequate absorption. Once patients can tolerate wound care and exercise with oral opioids, discharge from the hospital can be arranged. Controlled-release morphine sulfate is an excellent oral opioid preparation for the control of background burn pain. Studies of sustained-release morphine sulfate show analgesic qualities comparable to continuous morphine sulfate infusions (29). Sustained-release morphine sulfate has a long duration of analgesia (T1/2 = 14 hrs), and its predictable blood levels correlate well with the analgesic effect (29), which peaks at 1.4 hrs (3). In contrast, standard oral morphine sulfate analgesia lasts for 3 hrs and reaches its peak at .5 hrs (3).

Long-term use of opioids can result in tolerance, but rarely results in psychologic dependence particularly when used for the treatment of acute pain (30). A withdrawal response has been seen in some burn patients when sustained-release morphine is discontinued (29).

Other opioids, including methadone, meperidine, fentanyl, sufentanil, and alfentanil, have been used to treat the pain associated with burns. Methadone is effective, but it is important to take into account that increased clearance may necessitate increased dosing (31). Meperidine may be a good pain medication for procedural pain, but it is not recommended for background pain because of its short half life and the risk of normeperidine accumulation, a toxic metabolite that can cause seizures. This is a very real consideration in burn patients with decreased renal clearance (11). Fentanyl, a potent opioid, in combination with midazolam can be used for procedure-related pain. A transmucosal delivery (lollipop) of fentanyl is available and is a safe means of analgesia for children (11,32,33). Alfentanil, with its rapid onset (< 1 min) and its short duration of action (15 min), has recently been advocated for procedural pain. Using IV boluses of 10 micrograms/kg given every minute until analgesia is achieved has been used safely for dressing changes and wound debridement (7). Nalbuphine, an opioid agonist–antagonist, has been studied for burn pain, but its use is limited because of the *ceiling effect*, at which increasing doses do not provide increased analgesia (34). Intramuscular opioids are not widely used in the burn population because of variable systemic drug levels and because many patients, particularly children, may have increased anxiety associated with injections.

Patient Controlled Analgesia (PCA). Intravenous PCA is shown to be safe and effective in the burn population. PCA morphine can be used in similar amounts to those used for intermittent bolus analgesia, but produces better pain relief and patient satisfaction (4). The major benefit of PCA is that patients do not have to wait to receive pain relief, which can be a real problem in busy burn units. PCA is adaptable to individual patient needs and provides a consistent blood level of analgesic. A significant variability in patient requirements exists, and the dosing amount and interval must be adjusted accordingly. The side effects are similar to those seen with intermittent morphine. The downside of PCA includes the requirement for intravenous access and the need for switch modification for patients with significant hand burns. For patients who have marked functional limitations or who, for other reasons, are not able to fully operate a PCA, a nurse-controlled device can be used. This device allows the nurse to push the button for the patient, delivering a maximum dose over specific intervals. This is particularly useful in the intensive care unit, where patients are immobile and nurse availability to assist with analgesia is not a limiting factor (4).

Nonsteroidal Antiinflammatory Agents. Once the wounds are nearly healed, nonsteroidal antiinflammatory drugs (NSAIDs) or plain acetaminophen can be used (35). NSAIDs or aspirin-based products are not recommended during the acute burn stage because of their antiplatelet effect and its associated risk of increased blood loss and the possibility of gastric ulceration and gastrointestinal bleeding (35).

Anesthetic Techniques and Agents. Inhalation analgesia using 50 percent nitrous oxide may be administered with or without opioids. It is easy to administer, has a rapid onset of action, and gives the patient some control over dosing (5). The safety of prolonged use of nitrous oxide has been questioned, with particular concerns about bone marrow suppression and hepatotoxicity. Nitrous oxide is not recommended for patients with traumatic brain injury, chronic neurologic disease, asthma, COPD, or chest trauma. It is also not recommended for pregnant women, children younger than 6 years, or for patients who are unable to self-administer (36). Few side effects are seen; fewer than 10 percent of patients develop nausea or vomiting. There are some concerns about long-term staff exposure, which can be decreased with adequate ventilation. The potential for abuse by staff members necessitates tight control of access to nitrous oxide (36).

Conscious sedation with ketamine has been advocated by some, because it produces a "dissociate" anesthetic state with profound analgesia. Ketamine is advantageous because it produces intense analgesia combined with cardiovascular stimulation and the preservation of adequate ventilation and airway reflexes (6). Initial dosing begins at 1 mg/kg. Difficulties with ketamine include tolerance with repetitive administration and vivid dreams or unpleasant emergence reactions, which are seen in 5 to 30 percent of patients. The incidence of emergence reactions is less in children and can be decreased with the concomitant use of opioids or benzodiazepines. Ketamine increases secretions, which may require preprocedure prophylaxis. Anesthesiology or an airway management team should be present during conscious sedation with ketamine (37). Because of the additional precautions associated with conscious sedation, this technique may be considerably more expensive than traditional techniques.

Regional anesthesia has a limited role in the management of acute burn pain because of the risk of catheter infection. Spinal epidural anesthesia is not recommended for patients with large open wounds for the same reason. Brachial plexus blocks can be used for isolated extremity injuries (11) and for tissue reconstruction once all of the wounds have healed.

General anesthesia is usually reserved for major debridement or skin grafting, but it has been used during debridement within the burn unit (8,38). Concerns over repeated procedures with general anesthesia include anesthesia-induced side effects (hyperkalemia, nausea, vomiting) as well as the significant nutritional consequences of prolonged periods with no oral intake both pre- and postoperatively (8,38). From a rehabilitation perspective, significant losses in both range of motion and endurance are seen because of the bed rest and missed therapy sessions that follow general anesthesia.

Anxiolytics. Anxiety decreases pain tolerance. Methods to reduce anxiety minimize the interplay between acute pain and sympathetic arousal. Therefore, anxiolytics may help decrease anxiety and improve pain tolerance. However, anxiolytics do not actually provide analgesia and thus should not be used as a substitute for narcotics (9,39). Benzodiazepines can attenuate the anxiety associated with medical procedures (9,39). Lorazepam reduces burn pain when combined with opioids (39). Anxiolytics should be administered 30 to 45 minutes prior to procedures to decrease anticipatory anxiety (39). Anxiety is usually proportional to burn size; it decreases with wound healing and improves with relaxation techniques. The anxiety response is also related to personality, past experiences, and cultural background (9). Tension is the strongest predictor of pain during a procedure (22).

Behavioral Pain Reduction Techniques

Nociceptive input from the burn results in the pain experience. This is altered by the affective components that effect an individual's pain experience including emotional, cultural, and religious factors that contribute to the interpretation of the incoming sensory input. Alternative treatment approaches are very helpful in altering the affective component of procedure-related burn pain. The most commonly used techniques include behavioral modification, desensitization, imagery, modeling, stress reduction, and hypnosis (9). These techniques decrease the pain experience but are not a substitute for analgesics. A combined approach using a variety of different techniques can be individualized for each patient.

Distraction techniques involve refocusing attention from pain to a sensory stimulus that combines auditory and visual overload (10). This can involve the use of videos during dressing changes to reduce anxiety and pain intensity. Patients may become bored with scenic and melodic videos and therefore should be offered alternative video material particularly reflecting life interests such as sports, romance, comedy, pornography, and different types of music (10). One study of virtual reality imagery during wound care showed promise for decreasing pain. Unfortunately, the hardware for setting up a virtual reality experience remains prohibitively expensive (40).

The restructuring of thoughts is an approach where a person's thoughts can be treated as behaviors and modified. A burn patient's thoughts about the pain associated with procedures can be modified to decrease the affective experience.

Patients having avoidant personality styles want to know very little about their treatment. In contrast, patients classified as sensitizers require as much information as possible. Avoidant personalities can distract themselves from an unpleasant experience using imagery, distracting conversation, or individualized videos. Sensitizers, who want information, can use reappraisal techniques in which they focus on the experience but change the interpretation of incoming sensory information, such as interpreting a deep aching as a healing sensation (9).

Education for burn patients should include both procedural and sensory preparatory information. Procedural information includes explaining what will occur, such as describing donor-site harvest techniques and location and the pattern of meshing to be used. Sensory information should include characterization of donor-site pain and any other sensations that the patient might experience (41). Patient education should also include reassurance that they will not become addicted to pain medications and that using medication is not a sign of weakness (9).

Behavioral issues, including operant reinforcement, are seen with "as-needed" dosing schedules. As-needed dosing schedules may reinforce pain behaviors and acting out, and may actually potentiate pain. As-needed pain medications may also increase a patient's arousal and awareness of symptoms. Administering medications on a time-consistent schedule, based on individual drug half-lives, may facilitate a patient's ability to cope with pain (41). A consistent quota system using fixed-interval breaks can decrease pain and facilitate a patient's ability to cope with the overwhelming aspects of progressive, multiple, aggressive procedures and therapies each day (9).

Relaxation techniques and hypnosis have both been useful in the burn population. Unfortunately, relaxation and imagery are often difficult to use in the hectic setting of most burn units. In these settings, brief relaxation techniques such as deep breathing may be more appropriate. Hypnosis can be applied rapidly with posthypnotic suggestions geared toward subsequent procedures. In one study, hypnosis decreased pain sensation more than opioids alone and more than opioids combined with psychological attention (42).

Depression is relatively mild in most burn patients, with clinically significant depression occurring in fewer than one-third of patients. Those patients who have a clinically complicated course, require multiple surgical procedures, or who are in hospital longer than 3 weeks are more likely to be depressed (21).

Itching is a common problem following wound healing and may be related to a combination of dry skin, neuropathic changes, and nerve regeneration. Dysesthesias within the scarred areas are seen in as many as 80 percent of patients at 1-year post-burn (28). Persistent pain and itching may cause depression, inactivity, social withdrawal, and feelings of isolation (19).

PAIN MANAGEMENT PROTOCOLS

Because of the subjective nature of pain perception and the effects of an individual's background on pain interpretation and dosing, standardized pain protocols are rapidly becoming the standard of care for individuals following burn injury. These protocols facilitate adequate dosing while avoiding the risks of overdosing and its subsequent respiratory suppression (43). Because healthcare providers had a tendency to undermedicate a patient's pain in the past, extra diligence is essential to achieve the balance between appropriate analgesia and oversedation. Critical pathways have also been safely and effectively used to manage pain and anxiety in children (43).

Pediatric Burn Pain Management

As many as 20 percent of burn admissions are of children younger than 4 years of age (7). Many studies show that there is a tendency to undermedicate burn pain in children. A 1978 survey showed that only 8 percent of burn units used narcotics stronger than codeine, 68 percent used acetaminophen +/- codeine, and 24 percent of burn units used no routine pain medications for children prior to procedures (18). Younger children were less likely to be adequately medicated. These children can develop significant psychopathologic conditions after burn injury and require therapy, which may be directly related to the pain experienced in burn treatment (7,44). Aggressive analgesia using systemic opioids, with or without the use of sedatives, can be safely administered in closely titrated doses based on individualized patient response. It must be understood that some children may require doses similar to those given to adults (45). Intravenous administration is preferred over intramuscular administration because of the anxiety response associated with injections. Oral opioids can be safely used, and the availability of morphine drops has revolutionized pain management in children. Fentanyl, especially the fentanyl lollipop, is another safe opioid for the treatment of severe pain in children with burns. It is especially useful for the pain of dressing changes (32). General anesthesia is reserved for extremely painful procedures. Ketamine may also be a useful agent in children because of its decreased risk of side effects in children, when compared to adults (4).

PCA is effective in children as young as 4 years (46). Morphine requirements vary considerably. Tolerance may develop, but weaning is usually not a problem. PCA decreases patient dependence on staff, which may decrease anxiety and promote a sense of control. It avoids injections, which may cause significant anxiety in children. Continuous background infusion prevents fluctuations in blood levels, but patients may still need boluses for procedures. PCA is adaptable to individual patient needs. As in adult use, the downside of PCA for children includes the requirement for IV access and the need for switch modification for patients with significant hand burns (46).

Psychologic pain controlling techniques can be used in children, but they must be applied in a developmentally appropriate manner. Children have a tendency to be more suggestible than adults, are more likely to engage in escape behaviors, do well with distraction techniques, and may do well with hypnosis (42). Children respond better to procedural pain if given some control over circumstances, such as allowing them to remove their own dressings. Fixed-interval rest breaks may help with procedures. It is important to realize that children reflect their environment and a calm attitude in staff and family can facilitate coping. Aversive stimulation should be limited to a single environment, and the child's room and play area should be "safe" areas that are free from painful procedures. Play therapy in conjunction with a child-life specialist can facilitate coping with the pain and anxiety of a burn injury (9,41).

Parental participation can play a role in reducing a child's experience of pain during invasive procedures and may also improve parental coping strategies and long-term compliance with treatment (47). Another positive outcome of increased parental participation is increased parental understanding of the treatment program and decreased parental anxiety through increased exchange of information with staff. An improved understanding of the treatment program, includes explanations of wound care and healing, indications for surgical intervention, and the need for therapy and compression garments.

Burn Pain Management in the Elderly

An aging population, combined with improved survival following burn injury, has dramatically increased the number of geriatric burn survivors. Flame-related burns predominate in this population (17), usually related to difficulty in escaping from the scene of an accident. This situation also leads to the increased incidence of inhalational injuries (17). In the elderly, mortality is related to age, burn size, need for artificial ventilation, and in-hospital complications (17). Although it is clear that elderly individuals experience pain, they are often undermedicated because of concerns about oversedation and decreased drug clearance (48). A study of acute burns showed the effects of age on narcotic dosing: in this study, patients over 75 years of age received significantly less opioid medication than patients aged 66 to 75 years, who received less medication than patients aged 55 to 65 years. Although these findings may be based on staff interpretation that these patients experience less pain, unfortunately, this may instead reflect the underreporting of pain seen in this age group. It has been shown that drug metabolism is slower in the elderly, and therefore individual doses may last for a longer period of time. It may also be true that the elderly avoid narcotics because of the side effect profile, including sedation, mental status changes, and constipation (49). It is critically important that pain in the elderly is thoroughly assessed and that any bias is avoided so that adequate treatment can be provided. Careful attention is also important to avoid excessive dosing, which may cause respiratory suppression or other unacceptable side effects (49).

CONCLUSIONS

Burns are one of the most excruciatingly painful injuries known to man, both acutely and over the course of the rehabilitation period. During this period, it is essential to frequently reassess a patient's pain, which may vary over time and with changes in treatment. A comprehensive individualized approach to patient management should include the judicious use of opioids, particularly morphine, for management of both procedural and background pain. This, combined with anxiolytics and psychologic techniques, is essential to decrease the stress of burn injury. Careful monitoring for oversedation is critical for maximizing functional performance and facilitating early mobilization.

REFERENCES

1. Murray J. The history of analgesia in burns. *Postgrad Med J* 1972; 48:124–127.
2. Wilson G, Tomlinson P. Pain relief in burns—how we do it. *Burns* 1988; 14:331–312
3. Herman R, Veng–Pederen P, Miotto J, et al. Pharmacokinetics of morphine sulfate in patients with burns. *J Burn Care Rehabil* 1994; 15:95–103.
4. Kinsella J, Glavin R, Reid W. Patient-controlled analgesia for burn patients: A preliminary report. *Burns* 1988; 14:500–503.
5. Filkins SA, Cosgrove P, Marvin JA, et al. Self-administered anesthetic: A method of pain control. *J Burn Care Rehabil* 1981; 2:33–34.
6. Jarem BJ, Walker JA, Parks DA, et al. Current practice of anesthesia for pediatric burns. *Anesthesiology Rev* 1978; 5:16–2236.
7. Latarjet J, Choinere M. Pain in burn patients. *Burns,*1995; 21:344–348.
8. Dimick P, Helvig E, Heimbach D, et al. Anesthesia-assisted procedures in a burn intensive care unit procedure room: Benefits and complications. *J Burn Care Rehabil* 1993; 14:446–449.
9. Patterson DR. Non–opioid-based approaches to burn pain. *J Burn Care Rehabil* 1995; 16:372–376.
10. Miller A, Hickman L, Lemasters G. A distraction technique for control of burn pain. *J Burn Care Rehabil* 1992; 13:576–580.
11. Ashburn M. Burn pain. The management of procedure-related pain. *J Burn Care Rehabil* 1995; 16:365–371
12. Brigham PA, McLoughlin E. Piecing together a national burn profile [abstract 104]. In: American Burn Association Twenty–Sixth Annual Meeting, Orlando, 1997.
13. Levine JD, Fields HL, Basbaum AI. Peptides and the primary afferent nocioceptor. *J Neurosci* 13:2273–2286.
14. Treede RD, Meyer RA, Raja SN, Campbell JN. Peripheral and central mechanisms of cutaneous hyperalgesia. *Prog Neurobiology* 1992; 38:397–421.
15. Brandt CP, Yurko L, Coffee R, Fratianne R. Complete integration of inpatient and outpatient burn care: evolution of an outpatient burn clinic. *J Burn Care Rehabil* 1998; 19:406–408.
16. Feller I, Jones CA. Introduction: Statement of the problem. In: Fisher S, Helm P (eds.), *Comprehensive Rehabilitation of Burns*. Baltimore: Williams & Wilkins, 1984.
17. Still JM, Law EJ, Belcher K, Thiruvaiyaru D. A regional medical center's experience with burns of the elderly. *J Burn Care Rehabil* 1999; 20:218–223.
18. Hartford CE. In Fisher S, Helm P (eds.), *Comprehensive Rehabilitation of Burns*. Baltimore: Williams & Wilkins, 1984.
19. Marvin J, Heimbach D. Pain management. In: Fisher S, Helm P (eds.), *Comprehensive Rehabilitation of Burns*. Baltimore: Williams & Wilkins, 1984.
20. Marvin J. Pain assessment versus measurement. *J Burn Care Rehabil*, 1995; 16:348–357.
21. Charlton JE, Klein R, Gagliardi G, et al. Factors affecting pain in burned patients: A preliminary report. *Postgrad Med J* 1983; 59:604–607.
22. Geisser M, Bingham H, Robinson M. Pain and anxiety during burn dressing changes: Concordance between patients' and nurses' ratings and relation to medication administration and patient variables. *J Burn Care Rehabil* 1995; 16:165–171.

23. Perry S, Heidrich G, Ramos E. Assessment of pain by burn patients. *J Burn Care Rehabil* 1981; 2:322–326.
24. Saffle JR, Schnebly WA. Burn wound care. In: Richard R, Staley M (eds.), *Burn Care and Rehabilitation Principles and Practice*. Philadelphia: FA Davis, 1994.
25. Apfel LM, Irwin CP, Staley MJ, Richard RL. In: Richard R, Staley M (eds.), *Burn Care and Rehabilitation Principles and Practice*. Philadelphia: FA Davis, 1994.
26. Nothdurft D, Smith PS, LeMaster JE. In: Fisher S, Helm P (eds.), *Comprehensive Rehabilitation of Burns*. Baltimore: Williams & Wilkins, 1984.
27. Jonsson A, Cassuto J, Hanson B. Inhibition of burn pain by intravenous lignocaine infusion. *Lancet* 1991; 388:151–152.
28. Choiniere M, Melzack R, Rondeau J, et al. The pain of burns: Characteristics and correlates. *J Trauma* 1989; 29:1531–1539.
29. Alexander L, Wolman R, Blache C, et al. Use of morphine sulfate (MS Contin) in patients with burns: A pilot study. *J Burn Care Rehabil* 1992; 13:581–583.
30. Kealey G. Opioids and analgesia. *J Burn Care Rehabil* 1995; 15:363–364.
31. Denson D, Concilus R, Warden G et al. Pharmacokinetics of continuous intravenous infusion of methadone in the early post-burn period. *J Clin Pharmacol* 1990; 30:70–75.
32. Lind G, Marcus M, Mears S, et al. Oral transmucosal fentanyl citrate for analgesia and sedation in the emergency department. *Ann Emerg Med* 1991; 20:1117–1120.
33. Sharar SR, Bratton SL, Carrougher GJ, Edwards WT, Summer G, Levy FH, Cortiella J. A comparison of oral transmucosal fentanyl citrate and oral hydromorphine for inpatient pediatric burn wound care analgesia. *J Burn Care Rehabil* 1998; 19:516–521.
34. Lee J, Marvin J, Heimbach D. Effectiveness of nalbuphone for relief of burn debridement pain. *J Burn Care Rehabil* 1989; 10:241–246.
35. Kinsella J, Booth M. Pain relief in burns: James Laing Memorial Essay 1990. *Burns*, 1991; 17:391–395.
36. Helvig E, Heimbach D. Nitrous oxide in the management of burn pain. In :Pain management in the burn patient: A Workshop Review, 1992 p.15–18.
37. Demling RH, Ellerbee S, Jarrett F. Ketamine anesthesia for tangential excision of burn eschar: A burn unit procedure. *J Trauma* 1978; 8:267–270.
38. Powers P, Cruse C, Daniels S, et al. Safety and efficacy of debridement under anesthesia in patients with burns. *J Burn Care Rehabil*, 1993; 14:176–180.
39. Patterson DR, Ptacek JT, Carrougher GJ, Sharar SR. Lorazepam as an adjunct to opioid analgesics in the treatment of burn pain. *Pain* 1997; 72:367–374.
40. Hoffman HG, Doctor JN, Patterson DR, Carrougher GJ, Furness TA. Virtual reality as an adjunctive pain control during burn wound care in adolescent patients. *Pain* 2000; 85:305–309.
41. Patterson DR. Practical applications of psychological techniques in controlling burn pain. *J Burn Care Rehabil* 1992; 12:13–17.
42. Patterson DR, Everett J, Burns G, et al. Hypnosis for the treatment of burn pain. *J Consult Clin Psychol* 1992; 60:713–717.
43. Sheridan SL, Hinson M, Nackel A, Blaquiere M, Daley W, et al. Development of a pediatric burn pain and anxiety management program. *J Burn Care Rehabil* 1997; 18:455–459.
44. Crompton D, Raphael B, Pegg S. Burns. *Med J Aust* 1990; 52:509–511.
45. Watkins P. This One's for Billy. *J Burn Care Rehabil*, 1993; 14:58–64.
46. Gaukroger P, Chapman J, Davey R. Pain control in pediatric burns: The use of patient-controlled analgesia. *Burns* 1995; 17:396–399.
47. George A, Hancock J. Reducing pediatric burn pain with parent participation. *J Burn Care Rehabil* 1993; 14:104–107.
48. Melzak R. The tragedy of needless pain. *Sci Amer* 1990; 262:27–33.
49. Honari S, Patterson DR, Gibbons J, Martin-Herz SP, Mann R, et al. Comparison of pain control medication in three age groups of elderly patients. *J Burn Care Rehabil* 1997; 18:500–504.

14 | HIV Pain Management

Richard T. Jermyn, D.O.
Deanna M. Janora, M.D.
Barbara S. Douglas, M.D.

In 1997 the Joint United Nations Program on HIV-AIDS (UNAIDS) estimated that 30.6 million persons were infected with the human immunodeficiency virus (HIV) worldwide. An estimated 11.7 million persons throughout the world have died of acquired immune deficiency syndrome (AIDS) since the beginning of the epidemic (1).

It was originally believed that HIV primarily attacked homosexual men and intravenous (IV) drug users. Currently, however, there are at least four groups considered at risk for HIV/AIDS: men having sex with men, IV drug users, infected mothers vertically transmitting the disease to their fetus, and heterosexual persons, especially in minority communities (1,2).

Although patterns of transmission vary throughout the world, by 1996 trends in the United States showed a decrease of infection rate in the homosexual and IV drug–using population and an increase in the heterosexual population (3). An exception is the homosexual adolescent and young male population, which has demonstrated an increase in HIV/AIDS infection since 1996 (3). Blacks, females, and Hispanics are among the heterosexual populations that have demonstrated an increase in HIV/AIDS infection since 1996 (4). Perinatal transmission has declined significantly since 1997, primarily due to pharmacologic prophylaxis during pregnancy and the increased availability of prenatal care (5).

HIV is a lentivirus, a form of nervous system–attacking retrovirus that has a long latency period. It has a direct effect on the intestines, glial cells, and bone marrow (6). Secondary invasion occurs in conjuction with a lowered CD4 count and the destruction of lymphocytes (6). AIDS is the end-stage manifestation of a chronic HIV infection. AIDS is clinically defined as a decline of immune function, concurrent with a CD4 count below 200 cells per microliter of blood (7). The clinical manifestations of AIDS are recurrent pneumonias, pulmonary tuberculosis, and invasive carcinomas, neoplasms, and lymphomas (7). Transmission is via blood and body fluids, and can occur through unprotected sex and the sharing of IV drug needles, or through vertical transmission between an infected mother and her fetus.

Currently, more than $8 billion has been spent in combating this disease (8). The loss of income caused by AIDS approaches the combined cost of the Korean and Vietnam wars.

THE CHANGING VIRUS

Between 1996 and 1997, the death rate due to HIV/AIDS decreased 47.7 percent, reducing it from the eighth to the fourteenth leading cause of death in the United States (9). This decline is in part because of the advent of antiretroviral pharmacologic therapy (10). These medications, as outlined in Table 14.1 (11), can have very serious side effects that may both decrease the quality of life of the patient and cause pain syndromes. Common side effects include painful sensory neuropathy, nausea, vomiting, diarrhea, headaches, fatigue, pancreatitis, and central nervous system (CNS) symptoms (12).

In addition to the side effects of the antiretroviral medications, the HIV virus and secondary infections that result from an immunocompromised system can also manifest as chronic fatigue, painful sensory neuropathies, myelopathy, and myopathies. Depending on the population studied, 25 to 80 percent of patients infected with HIV have at least one type of pain (13,14,15).

Pain is a leading factor in a patient's decreased quality of life and ability to function (13). The prevalence of pain in the HIV-infected population varies from 20 to 80 percent and generally increases as the disease progresses (12,13,14). Generally, patients usually suffer from more than one source of pain. Unfortunately, pain in the HIV/AIDS population is highly underdiagnosed and usually undertreated (15,16,17). Larue et al. studied 315 patients, both hospitalized and ambulatory. They compared patients' reports of pain to treating physicians' perception of the pain. They concluded that physicians underestimated the severity of the pain in at least half of the patients. Fifty-seven percent of the patients with moderate to severe pain received no analgesics (18).

An expert panel of the United States Agency for Health Care Policy and Research (AHCPR) has recommended that the guidelines established for cancer pain be adopted for HIV/AIDS–related pain (18,19). However, although there are many similarities between cancer pain and HIV/AIDS pain, the characterization of pain differs in several important areas. People with HIV/AIDS may be struck during their younger, more productive years. Minorities may not have access to medical care because of financial constraints. Family or social support may be minimal or nonexistent. Drug abuse may be a major factor in both pain treatment and the progression of the disease. Finally, the societal stigma against people infected with HIV/AIDS is still very prevalent in both the general and medical communities.

ROLE OF PHYSICIAN IN HIV PAIN MANAGEMENT

The role of the physician becomes increasingly important as HIV survival rates increase and federal funding decreases. By 1998, the estimated monthly cost of medications and HIV viral load-testing surpassed $1,500 a month, and this figure is pro-

Table 14.1. Clinical Glossary of Antiretroviral Drugs

	Drug	Commercial Name	Dose	Toxicity	Comments
Nucleoside Analogs	Zidovudine	ZDV, AZT, Retrovir	200 mg tid or 300 mg bid	Anemia, neutropenia, nausea, vomiting, fatigue, malaise	May prevent AIDS dementia complex. Prevents perinatal transmission; may reduce transmission after occupational exposure.
	Didanosine	ddI, Videx	200 mg bid (fasting); 400 mg once daily under evaluation	Gastrointestinal (GI) disturbances, pancreatitis, peripheral neuropathy	Less neurotoxic than zalcitabine. Requires gastric neutralization with antacids, which can interfere with absorption of other drugs. Avoid use in patients with high potential for pancreatitis (use of drugs, alcohol, prior history).
	Zalcitabine	ddC, HIVID	0.75 mg tid	Oral ulcers, peripheral neuropathy, pancreatitis	Most effective in previously untreated patients, particularly in combination with zidovudine.
	Stavudine	d4T, Zerit	40 mg bid	Peripheral neuropathy	Less neurotoxic than didanosine or zalcitabine; generally well tolerated.
	Lamivudine	3TC, Epivir	150 mg bid	None	Resistance develops rapidly but may restore zidovudine sensitivity. No clear side effects.
	Abacavir	ABC, Ziagen	300 mg bid	Nausea, hypersensitivity reaction	More potent than other nucleoside analogs. Patients who experience a hypersensitivity reaction to abacavir should never be rechallenged.
Protease Inhibitors	Saquinavir	Fortovase	1200 mg tid with food	Nausea, abdominal cramping, diarrhea	Often used in combiniation with ritonavir or nelfinavir.
	Indinavir	Crixivan	800 mg every 8 h fasting	Nephrolithiasis, hyperbilirubinemia	Elevated bilirubin common and typically benign. Aggressive hydration recommended to prevent renal stones. May be given with low-fat, low-protein snacks.
	Ritonavir	Norvir	600 mg bid with food	Circumoral parestuesias, nausea, headache, fatigue, taste disturbance	Dose escalation recommended (see package insert). Liquid formulation associated with significant taste disturbances; it may be mixed with chocolate milk or nutritional supplements to improve tolerability.
	Nelfinavir	Viracept	750 mg tid (with meals)	Diarrhea	Nelfinavir is commonly dosed twice daily (1250 mg twice daily).
	Amprenavir	Agenerase	1200 mg bid	Rash, GI side effects	
Non-nucleoside Reverse Transcriptase Inhibitors	Nevirapine	Viramune	200 mg bid	Rash	Rapid resistance. Dose escalation commonly recommended to prevent rash (200 mg qd × 14 days, then 200 mg bid).
	Delavirdine	Rescriptor	400 mg tid	Rash	Rapid resistance. Dose escalation to prevent rash is not recommended.
	Efavirenz	Sustiva	600 mg qd	Central nervous system (CNS) symptoms, rash	Rapid resistance. CNS symptoms generally resolve after first few weeks of dosing.

In: Sande M, Volberding P. *The Medical Management of AIDS*, 6th ed. Philadelphia: WB Saunders, 1999: 98.

jected to continue to rise (20). Optimal services are required at a minimal cost. The role of the physician in managing HIV/AIDS pain is outlined as follows:

- Diagnose pain syndromes; it has been demonstrated that physicians are more aggressive with pain management in HIV/AIDS patients when they have a known diagnosis (18).
- Rule out or treat life-threatening pain syndromes appropriately.
- Screen for depression and drug and alcohol abuse, and refer the patient to the appropriate treatment professional.
- Perform a functional status assessment. If the patient is hospitalized, assist him in making decisions about returning home or entering a rehabilitation or long-term care facility.
- Determine what support systems are needed, such as physical and occupational therapy services, a home health aide, or hospice services
- Provide for assistive and adaptive equipment such as canes, walkers, and orthotics.

In managing the patient with HIV/AIDS pain, a team of healthcare professionals is required. This primary-care team consists of infectious disease specialists, physical medicine and rehabilitation specialists, psychiatrists, physical and occupational therapists, pain counselors, and drug and alcohol detoxification specialists. Consultations may be required from neurosurgery, neurology, dermatology, obstetrics and gynecology, gastroenterology, and podiatry.

ASSESSMENT OF PAIN

The initial treatment of pain begins with a complete pain history and physical examination. The history should include a description of pain characteristics (22). The physician should be aware of how long the patient has been diagnosed with HIV/AIDS, since some pain syndromes are more prevalent in different stages of the disease. Critical laboratory studies include a recent viral load test, a CD4 count, hepatitis profile, and liver and renal function studies. At the initial visit, a complete blood count (CBC) and electrolytes should be performed, as well as tests for folate and B12 levels, and thyroid function. These results establish baseline levels that can be used to monitor disease progress.

Any deletion, addition, or change in medications, especially antiretroviral medications, should be reviewed. Because these medications may cause pain syndromes as a side effect, patients may choose to stop or change the dosages of the medications. Many times the physician managing pain is the first to be aware of these changes.

A detailed past medical history specifically inquiring on hepatitis, renal disease, past bacterial or viral illnesses, and injuries or traumas should be obtained. Some bacterial and viral illnesses such as herpes zoster can resurface and should be investigated.

A psychosocial screen should be obtained. There exists a significant correlation between the presence and intensity of pain and psychologic distress, depression, hopelessness, and a decreased quality of life (23). All patients must be screened for drug or alcohol abuse.

A complete functional exam should be obtained. This should include questions about activities of daily living (ADLs), assistive devices used for ambulation and ADLs, current occupation or last occupation held, and the home physical environment. All social support systems should be investigated. It is also important to know what recreational activities the patient enjoys.

A thorough neuromuscular examination should be completed, with particular attention paid to all areas of patient complaints, such as the mouth, abdomen, or feet. The neurologic examination should consist of cranial nerve testing, identification of corticospinal tract signs, evaluation of Babinski and deep-tendon reflexes, and a sensory examination for pin prick, light touch, and vibration in all sensory dermatomes and peripheral nerve distributions. Special attention should be paid to the sensory examination in the feet, so that sensory peripheral neuropathy is not missed. Cerebellar testing and gait analysis are extremely important, especially on patients in advanced stages of the disease. Manual muscle testing should be performed. Proximal muscle weakness can be a sign of an acute myopathy; therefore, dynamic muscle testing should also be performed, using squatting or stair climbing routines.

The patients' skin should be examined for evidence of herpes zoster or Kaposi's sarcoma. An examination of the mouth should look for evidence of oral thrush. All painful lymph nodes should be palpated for evidence of an acute infection or lymphoma.

A patient with peripheral sensory neuropathy should have a detailed foot examination. The physician should look for evidence of ingrown toenails, hyperpronation syndrome, and fractures that could lead to charco joint deformities. Foreign bodies in the foot or evidence of infection should be treated. The patient's gait pattern should be evaluated with and without shoes. An examination of the shoes for wearing patterns is important.

The first step in diagnosing pain syndromes is to determine whether the patient is or is not immunocompromised. The evaluation of the immunologic status of the patient is done by measuring CD4 cells and viral load. CD4 cells respond to class II major histocompatibility complex antigens. They release inflammatory proteins called cytokines that augment the immune response. CD4 lymphocytes are the primary target of HIV infection (24), hence the loss of CD4 cells are an important clinical measurement of immunocompromise.

Viral RNA and DNA assays, or viral load tests, are also commonly used in clinical practice. The sensitivity of viral RNA assays is very high and continues to improve. Plasma HIV RNA levels should be obtained every 3 to 4 months, usually in combination with CD4 counts, to determine the effectiveness of pharmacologic treatment (24).

A patient who is found to be immunocompromised may require an extensive work-up for his pain syndromes. He may have a life-threatening disease such as infectious meningitis, lymphoma, cancer, or inflammatory myopathy that will require immediate treatment.

PAIN SYNDROMES IN HIV/AIDS

A patient infected with HIV/AIDS may present with pain caused by the direct effect of the virus, as a result of immunosuppression from opportunistic infections, from side effects of the medications used to treat HIV infection (such as antiretrovirals and chemotherapy), or from preexisting syndromes not related to HIV infection (see Table 14.2) (25).

The pain symptoms in the HIV/AIDS patient can be varied. In 1989, Leibowitz published a retrospective study of hospitalized patients with HIV/AIDS and discovered that pain was the second most common reason for hospitalization, accounting for 30 percent of the admissions. Pain symptoms on admission were: chest pain (22 percent), headache (13 percent), and oral cavity pain (11 percent) (14). In 1993, Singer did a large prospective, longitudinal study of ambulatory patients in all stages of the disease and reported the most common painful syndromes were headaches, herpes simplex infection, painful peripheral neuropathy, back pain, herpes zoster infection, zidovudine (AZT)-induced headaches, and arthralgias (15).

Because the presenting symptoms of HIV/AIDS can be so variable, attempts have been made to classify these symptoms. HIV/AIDS-related symptoms have been classified as having somatic, visceral, or neuropathic origins (15,25–28). Pain of somatic pathophysiology is related to a localized region of tissue injury. This can occur in the muscle, skin, or bone. Pain of visceral pathophysiology is related to a damaged viscus or mesenteric structure, such as the gastrointestinal or esopharyngeal systems (see Table 14.2) (26). Finally, neuropathic pain is defined as a dysfunction in the central or peripheral nervous system.

As seen in Table 14.3, somatic pain syndromes can be the direct result of either viral infection or of side effects from antiviral medications. (Somatic pain syndromes are covered in the Rheumatologic Manifestations section later in this chapter.)

The visceral pain syndromes can also be quite varied. Chronic throat pain may be the result of oropharyngeal infection such as that caused by oral thrush or, less commonly, intraoral Kaposi's sarcoma. Chest pain may be the result of pneumonia, pleuritis, pericarditis, or esophagitis, or musculoskeletal dysfunction from prolonged coughing (29,26). Abdominal pain may be caused by enteritis, colitis, pancreatitis, tumor invasion, or hepatitis (26,30,31). Coinfection with hepatitis B (HBV) and hepatitis C is increasingly an issue as patients survive longer with HIV. As many as 95 percent of HIV/AIDS patients have serologic markers of past HBV infection (32–34), and the presence of HIV can increase the severity of chronic hepatitis (35). Liver failure can lead to painful abdominal distension, leg swelling, and mental status changes.

Neurologic Manifestations

Neurologic involvement is the most frequent complication that occurs with HIV infection (36,37). Table 14.4 lists the most common neurologic complications in

Table 14.2. AIDS-Related Pain Syndromes

Somatic Pain Syndromes Caused by HIV or AIDS-defining Illnesses
Skin pain caused by Kaposi's sarcoma
Arthritis/arthralgia syndromes
- Nonspecific arthralgias
- HIV-associated arthritis
- Psoriatic arthritis
- Painful articular syndrome
Myositis/myalgia
- HIV-associated myositis
- Septic myositis
Somatic pain caused by neoplasms

Somatic Pain Syndromes Caused by Treatment
Arthralgia/rnyalgia caused by antiviral drugs
- zidovudine-associated myopathy
Somatic pains related to antineoplastic therapies

Visceral Pain Syndromes Caused by HIV or AIDS-Defining Illnesses
Painful pharyngitis
Painful esophagitis
- Related to Candida, cytomegalovirus (CMV), or other opportunistic infection
- Related to neoplasm
Painful enteritis/colitis
- Related to HIV
- Related to opportunistic infection
- Related to neoplasm
Diseases of the biliary tract, liver and pancreas
- Infectious or neoplastic cholecystitis
- Infectious hepatitis
Abdominal pain caused by organomegaly
Abdominal/pelvic pain caused by intestinal Kaposi's sarcoma or other neoplasm

Visceral Pain Syndromes Caused by Treatment
Painful enteritis/colitis caused by antiviral therapy

Neuropathic Pains Caused by HIV or AIDS-Defining Illnesses
HIV neuropathy
- Predominantly sensory neuropathy
- Chronic inflammatory demyelinating polyneuropathy
HIV myelopathy
Cytomegalovirus polyradiculopathy
Cytomegalovirus multiple mononeuropathy
Herpes zoster/postherpetic neuralgia
Neuropathic pain caused by neoplasms

Neuropathic Pains Caused by Treatment
Painful neuropathy caused by antiviral therapy
- Antiretrovirals: ddl (didanosine), ddC (zalcitabine), d4T (stavudine)
- Antivirals: foscarnet
Painful neuropathy caused by other anti-infectives
- PCP prophylaxis: dapsone
- Antibacterial: metronidazole
- Antimycobacterials: isoniazid
Painful neuropathy caused by antineoplastic therapy

Other HIV-Related Pain Syndromes
Headache
- Related to meningitis
- Related to neoplasm
- Related to therapy

In: Portenoy, R. Contemporary Diagnosis and Management of Pain in Oncologic and AIDS Patients. Newtown, PA: Handbook in Health Care, 1997: 64–65.

Table 14.3. Sources of Nociceptive Pain in HIV/AIDS (Lefkowitz, 1994)

Cutaneous causes	*Deep somatic causes*
• Kaposi's sarcoma	• Rheumatologic (e.g., arthralgias)
• Oral cavity pain	• Back pain
	• Myopathies
Visceral causes	
• Tumor	*Headache*
• Gastritis	• HIV-related (e.g. meningitis, encephalitis, neoplasm)
• Pancreatitis	
• Infection	• HIV-unrelated (e.g. tension, migraine)
• Biliary tract disorders	• Iatrogenic (e.g. AZT)

In: Portenoy, R. *Contemporary Diagnosis and Management of Pain in Oncologic and AIDS Patients.* Newtown, Pa.: Handbook in Health Care, 1997; 64-65.

HIV-infected patients. HIV enters the brain shortly after initial infection and remains throughout the course of the disease. Central and peripheral nervous system complications may be a direct effect of HIV infection itself, from secondary infections resulting from an immunocompromised state, or as a side effect of antiretroviral medications. Space-occupying lesions in the brain or spinal cord can be the result of a lymphoma or cancer. Because neurologic complications are frequently misdiagnosed in the HIV population, the physician must perform a thorough neuromuscular examination (38). Symptoms and physical findings can be classified as involving either the lower or the upper motor neuron.

Lower Motor Neuron Involvement

Peripheral Neuropathy. According to the Multicenter AIDS Cohort Study data, peripheral neuropathy is the most common neurologic disorder associated with HIV infection (37). Distal sensory polyneuropathy (DSP) is the most common form of peripheral neuropathy seen in the HIV-infected population (39). DSP is present in 25 to 50 percent of patients with AIDS (27,39–43). The most common symptoms of DSP are numbness, burning, and paresthesias in the symmetric lower extremities; these symptoms start in the toes and ascend proximally. In severe cases, symptoms may exist in the upper extremity, accompanied by associated muscle weakness. Neurologic findings on physical examination are depressed or absent distal reflexes, increased vibratory thresholds at the toes and ankles, and reduced pain and temperature sensation in a "stocking" and "glove" distribution (44). A gait evaluation shows mild to moderate lower extremity ataxia, depending on the severity of the peripheral neuropathy. Sural nerve biopsy and autopsy has revealed that distal axonopathy exists in almost every patient with AIDS (45). Electrodiagnostic studies describe peripheral nerve axonal loss, demyelination, and muscle denervation (40). A recent electrodiagnostic study examined 251 HIV-seropositive patients and found that low CD4 counts correlate with decreases in amplitude and conduction velocity, and increases in distal latencies in selected motor and sensory nerves. Researchers also concluded that age and nutritional deficiencies contribute significantly to the electrophysiologic changes of DSP in

Table 14.4. Neurologic Complications in HIV-1 Infected Patients

Predominantly nonfocal
    AIDS dementia complex (subacute-chronic HIV encephalitis)
    Acute HIV-related encephalitis
    Cytomegalovirus encephalitis
    Herpes simplex virus encephalitis
    Metabolic encephalopathies
Predominantly focal
    Cerebral toxoplasmosis
    Progressive multifocal leukoencephalopathy
    Cryptococcoma
    Varicella-zoster virus encephalitis
    Tuberculous brain abscess/tuberculoma
    Neurosyphilis (meningovascular)
    Vascular disorders-notably nonbacterial endocarditis and cerebral hemorrhages
      associated with thrombocytopenia
    Primary CNS lymphoma
Spinal cord
    Vacuolar myelopathy
    Herpes simplex or zoster myelitis
Meninges
    Aseptic meningitis (HIV)
    Cryptococcal meningitis
    Tuberculous meningitis
    Syphilitic meningitis
    Metastatic lymphomatous meningitis
Peripheral nerve and root
    Infectious
        Herpes zoster
        Cytomegalovirus polyradiculopathy
    Virus or immune related
        Acute and chronic inflammatory HIV polyneuritis
        Mononeuritis multiplex
        Sensorimotor demyelinating polyneuropathy
        Distal painful sensory polyneuritis
    Muscle
        Polymyositis and other myopathies

In: Adams RD, Victor M. *Principles of Neurology*, 5th ed. New York: McGraw-Hill, 1993; 663.

AIDS (40). DSP is demonstrated to significantly affect the quality of life of a patient, and it may limit the use of antiretroviral medications (46).

The cause of peripheral neuropathy in patients with HIV is not known. Several mechanisms have been proposed, including advanced HIV disease, cytomegalovirus (CMV) infection, nutritional deficiency, age, weight loss, vitamin B12 deficiency, and cytokine-mediated neurotoxic effects (39,40,47–52). One hypothesis is that HIV damage to dorsal root ganglion neurons may lead to central–peripheral axonal degeneration (48).

Pharmacologic therapies that are known to cause DSP include the use of vincristine, isoniazid, and thalidomide (53–55). In HIV-infected patients, the use of the dideoxynucleotide analogs ddI, ddC, and d4T can cause DSP (54–56). It is believed that the neurotoxicity of the dideoxynucleotides may be the result of interference with mitochondrial DNA synthesis, possibly associated with reduced levels of acetyl-carnitine (57).

An appropriate diagnosis of DSP is made through a thorough neuromuscular history and physical examination. The history should exclude other causes of DSP including diabetes mellitus, neurotoxin exposure, alcoholism, vitamin deficiencies, and metabolic inflammatory diseases such as hepatitis. Any additions or dosage changes in the antiretroviral medications should be examined. The clinical features of toxic neucleoside DSP are indistinguishable from viral-induced DSP. A DSP diagnosis can usually be made through neurologic examination and without electrodiagnostic studies (37). In complex cases, however, electrodiagnostic studies will demonstrate a distal sensory and motor polyneuropathy (40).

If a toxic drug effect is suspected, the treatment for DSP begins with the withdrawal of the suspect medication. Symptoms can persist for 8 to 16 weeks after withdrawal of the agent (56). Aggressive pain management utilizing pharmacologic therapies and rehabilitation interventions is recommended. (This treatment is covered later in this chapter.)

Inflammatory Demyelinating Polyneuropathy. Inflammatory demyelinating polyneuropathy (IDP), although rare, can occur very early in the disease process. IDP resembles subacute Guillain–Barré syndrome. The clinical findings of IDP are rapidly progressive muscle weakness involving two or more extremities, decreased or absent reflexes, and cranial nerve involvement (58). The pathophysiology is unknown, but it is believed to have an autoimmune component because cerebral spinal fluid (CSF) exhibits antiperipheral nerve myelin antibodies (59). Acute inflammatory demyelinating polyneuropathy (AIDP) can have an acute onset and may be the only symptom for the disease. Chronic inflammatory demyelinating polyneuropathy may have a more gradual onset. In advanced disease, CMV can infiltrate the peripheral nerves and act as an agent for IDP (60).

Diagnosis of IDP is made through CSF analysis, which will exhibit a lymphocytic pleocytosis that is unique to patients with HIV/AIDS (61). There is also an elevation of CSF protein (61). Electrodiagnostic studies demonstrate acquired demyelination and axonal degeneration (44).

The treatment for IDP is primarily immunomodulation therapy with corticosteroids (60 to 80 mg of prednisone to start, then tapered), plasmapheresis, and high-dose intravenous immunoglobulin (0.2 to 0.4 gm/kg IV daily for 5 days) (43,62). The prognosis for IDP in the HIV/AIDS patient is not as good as that for patients in the noninfected population (43,62).

Progressive Polyradiculopathy. Progressive polyradiculopathy usually presents in later stages of the disease (63,64). Presenting symptoms usually include radicular-type pain in the cauda equina distribution, hyporeflexia in the lower extremities, mild sensory loss, and sphincter dysfunction. Patients demonstrate a rapidly progressive flaccid paraparesis and may present with urinary retention (63).

HIV-related progressive polyradiculopathy is usually caused by CMV infection, but neurosyphilis and lymphomatous meningitis must also be considered as causes (44). Diagnosis is made through CSF examination, which is characterized by marked polymorphonuclear pleocytosis, elevated protein, and hypoglycorrachia (44). Electrodiagnostic studies using needle electromyography (EMG) reveal widespread denervation in the lower extremity and lumbar paraspinal muscles (44).

Patients having suspected HIV-related progressive polyradiculopathy should be aggressively treated with ganciclovir, foscarnet, or cidofovir (65).

Mononeuropathy Multiplex. Mononeuropathy multiplex (MM) can manifest as a focal sensory neuropathy of a cranial, peripheral motor, sensory, or mixed motor sensory nerve (66). It can occur both early and late in the HIV disease process. MM in relatively nonimmunocompomised patients is usually relatively benign and involves only a few nerves. MM may remit spontaneously or with the use of oral corticosteroids (66). Its pathogenesis is believed to have an autoimmune, vasculitic characteristic.

In patients who are immunocompromised, a more aggressive form of MM occurs, which can lead to progressive paralysis and even death. It is usually caused by a focal nerve CMV infection (67). Diagnosis is usually made by physical examination. Electrodiagnostic studies reveal multifocal and asymmetric pathology of cranial, sensory, and motor nerves with axonal demyelination. CSF analysis and sural nerve biopsy may demonstrate evidence of CMV infection (68). Because MM can be a difficult diagnosis, empirical treatment is recommended if MM is even suspected. Treatment with anti-CMV therapy such as oral or intravenous ganciclovir is recommended (69).

Diffuse Upper Motor Neuron Processes. Diseases of the upper motor neuron in HIV/AIDS can generally be classified as diffuse processes or focal processes (see Table 14.4) (70). Patients with diffuse brain processes usually present with an impairment of alertness and cognition. This is in exception to AIDS dementia complex (ADC), which generally spares alertness but affects cognitive, motor, and behavioral functions.

AIDS Dementia Complex (ADC). Although ADC is not a pain syndrome, it is a major neurologic finding in the HIV/AIDS patient population. The level of ADC-caused cognitive impairment influences both pain management and rehabilitation for the patient. ADC is characterized by a triad of cognitive, motor, and behavioral dysfunctions. It is the most common CNS complication of HIV infection. The clinical findings of ADC are summarized in Table 14.5 (71). Early symptoms generally include difficulties with concentration and memory. Multistep tasks and concentration become difficult. Early in the course of the disease, mental status exams are normal but this changes as the disease progresses. Symptoms of motor dysfunction can consist of gait dysfunction and slower, less precise movements. As the disease progresses, ataxia, weakness, spasticity, and bowel and bladder incontinence can occur (72). Computed tomography (CT) or magnetic resonance imaging (MRI) usually show cerebral atrophy with widened cortical sulci and enlarged ventricles (73).

Table 14.5. Management of the Neurologic Complications of HIV-1 Infection and AIDS

	Comparison of AIDS Dementia Complex Staging and WHO/AAN Classifications	
AIDS Dementia Complex Staging	WHO/AAN Classification: HIV-Associated Cognitive-Motor Complex	
Stage 0: Normal	No corresponding designation	
Stage 0.5: Subclinical or Equivocal Minimal or equivocal symptoms Mild (soft) neurologic signs No impairment of work or activities of daily living (ADL)		
Stage 1: Mild Unequivocal intellectual or motor impairment Able to do all but the more demanding work or ADL	HIV-1 -Associated Minor Cognitive-Motor Disorder Symptoms: Two of five types in cognitive, motor, behavioral spheres Examination: neurologic or neuropsychological abnormalities Mild impairment of work or ADL HIV-Associated Dementia and HIV-Associated Myelopathy	
Stage 2: Moderate Cannot work or perform demanding ADL Capable of self-care Ambulatory but may need a single prop	*Mild* Impaired work and ADL Capable of basic self-care Ambulatory but may need a single prop	
Stage 3: Severe Major intellectual disability or Cannot walk unassisted	*Moderate* Unable to work or function unassisted or Cannot walk unassisted	
Stage 4: End Stage Nearly vegetative Rudimentary cognition Para- or quadriplegic	*Severe* Unable to perform ADL unassisted Confined to bed or wheelchair	

In: Sande M, Volberding P. *The Medical Management of AIDS*, 6th ed. Philadelphia: WB Saunders, 1999; 223.

Table 14.6. Possible Mechanisms for Rheumatic Manifestations of HIV Infection

Direct effect of HIV on endothelial, synovial cells, and other hematopoietic cells resulting in:
    Destruction of CD4+ T cells
    Increased cytotoxic cell activity
    Increased expression of autoantigens
  Polyclonal activation of B cells:
    Increased serum immunoglobulins
    Immune complex formation
    Production of autoantibodies
    Anti-idiotypic antibodies
  Increased expression and release of cytokines: Th I to Th2 switch
  Genetic factors: HLA-B27 and non-HLA factors
  Environmental factors:
    Infection with arthritogenic organisms
    Superantigen activation immunocytes
    Molecular mimicry

In: Cuellar ML. HIV infection-associated inflammatory musculoskeletal disorders. *Rheum Dis Clin N Am* 1998:24, Number 2.

RHEUMATOLOGIC MANIFESTATIONS OF HIV/AIDS

There are many potential rheumatologic manifestations of HIV infection. The etiology is thought to be multifactorial and diffuse (see Table 14.6) (74). The most common rheumatologic manifestation associated with HIV infection is arthralgia (see Table 14.7) (74). Other manifestations include painful articular syndrome, Reiter's syndrome, psoriatic arthritis, HIV-related arthritis, Sjögren's syndrome, vasculitis, septic arthritis, and fibromyalgia.

Arthralgia

Arthralgia is common and can occur at any stage of HIV infection. Arthralgia is usually oligoarticular, and mild to moderate in intensity (74). Joint pain can be a manifestation of acute seroconversion. Arthralgia may accompany initiation of zidovudine therapy, but in that setting the pain is characteristically self-limited and resolves within a few weeks of starting the medication (75).

    Painful articular syndrome is characterized by severe intermittent pain and involvement of less than four joints, without evidence of synovitis. It usually lasts less than 24 hours and generally occurs late in the disease process (74). This syndrome is generally uncommon, with an unclear etiology (75).

Reiter's Syndrome

Reiter's syndrome is seen in as many as 10 percent of HIV-infected people who develop arthritis. An additional 10 to 20 percent of patients are categorized as having "reactive arthritis" because they lack the nonarticular features of Reiter's

Table 14.7. Clinical Spectra Of HIV-Associated Rheumatic Disorders

Manifestation	Prevalence
Arthralgia	3.9–40.0
Painful articular syndrome	4.1–10.0
HIV arthropathy	5.0–12
Reiter's syndrome	2.1–10.8
Psoriatic arthritis	1.7–2.0
Undifferentiated spondyloarthropathy	1.0–15
Tendinitis	2.0–5
Myositis	0.5–1.1
Vasculitis	1.0–40
Raynaud's syndrome	1.0–17
Sicca syndrome	0.5–50
Septic arthritis	0.0–3.5
Other: Sweet's syndrome, uveitis, Behcet's, fibromyalgia	< 1.0

In: Cuellar ML. HIV infection-associated inflammatory musculoskeletal disorders. *Rheum Dis Clin N Am* 1998:24, Number 2.

syndrome (75). These include enthesitis, nail involvement, oral ulcers, and uveitis. Most patients with HIV infection develop an incomplete form of Reiter's syndrome, but the classic presentation of urethritis, conjunctivitis, and arthritis may also occur (74). The arthritis of Reiter's syndrome is typically severe and oligoarticular. Clinical manifestations usually follow the onset of immunodeficiency. Notably, 65 to 75 percent of HIV-positive patients with Reiter's syndrome are HLA-B27 positive (75).

Psoriatic Arthritis

HIV infection may exacerbate underlying psoriasis or induce psoriasis de novo. The prevalence of psoriasis in HIV-infected patients ranges from 1 to 20 percent, whereas the prevalence of psoriatic arthritis may be somewhat higher. Psoriasis and psoriatic arthritis may precede or follow the clinical onset of immunodeficiency. The pattern of joint involvement in psoriatic arthritis is more frequently polyarticular and asymmetric, accompanied by enthesopathy and dactylitis. SI joint and spinal involvement rarely occur. The clinical course of the disease is variable (74).

HIV-arthritis has an acute onset of severe oligoarticular and asymmetric involvement affecting mainly the knees and ankles. The presentation is typically late in the course of the disease and the course is usually self-limiting (74). The symptoms are reported as lasting from weeks to months (74,75).

Sjögren's Syndrome

Sjögren's syndrome can present with the initial symptoms of dry eyes and dry mouth, both of which are reported with increasing frequency in AIDS patients.

The combined features of male predominance, the absence of a well-defined connective tissue disease, an age of less than 40 years, and generalized lymphadenopathy distinguish the HIV-related disease from the idiopathic variant of Sjögren's syndrome (74,75).

Other Arthritic Conditions

Multiple types of vasculitis are associated with HIV infection, the most common appearing as necrotizing vasculitis of the polyarteritis nodosa type. This often presents as peripheral sensory or sensorimotor neuropathy. Drug-induced hypersensitivity vasculitis typically presents as a cutaneous disease and has been reported in association with multiple medications (75).

Septic arthritis in the HIV-positive population is seen more frequently in patients having the risk factors of IV drug use and hemophilia. Involvement is generally monoarticular, with the hip joint most commonly affected. Sternoclavicular joint involvement is common in patients with a history of IV drug use.

The prevalence of fibromyalgia in association with HIV infection may exceed its prevalence in the non-HIV–infected population (76). Diagnoses are made using the American College of Rheumatology criteria (77). Fatigue is the predominant symptom and may be incapacitating.

MANAGEMENT OF PAIN DISORDERS IN THE HIV-INFECTED POPULATION

The rehabilitative team approach has particular applicability in the treatment of patients with HIV infection. The team must be well versed in managing the spectrum of painful manifestations of HIV, skilled in diagnosing them, and comfortable with designing analgesic protocols and comprehensive therapeutic programs. The goal of treatment must be an optimization of functional status and safety.

Any review of rehabilitation efforts in patients with painful HIV-related disorders would be remiss without a discussion of the role of aquatic therapy. The aquatic environment is often uniquely suited to provide pain relief as well as the opportunity for enhanced range-of-motion, strength, and mobility exercises. Therefore, an aquatic program can often serve as the cornerstone of a multifaceted treatment program.

HIV-infected patients may be unable to tolerate land-based physical therapy for a number of reasons including pain, incapacitating fatigue, and weakness. These factors may lead to an inability to stabilize joints to the extent that exercise can be tolerated. Pain is often diminished in the pool setting. The water's turbulence, pressure, and temperature serve to increase sensory input. The water's buoyancy leads to decreased joint compression and decreased muscle activity, and the aquatic environment's milieu of increased mental and social stimulation may serve as a pain distractor. Through water's buoyant effects, the patient may develop a sense of relaxation, which further helps to decrease pain. With less pain-limited movement, range-of-motion exercises can be undertaken with greater ease. In essence, water itself acts as an active-assistive device. Distractive devices can also enhance range-of-motion activities (78). Once the range of motion is adequate, resistance training can usually be incorporated as a means to increase strength. Often, land-based resistance training is not feasible. This is true particularly during exacerbations of rheumatologic manifestations such as inflammatory arthritis, when a patient is unable to tolerate anything other than joint rest.

There are no clearly established guidelines for the initiation of range-of-motion exercises and strength training in the aquatic environment for myopathic patients with elevated serum creatinine phosphokinase (CPK). Generally, in a land-based program, once CPK falls to near-normal levels in the myopathic patient, starting active range-of-motion or isometric exercises carries a minimal risk (79). No documentation was found on the impact of an aquatic strengthening and range-of-motion program on already elevated muscle enzyme levels. However, whether myopathic patients are training in water or on land, CPK levels should be closely monitored.

Water's viscosity provides an innate resistive element. Limb movement through water is smooth, and does not produce strong torque at the end of an extremity. Therefore, there is significantly less local stress to joints and soft tissue. Resistance can be increased through altering the speed or direction of movement. Additional resistance can be incorporated through devices such as hand paddles, gloves, or foot flippers.

Water's viscosity also serves to make the aquatic setting a wonderful place for proprioceptive training. This may be particularly beneficial for patients with impaired proprioception secondary to peripheral neuropathy. Training should focus on using submaximal effort to achieve maximal sensory input. Viscosity provides a slow-motion, three-dimensional environment that facilitates proprioceptive feedback through functional movements. The key is the use of repetitive movement patterns, which promote neuromuscular control on a subconscious level. The patient becomes more aware of what elements are necessary for functional movements. Aquatic therapy may also benefit the patient with fibromyalgia, both in terms of pain control and normalization of sleep cycles. Diminished pain, thus allowing for participation in an exercise program, may lead to improved sleep–wake patterns enhanced by physical exertion. In general, aquatic therapy may heighten the functional status of many patients with painful conditions related to HIV, through pain relief, strengthening, and improved mobility.

Unfortunately, some patients are poor candidates for a pool-based regimen (78). These include patients with incontinence of bowel or bladder, possibly secondary to myelopathy, those with dementia so significant that they are at risk of injury even in a supervised environment, and those with decubiti (possibly related to a combination of immobility and suboptimal nutrition).

Land-based physical and occupational therapies are appropriate interventions for painful disorders in HIV patients who are able to tolerate a more intense regimen. A recently published study (80) examined the effects of testosterone replacement, with or without a program of resistance exercise, on muscle strength and body composition in HIV-infected males with weight loss and low testosterone levels. Resistance training took place through the leg press, bench press, leg curl, latissimus pull, and overhead press. The authors concluded that, in HIV-positive males with moderate weight loss and low testosterone levels, both resistance exercise and testosterone replacement was associated with significant gains in muscle strength, muscle size, and body weight. The effects of testosterone and exercise training combined were not additive.

Pain Management and Rehabilitation Issues in Neurologic Disorders

The rehabilitation program for DSP begins with patient education. Patients with impaired lower extremity sensation must be taught to examine their feet on a daily basis for evidence of ulceration, trauma, or unequal distribution of pressure. Patients with neuropathy require protective footwear such as orthotic shoes with, ideally, a large toe box and plastizote inserts (for details, see Chapter 8, on peripheral neuropathy). Those with evidence of unequal pressure distribution in the feet or areas of callus or breakdown may require custom-molded shoes to redistribute pressure. Neuropathic patients with bony foot deformities may warrant extra-depth orthotic footwear with a wide toe box to safely accommodate the deformities.

Neuropathic patients who employ modalities of heat or cold in an attempt to manage pain must be advised of the dangers of direct heat or cold on their insensate feet. With their sensory impairments, patients may initially see rather than feel burns caused by heating pads or radiators. In addition, prolonged cold can lead to neural hypoxia. All applications of heat or cold must be time-limited and must be supervised if the patient does not have the cognitive capacity to comply with temporal constraints. Skin examination should be undertaken before and after the application of the modality.

For patients suffering from a myelopathic process, symptomatic treatment is appropriate. Attempts should be made to reduce spasticity if it is considered to be a pain-causing factor. Antispasticity agents such as baclofen are advocated for the treatment of spasticity (81), but the physician must be alert for increased patient fatigue when employing this agent. Orthotics should be considered for patients with foot drop, and if impaired sensation is an issue, an ankle–foot orthosis with double-metal uprights may be more prudent than a molded ankle–foot orthosis. Physical and occupational therapies may help to preserve function or to allow the patient to safely adapt to his new functional constraints.

For patients suffering from ADC, rehabilitation interventions can be very helpful. Patients should be instructed to use a daily calendar and memory book. Pill boxes can be helpful for patients having difficulty taking their medications on time. Pharmacologic intervention, such neurostimulants, may help with both fatigue and memory loss (82,83). Assistive devices such as canes and walkers may be needed in later stages of the disease. A bowel and bladder program may be undertaken in later stages of the disease as well.

Rehabilitation of Rheumatologic Disorders

Acute rheumatologic manifestations of HIV are managed with joint rest, isometric exercise, relative immobilization, and orthoses (76). Selectively resting individual joints by the use of orthoses can help relieve pain and prevent the contracture of severely inflamed joints, especially those too swollen to exercise. The principle is to maintain the joint in its physiologic position, especially during periods when the joint is stressed (84). The time-limited application of cold can be utilized as an analgesic modality in inflammatory conditions. Physical and occupational therapies should provide a forum for patients to learn the practical applications of energy conservation and joint conservation techniques. Therapists may choose to reduce the functional demands of an activity either temporarily (as during periods of acute inflammation or limited weight bearing), or permanently by incorporating a variety of assistive devices for ADLs and generalized mobility that substitute for lost range of motion and strength. These devices might include long-handled appliances and utensils or other devices with built-up handles (85).

Progressive resistance exercise with further joint mobilization begins as acute synovities resolve (76). Pain-limited weight bearing may more easily be addressed in water than on land, with a progression of weight bearing accomplished mainly by decreasing the water depth at which an exercise is performed (78).

In general, arthralgias respond to nonsteroidal antiinflammatory drugs (NSAIDs) (75). Narcotics are often required for painful articular syndrome (74), but may be unable to provide adequate analgesia (75). Patients with Reiter's syndrome may not respond to NSAIDs. Unfortunately, immunosuppressive analgesic medications like methotrexate and azathioprine may promote opportunistic diseases and Kaposi's sarcoma (75). A case report describes an AIDS patient with Reiter's syndrome whose arthritis and skin lesions responded poorly to nonsteroidals and topical corticosteroids. He responded dramatically to acitretine initially and on recurrence many months later (86).

Symptoms in mild cases of psoriatic arthritis can often be controlled with NSAIDs. More severe disease may require the use of immunosuppressive agents, but these are considered poor choices for patients with HIV (87). For symptoms of HIV-arthritis, nonsteroidal agents may provide analgesia, and intraarticular steroid injections may be beneficial (75).

For patients suffering from pain related to fibromyalgia, nonsteroidal use, trigger-point injections, and tricyclic antidepressants (TCAs) such as cyclobenzaprine and amitriptyline can be utilized as therapeutic options. Aerobic exercise is an important therapeutic activity (76); as discussed earlier, aquatic therapy may play a critical role in symptomatic relief.

PHARMACOLOGIC PAIN MANAGEMENT

The AHCPR has recommended that HIV-related pain be treated similarly to cancer-induced pain. The World Health Organization (WHO) "analgesic ladder" is the foundation for treatment of pain syndromes (for details, see Chapter 12 on

Table 14.8. Medications with High Protein Binding

Celecoxib	97%
Rofecoxib	87%
Carbamazepine	76%
Mexiletine	55%
Lamotrigene	55%
Fluoxetine	
Paroxetine	

cancer pain). People who suffer from HIV may suffer from several different types of pain. The goal is to treat the most significant pain initially, then address other pain symptoms. Neuropathic pain, usually caused by peripheral sensory polyneuropathy, is the most common pain syndrome seen in the HIV-infected population.

The occurrence of malnutrition and AIDS wasting syndrome and the increased incidence of liver and kidney damage by concomitant disease processes are specific issues of concern when prescribing pain medications in the HIV-infected population. If any of these conditions are present, it affects the choice of medications and dosages that can be prescribed. Malnourished patients have lower levels of serum proteins, hence medications that are highly serum protein–bound will not have enough protein to which to bind (see Table 14.8). The serum levels of these medications may thus be higher than intended with a usual dose. This may increase the risk for adverse effects or toxicity. If the liver or kidneys are not functioning optimally, drugs that are metabolized through these organs may not be as effective or may have higher-than-normal serum levels (see Tables 14.9 and 14.10) Certain medications require ongoing laboratory monitoring tests for safety (see Table 14.11). In addition, HIV-infected patients are often using several medica-

Table 14.9. Medications Metabolized in the Liver

Acetominophen
Aspirin
Codeine
Hydrocodone
Morphine
Rofecoxib
Celecoxib
Tramadol*
Amitriptyline*
Desipramine*
Paroxetine*
Carbamazepine*
Mexiletine

* Indicates drugs primarily using the cytochrome P450 system.

Table 14.10. Commonly Used Pain Medications That Require Adjustment of Dose with Renal Disease

Acetaminophen
Aspirin
Codeine
Propoxyphene (avoid with hemodialysis)
Morphine
Fentonyl
Meperidine
Ketorolac
Paroxetine
Gabapentin (200-300mg after hemodialysis)

tions, and the potential for drug interaction is significantly increased with the addition of any new medications (see Table 14.12).

Nonopioid Analgesics

Nonopioid analgesics including acetaminophen, aspirin (acetylsalicylic acid), and NSAIDs, must be used with caution in patients with HIV infection because of potential drug interactions and the increased risk of adverse events, such as gastrointestinal ulceration.

Acetaminophen is metabolised through the liver and may interfere with the metabolism of AZT, a common medication used by patients with HIV infection. There is also a dose-dependent risk of hepatotoxicity with acetaminophen, which

Table 14.11. Recommended Laboratory Tests

Liver Function Tests
      Hydrocodone
      Rofecoxib
      Tramadol
      Amitriptyline
      Paroxetine
      Carbamazepine
      Mexiletine

Complete Blood Count
      Desipramine
      Carbamazepine
      Mexilitine

Glucose
      Desipramine

Table 14.12. Drug–Drug Interaction

Cimetidine (Tagamet) inhibits the cytochrome P450 system, therefore may increase plasma levels of medications metabolized through this enzyme pathway.

Phenobarbital induces the cytochrome P450 pathway, therefore may decrease plasma levels of medications metabolized through this enzyme pathway.

Active serum levels of Norvir, an HIV protease inhibitor, are increased by concomitant administration of fluoxetine or desipramine. Norvir levels are decreased by interactions with meperidine or methadone.

is increased further in patients with a history of previous liver disease or alcohol abuse.

Aspirin is a highly protein-bound compound, metabolized through the liver and eliminated through the kidneys. The use of aspirin should be avoided in patients with end-stage renal disease, and the usual dosage should be decreased in patients with malnutrition or liver disease. Overdosage of aspirin may produce tinnitus, drowsiness, vomiting, and diarrhea.

Long-term use of NSAIDs in the HIV-infected population is ill-advised because of the increased risk of gastrointestinal and renal morbidity (88). Because of the decreased incidence of gastrointestinal side effects (including gastric ulceration) associated with their use, the COX-2 inhibitors may be of more benefit in the HIV population. However, there are no studies to confirm this. Because of the multiplicity of other medications already in use to treat their primary disease, patients with HIV infection may be more likely to comply with the once or twice daily dosing of these new NSAIDs. It must be noted that celecoxib (Celebrex®) has a sulfa group attached as part of its chemical structure. Patients with HIV infection have a higher incidence of sulfa allergy than the general population. Before starting celecoxib, patients should be specifically questioned about previous allergic reactions to medications containing sulfa, such as trimethoprim and sulfamethoxazole (Bactrim®) used to treat *Pneumocystis carinii* pneumonia in HIV patients.

Opioid Analgesics

The use of sustained-release morphine for severe chronic pain in patients with AIDS has been supported in a controlled clinical trial by Kaplan (89). A patient–physician medication contract is recommended to help monitor the legal, psychosocial, and medical issues involved in the use of chronic opioids for pain (90). Pain continues to be remarkably undertreated in the AIDS/HIV-infected population even when in hospice care (91). Potential patient-reported barriers to pain management were surveyed by Breitbart et al. (92). They found that the primary concerns of nearly 200 ambulatory AIDS patients in New York City were addiction potential of the pain medication, potential discomfort associated with administration (primarily injection), or fear of adverse effects such as nausea and vomiting. In a related survey of AIDS care providers in five major U.S. cities, Breitbart et al. (93) revealed similar patient concerns of potential abuse or addiction, in addition to a provider barrier in the form of lack of knowledge about the medications used to treat pain or access to pain management experts.

Transdermal delivery systems or "patches" of fentanyl (Duragesic®), a strong opioid analgesic, can provide 48 to 72 hours of continuous pain relief. They can be especially helpful in patients who have difficulty taking oral medications because of oral thrush, dysphagia from brainstem damage, or during the end stages of the disease. Transdermal patches should be used with caution in the HIV-infected patient, because fentanyl is highly protein bound and this method of medication is not easily titrated. Because of a long drug half-life, it takes 12 to 24 hours for the serum concentration of fentanyl from transdermal patches to stabilize. Initial use of any transdermal medication must be accompanied by a shorter acting form of medication to achieve pain relief until the serum concentration reaches appropriate levels. Fever, not uncommon in the HIV-infected population, can increase absorption of transdermal medications. Increased absorption of these potent medications can lead to a shorter duration of action and a higher risk of toxicity, including respiratory depression.

Intrathecal or epidural administration of morphine may be indicated in patients who have had some relief with oral opioids but cannot tolerate the higher dosages needed to achieve significant pain control because of associated side effects. Surgical placement of a catheter delivers the medication from an implanted reservoir directly to the spinal cord, the site of opioid receptors. This allows the patient to reduce his oral medication and maintain a steadier level of pain control. When using intrathecal or epidural administration routes, it is not possible for the patient to self-adjust, overuse, or abuse his dosage of medication. Because intrathecal or epidural administration requires a surgical procedure, there is a risk of infection, and the patient must be able to properly care for his surgical site. The medication reservoir must be refilled periodically via an injection delivered by a qualified healthcare provider.

Other routes of injection, such as intramuscular (IM), subcutaneous (SQ), and intravenous (IV) (including patient-controlled analgesia [PCA]), are used primarily during late stages of the disease and during hospice treatment, because of the training and assistance needed for administration, the high cost, and the potential for abuse.

The side effects of all opioid analgesics include sedation, nausea, vomiting, constipation, delirium, attention deficits, and disorientation. Certain medications such as meperidine (Demerol®) can also lead to renal failure and seizure disorders. The highest incidence of respiratory depression when dosing opioid analgesic occurs when switching between analgesics. The rule of thumb when switching from one opioid analgesic to another is to use one-half to three-quarters of the equivalent dose and titrate as needed. When dosing an opioid, the physician must always be aware of the drug's half-life. The longer half-life medications can take up to several days to be eliminated from the system after discontinuing or changing the opioid analgesic. Combinations of opioid and nonopioid medications can be used to achieve better pain control and allow lower doses of opioids, thus decreasing the risk of opioid-related side effects.

Adjuvant Analgesics

Adjuvant analgesics, including antidepressants and anticonvulsants, can be utilized at any stage in the analgesic ladder for treatment of pain in patients with HIV infection. In addition to enhancing the efficacy of opioid medications, these drugs may also provide some independent pain relief.

Antidepressant Medications.   Antidepressant medications work on both serotonergic and noradrenergic pathways in the cortical pain centers of the brain and can potentiate the analgesic affects of opioids. Commonly used TCAs include amitriptyline (Elavil®), nortriptyline (Pamelor®), imipramine (Tofranil®), desipramine (Norpramin®), and doxepin (Sinequan®). Although not studied as extensively as the TCAs, other classes of antidepressants such as trazodone (Desyrel®), and serotonin-specific reuptake inhibitors (SSRIs) such as fluoxetine (Prozac®), paroxetine (Paxil®), and sertraline (Zoloft®), are also used for adjuvant pain control with some clinical success. It was previously believed that when using these medications, doses lower than those used to treat depression were adequate to treat pain. Newer evidence suggests that pain relief is most likely related to adequate serum levels, and that antidepressant medications should be titrated to the achieved level of pain relief. Breitbart et al. states that the use of psychotropic analgesic drugs in patients with AIDS is not only beneficial in the treatment of the psychiatric complications of the disease process, but also as an adjuvant analgesic agent in the management of pain (94). In a crossover study by Zampini et al. (95), the efficacy of amitriptyline (15.5 mg tid for 4 weeks) was related to the motor conduction velocity of the peroneal nerve in painful axonal and mixed peripheral polyneuropathies. The efficacy of amitriptyline in this study was inversely correlated with the amplitude of sural nerve sensory action potential and directly correlated with tibial nerve F-wave latencies in pain produced by demyelinating neuropathies. Contrasting evidence continues to appear, such as the comparison of amitriptyline (75 mg/d for 14 weeks) with placebo by Shlay et al. (96). No difference was found in their effectiveness at relieving pain caused by HIV-related peripheral neuropathy for the eleven patients in the direct comparison arm of the study. Newer antidepressants do not appear to be as effective in treating neuropathic pain (97).

Anticonvulsant Medications. Medications originally designed to treat seizure disorders, such as carbamazepine (Tegretol®) and gabapentin (Neurontin®), have been demonstrated to be helpful in the treatment of neuropathic pain and other types of pain (98). Gabapentin, at doses of 300 mg to 3,600 mg/day can relieve neuropathic pain in the HIV-infected population (99). Gabapentin is not highly protein bound, so the serum level is not affected in malnourished patients. It is not metabolized through the enzymatic pathways of the liver, so there are no significant drug–drug interactions. Initial reports regarding the use of lamotrigene (Lamictal®) show that it is helpful in decreasing the pain symptoms of AIDS-related neuropathy (100). Doses of lamotrigene were started at 25 mg per day and gradually increased to 300 mg per day over a 6-week period. This gradually increasing dosage schedule was used in an attempt to reduce the appearance of skin rash, which is the most common side effect of this medication.

In addition to helping alleviate pain, antidepressants and antileptics may also potentiate the effect of opioid medications. Antidepressants and anti-epileptics may also act as powerful mood stabilizers and, if titrated at nighttime, their sedating effect can help improve sleep.

Psychostimulants. Psychostimulants can be used to diminish sedation and can act as an adjunctive to analgesics. Methylphenidate (Ritalin®) is shown to decrease sedation for patients with pain, improve function in neurophysiological testing, stimulate appetite, and improve mood. Fatigue, as mentioned earlier, is a major symptom in the HIV-infected population.

Antiarrhythmics. In one study by Zampini et al. (95), mexilitine (200 mg bid), an oral antiarrhythmic, was found to be effective against neuropathic pain associated with mixed and axonal types of HIV-related neuropathy.

New and Developing Treatments for Pain

Acetyl-L-carnitine has been used with some success in trials for HIV-infected patients with neuropathic pain (101). Zampini et al. (95) found that the success of acetyl-L-carnitine (1 gr tid) correlated with a higher CD4+ count and was most useful in the early stages of HIV neuropathy.

Other pilot studies have not been as promising. Initial work by Simpson et al. (102), reveal that intranasal peptide T was safe but ineffective for HIV-related peripheral neuropathic pain.

Experimental models of the peptide SNX-111, which is produced by the conch (*Strombus alatus*), indicate high analgesic potency (103). SNX-111 appears to act by blocking calcium channels on nerve cell membranes, thus decreasing pain signal transmission (104). Because this peptide is not able to cross the blood–brain barrier, it must be administered intrathecally. Trials using SNX-111 for intractable pain in AIDS patients are underway.

All the therapies listed thus far have addressed the treatment of the symptoms of pain, not the cause—specific damage to the nerves themselves. Laboratory in vitro testing of nerve growth factor (NGF) stimulated the growth and repair of nerves (105). Pain from HIV-related peripheral sensory polyneuropathy is being studied using a twice-weekly subcutaneous injection of recombinant human NGF. The future use of NGF as an intrathecal agent is possible as well.

Pain Management in the HIV Patient with Drug Abuse History

HIV-infected patients who suffer from a history of drug abuse are among the largest groups inadequately or inappropriately treated for pain. Patients with a history of injectable drug use report that they were more likely to receive inadequate pain medication, resulting in less pain relief and a higher degree of psychologic distress (106). There are specific principles to guide the treatment of this subgroup. Only long-acting opioid agents should be prescribed for patients with a previous addiction. This eliminates many of the factors, such as an immediate euphoria, that short-acting agents provide and that reinforce addictive behavior. If a patient's pain is being treated appropriately, their functional level should increase, reinforcing the benefit of using the chosen medication, including opioids. The functional level of patients who are drug seeking or addicted is likely to significantly decrease when given these medications. Kaplan et al. (107) compared the dose and effectiveness of oral sustained-release morphine between AIDS patients with and without a prior substance abuse history. The dose of required medication was titrated to an overall 50 percent decrease of pain and a decline in use of immediate-release morphine for breakthrough pain to twice or less per day. Patients with a history of substance abuse required significantly higher dosages (177.4 mg) when compared to nonusers (84.9 mg), but both groups achieved beneficial pain reduction.

Complementary or Alternative Pain Treatments

According to the Center of Alternative Medicine and Research, patients choose to try unproved alternative or complementary treatments for a serious, life-threatening disease such as HIV when:

- conventional therapies have been exhausted,
- conventional therapies have questionable efficacy or are associated with significant adverse effect, or
- no conventional therapy exists to relieve the patient's condition.

Patients with HIV infection may view the options of alternative therapies with more optimism because of the lesser degree of side effects expected, or because of an attitude of "What harm can it do?" In addition, alternative medicine is now viewed as quite socially acceptable, whereas the stigma of taking medications for HIV is still present. The cost of alternative medicine and supplements may also be less than traditional medications, despite the fact these new treatments are not routinely covered by insurance plans. However, patients must be cautioned that there can be potentially serious interactions between alternative oral supplements and conventional medications, such as protease inhibitors, which could decrease their effectiveness against HIV. The exact method of metabolism for most alternative treatments is unclear. For example, the cytochrome P450 pathway of hepatic metabolism is critical in the effectiveness of protease inhibitor medication. If an alternative medication affects this pathway, there may be an increased risk of toxicity or a decreased effectiveness of the protease inhibitor (108). Most patients do not voluntarily report the alternative therapies they are using to their physicians. Therefore, it is critical for the treating physician to specifically ask the patient about alternative therapies being used. To obtain the most honest answers, it is vital to ask this question in a neutral, nonjudgmental manner. Documentation of these therapies must be included in the patient record. In addition, the cost of alternative therapies must be considered. Most insurance carriers will not reimburse for many alternative therapies, so it is necessary for patients who want to use them to pay privately. The cost of alternative treatments can escalate quickly and even surpass the costs of traditional treatments (109). Because many of these patients have limited incomes, it is vital to know if the costs of their alternative treatments are preventing them from obtaining traditional, physician-prescribed medication.

Despite being untested in clinical studies, positive anecdotal reports continue to circulate concerning the use of transcutaneous nerve stimulation (TENS) and behavioral techniques, such as biofeedback, hypnosis, and relaxation techniques as means of pain management for patients with HIV infection. International efforts to bring relief to Third World and rural countries have included training people to provide reflexology as a means of pain relief for patients with AIDS (110).

Acupuncture. Although anecdotal reports of pain relief from acupuncture abound, to date there have been no controlled research trials regarding its use and effectiveness to treat pain. A recent study showed no difference in pain relief between the use of standard acupuncture points and control points for 239 patients with HIV-related peripheral neuropathy (111). Aside from the maintenance of universal precautions with acupuncture needles, no contraindications exist to limit a trial of acupuncture in patients with HIV infection. A small group of patients reported improvements after the application of low-voltage noninvasive electroacupuncture that utilized skin electrodes over leg acupuncture points (112). Despite the lack of hard scientific evidence, some insurance carriers are beginning to include acupuncture as a covered service. This decreased financial pressure is likely to increase the use of acupuncture by all patients with pain unrelieved by traditional methods.

Vitamins, Herbs, and Nutritional Supplements. In addition to the prescription medications previously discussed, nutritional supplements including vitamins, minerals, and antioxidants, as well as herbs and other supplements, may play a role in helping to decrease pain (113). Patients in non-Western and developing countries, where access to medication may be significantly more difficult, have reported some benefit in the use of herbal or "traditional" medicines in treating pain related to HIV neuropathy as well as associated herpes zoster infections (114). The degree of pain relief achieved with these treatments is variable, but the physical side effects are minimal. For example, vitamin B complex, including 25 to 50 mg daily each of vitamins B1, B2, and B3 is recommended for the treatment of neuropathic pain (115). Extra vitamin B6, in addition to B complex supplements, may help further relieve neuropathic pain within a few weeks. The usage limit for vitamin B6 supplement is 100 mg, taken orally with meals, three times a day for 8 to 12 weeks. Excessive amounts of vitamin B6 may actually cause further damage to the nerves, so that continued ongoing use should be avoided (116).

Deficiencies of vitamin B12 may lead to or worsen neuropathic pain. Vitamin B12 is believed to be poorly absorbed in HIV/AIDS patients. For patients with malabsorption problems, 1 mg injections of vitamin B12 can be prescribed one or two times per week to supplement low serum levels (116). Folate should be taken in a dose of 400 mcg per day. Other vitamins thought to have some benefit in the treatment of pain are vitamin E (400 IU p.o. daily), pantothenic acid (100 mg p.o. daily), and niacinamide (25 mg p.o. daily) (115). Goldberg recommends adding daily doses of vitamin C to the level of the patients' tolerance, which is usually limited by diarrhea. Daily supplements of calcium, magnesium (400 mg qD for 2 months) (116), and phosphorus are currently under investigation for their contributions to pain control. Glucosamine sulfate has seen an incredible rise in popularity based on its claims to reduce pain and regenerate new connective tissue in affected joints (117). An 8-week study comparing the use of glucosamine to NSAIDs showed no difference in efficacy between the two treatments (118) .

For neuropathic pain, the amino acid L-carnitine and the antioxidant alpha-lipoic acid are thought to repair injured nerve cells. Twenty-five percent of HIV-positive people have low blood levels of carnitine (116). The recommended dosage of L-carnitine is 2 grams daily. For persons taking the drug adefovir or PMEA, an additional 500 mg daily is needed. Symptoms of diabetic neuropathy were improved after 3 to 4 weeks of receiving 300 to 400 mg of alpha-lipoic acid per day. It is hoped the same affect can be achieved for those with the painful peripheral polyneuropathy caused by HIV infection.

Several herbs, including willow bark, black haw, and meadowsweet, contain small amounts of aspirinlike chemicals—salicins—which are converted to salicylic acid in vivo and can help decrease local inflammation (115). Evening primrose oil is a source of tryptophan, an essential fatty acid, and it has been shown to decrease pain in doses of 1 gram taken four times a day (119). Kava-kava leaves release dihydrokavain and dihydromethylglu when chewed. These compounds produce oral numbness and may be a relief in a sore mouth, such as that experienced with oral thrush infection (119). Turmeric taken orally at a dose of 400 mg three times a day is reported to relieve pain (119). Because sunflower seeds contain phenylalanine, which decreases the breakdown of enkephalins—substances produced by the body and thought to decrease pain—they may be consumed to alleviate HIV-related pain (119).

Caution must be used when ingesting any herbal agents. Because these are natural substances does not mean that they cannot have side effects and adverse reactions similar to those experienced with the use of prescription pain medications. For example, vervain, an herb that was shown in 1964 to decrease inflammation, also causes decreased heart rate and can constrict breathing passages (115,120). The drug–drug interactions of nutritional supplements with antiviral medications is unknown at this point.

Topical Agents

The burning electrical pain of peripheral sensory polyneuropathy is often addressed with topical agents. Initially, capsaicin depletes substance P from the unmyelinated C fibers. Other nerve impulses that carry the sensations of touch, temperature, and pressure are unaffected. It is believed that this action is accompanied by a decrease in local inflammation. In addition, the actions of certain pain-reducing prostaglandins may be increased by the use of topical capsaicin. Initial research suggests that a 5 percent topical lidocaine solution (Lidoderm,) was an effective pain reducer (121). Ongoing studies regarding the use of subcutaneous recombinant human NGF show pain reduction that was better than placebo during an initial 18-week trial (122).

A pilot study using an application of 5 percent lidocaine gel to the painful skin of patients with HIV peripheral neuropathies found a 46 percent reduction of mean pain scores on a patient description instrument.The only significant side effects were dry skin and blisters (121).

The use of ginger is also thought to block local release of substance P andcertain prostaglandins and leukotrienes. Oral doses of 2 to 4 teaspoons per day achieved a 75 percent decrease in chronic pain reported by 56 patients (123). Lavender oil, which contains linalol and linalyl aldehyde, can be used to massage sore muscles (119). Peppermint oil contains menthol, which has local anesthetic properties (119) . Allspice and tarragon oil contain eugenol, which is a constituent of anesthetic clove oil. These spices can be crushed and blended for application to painful joints (120). Gel from the aloe plant, either extracted directly from leaves or in a commercial preparation, can be used topically to soothe skin ailments that are causing pain. The aroma of eucalyptus is also thought to help decrease the perception of pain.

CONCLUSIONS

It is currently estimated that 30.6 million people are infected with HIV/AIDS. Pain has been demonstrated in 20 to 50 percent of patients living with HIV infection, yet pain in this population is highly underdiagnosed and undertreated. The AHCPR recommends that the same guidelines established for cancer pain be adopted for HIV/AIDS-related pain. The role of the physician in pain management is to diagnose, aggressively treat, and manage pain syndromes associated with HIV infection. Other symptoms such as depression, functional issues, and detoxification also must be addressed.

HIV pain may be the direct result of the virus, secondary to the immunocompromised state, or associated with the medications used to treat the disease. Generally, patients suffer from more than one type of pain syndrome. HIV/AIDS pain is manifested in both the neuromuscular and rheumatologic systems. Neuropathic pain and functional deficits occur from pathology in both the upper and lower motor neuron. DSP accounts for 50 percent of the pain associated with HIV/AIDS. Other lower motor neuron syndromes are mononeuropathy multiplex, autonomic neuropathy, and myopathy. Upper motor neuron pathology includes ADC, CMV encephalitis, progressive multifocal leukoencephalopathy, toxoplasmosis, primary CNS lymphoma, and myelopathy.

Arthralgia accounts for the most common rheumatologic manifestation of HIV-related pain. Other syndromes include painful articular syndrome, HIV arthropathy, Reiter's syndrome, psoriatic arthritis, undifferentiated spondyo-arthropathy, tendonitis, Raynaud's syndrome, Sicca's syndrome, septic arthritis, and myositis. The treatment of pain syndromes is critical for both pain relief and restoration of function. Proper footwear is an essential prophylaxis for peripheral neuropathy. Aquatic rehabilitation may be the best medium to rehabilitate both neuropathic and myopathic pain syndromes.

The WHO's analgesic ladder is the foundation of the pharmacologic management of patients with HIV/AIDS-related pain. The COX-2 inhibitors may be the safest NSAID to use in the HIV/AIDS population. Antidepressants, anticonvulsants, and neurostimulants can be of great benefit to the patient with neuropathic pain. Alternative and complementary modalities may prove helpful in alleviating some forms of pain.

REFERENCES

1. Joint United Nations Programme on HIV/AIDS and World Health Organization. *Report on the Global HIV/AIDS Epidemic*. Geneva: World Health Organization, 1997.
2. Centers for Disease Control and Prevention. Update: Trends in AIDS incidences—United States, 1996. *MMWR Morb Mortal Wkly Rep* 1997; 46:861.
3. Denning PH, Jones JL, Ward JW. Recent trends in the HIV epidemic in adolescent and young adult gay and bisexual men. *J Acquir Immune Defic Syndr Hum Retrovirol* 1997;16:374.
4. Centers for Disease Control and Prevention. *HIV/AIDS Surveillance Report* 1998; 2: 1–39.
5. Centers for Disease Control and Prevention. Update: Perinatally acquired HIV/AIDS—United States, 1997. *Morb Mortal Wkly Rep* 1997; 46:1096.
6. Levy JA. Pathogenesis of human immunodeficiency virus infection. *Microbiol Rev.* March 1993; 57:183–289.
7. Centers for Disease Control and Prevention. 1993 revised classification system for HIV infection and expanded surveillance case definition for AIDS among adolescents and adults. *Morb Mortal Wkly Rep* 1992; 41: 1–19.
8. Mother-to-Child HIV Transmission and Its Prevention. In:HIV/AIDS Clinical Management, Volume 16. Medscape, Inc., 1999. [http://www.medscape.com/medscape/HIV/Clinical Mgmt/CM.v16/CM.v16-04.html]
9. Centers for Disease Control and Prevention. *National Vital Statistics Reports* 1999; 19:1–10.
10. Palella F, Delaney K, Moorman A, et al. Declining morbidity and mortality among patients with advanced human immunodeficiency virus infection. *N Engl J Med* 1998; 338:853–860.
11. Sande M, Volberding P. *The Medical Management of AIDS*, 6th ed. Philadelphia: WB Saunders Company, 1999; 98.
12. Sande M, Volberding P. *The Medical Management of AIDS*, 6th ed. Philadelphia: WB Saunders Company, 1999; 97–115.
13. Breitbart W, McDonald MV, Rosenfeld BD, et al. Pain in ambulatory AIDS patients. I: Pain characteristics and medical correlates. *Pain* 1996; 68:315–321.
14. Lebovits AH, Lefkowitz M, McjCarthy D, et al. The prevalence and management of pain in patients with AIDS: A review of 134 cases. *Clin J Pain* 1989; 5:245–248.
15. Singer, E, Zorilla C, Fahy-Chandon B, Chi S, Syndulko K, Tourtelotte WW. Painful symptoms reported for ambulator HIV-infected men in a longitudinal study. *Pain* 1993; 54:15–19.

16. Brietbart W, Rosenfeld BD, Passik SD et al. The undertreatment of pain in ambulatory AIDS patients. *Pain* 1996; 65:243–249.

17. McCormick J, Li R, Zarowny D, et al. Inadequate treatment of pain in ambulatory HIV patients. *Clin J Pain* 1993; 9:279.

18. Larue F, Fontaine A, Colleau S. Underestimation and undertreatment of pain in HIV disease: Multicentre study. *BMJ* 314:23; 1997.

19. World Health Organization. *Cancer Pain Relief and Palliative Care*. Geneva: World Health Organization, 1996.

20. Hellinger F. Cost and financing of care for persons with HIV disease: An overview. *Health Care Financing Rev*1998; 19: 1–14.

21. AHCPR Publication No. 94–0592, U.S. Department of Health and Human Services, Public Health Service, 1994.

22. Portenoy, Russell. *Contemporary Diagnosis and Management of Pain in Oncologic and AIDS Patients*. Newtown, Pa.: Handbook in Health Care Co., 1997; 16.

23. Rosenfeld B, Breitbart W, McDonald M, et al. Pain in ambulatory AIDS patients. Pt II: Impact of pain on psychological functioning and quality of life. *Pain* 1996; 68:323–328.

24. Davey RT Jr, Lane HC. Laboratory methods in the diagnosis and prognostic staging of infection with human immunodeficiency virus type 1. *Rev Infec Dis* 12:912, 1990.

25. Breitbart, W, McDonald, M. Pharmacologic pain management in HIV/AIDS: FDA's Antiviral Drugs Advisory Committee recommended approval of the first non-nucleoside RT inhibitor, in combination with nucleosides. *J Internat Assoc Physicians in AIDS Care*; 1996.

26. Portenoy, R. *Contemporary Diagnosis and Management of Pain in Oncologic and AIDS Patients*. Newtown, Pa.: Handbook in Health Care Co., 1997; 64–65.

27. Hewitt DJ, McDonald M, Portenoy RK, et al. Pain syndromes and etiologies in ambulatory AIDS patients. In: Proceeding of the 13th Annual Meeting of the American Pain Society, Miami, Florida, 1994.

28. O'Neill WM, Sherrard JS. Pain in human immunodeficiency virus disease: A review. *Pain* 1993; 54:3–14.

29. Bonacini M, Young T, Laine L. The causes of esophageal symptoms in human immunodeficiency virus infection: A prospective study of 110 patients. *Arch Intern Med* 1991; 151:167–172.

30. Bonacini M. Hepatobiliary complications in patients with human immunodeficiency virus infection. *Am J Med* 1992; 92:404–411.

31. Barone JE, Gingold BS, Arbantis, ML, et al. Abdominal pain in patients with acquired immune deficiency syndrome. *Ann Surg* 1986; 204:619–623.

32. Gordon SC, Reddy KR, Gould EE, et al. The spectrum of liver disease in the acquired immunodeficiency syndrome. *J Hepatol* 2:47, 1986.

33. Lebovics E, Dworkin BM, Heier SK, et al. The hepatobiliary manifestations of human syndrome: A clinical and histologic study. *Hepatology* 1985; 5:293.

34. Lebovics E, Thung SN, Schaffner R, et al. The liver in the acquired immunodeficiency syndrome: A clinical and histologic study. *Hepatology* 1985; 5:293.

35. Vandercam B, Cornu C, Gala JL, et al. Reactivation of hepatitis B virus in a previously immune patient with human immunodeficiency virus infection. *Eur J Clin Microbiol Dis* 1990; 9:701.

36. Snider WD, Simpson DM. Neurologic complications of acquired immunodeficiency syndrome: Analysis of 50 patients. *Ann Neurol* 14:404–418

37. Bacellar H, Munoz A, Miller E. Temporal trends in the incidence of HIV-related neurologic diseases: Multicenter AIDS Cohort Study, 1985–1992. *Neurology* 44: 1892–1900.

38. Simpson DM, Katzenstein DA. Neuromuscular function in HIV infection: Analysis of a placebo-controlled combination antiretroviral trail. AIDS Clinical Group 174/801 Study Team. *AIDS* 12: 2425–2432.

39. So YT, Holtzman DM, Abrams DI. Peripheral nerve associated with acquired immun-odeficiency syndrome: Prevalence and clinical features from a population-based survey. *Arch Neurol* 45: 945–948.

40. Tangliati M, Grinnell J. Peripheral nerve function in HIV function: Clinical, electro-physiological, and laboratory findings. *Arch Neurol* 56: 84–89.

41. Dalakas MC, Pezeshkpour GH. Neuromuscular diseases associated with human immunodeficiency virus infection. *Ann Neurol* 1988; 23(Suppl):S38–S48.

42. Fuller GN, Jacobs JM. Nature and incidence of peripheral nerve syndromes in HIV infection. *J Neurol Neurosurg Psychiatry* 1993; 56:372–381.

43. Simpson DM, Olney RK. Peripheral neuropathies associated with human immunodefi-ciency virus infection. *Neurol Clin* 1992; 10:68–711.

44. Wulff EA, Simpson DM. HIV-associated neuropathy: Recent advances in management. *HIV Advances in Research and Therapy* 8:23–29.

45. Griffin JW, Crawford JO. Predominantly sensory neuropathy in AIDS: Distal axonal degeneration and unmyelinated fiber loss. *Neurology* 1991; 41(Suppl):374. Abstract 900S.

46. Simpson DM, Tagliati M. Nucleoside analog-associated peripheral neuropathy in human immunodeficiency virus infection. *J AIDS* 1995; 9:153–161.

47. Fuller GN, Jacobs JM, Gulloff RJ. Association of painful peripheral neuropathy in AIDS with cytomegalovirus infection. *Lancet* 1989; 2:937–941

48. Rance N, McArthur JC, Cornblath DR. Gracile tract degeneration in patients with sen-sory neuropathy and AIDS. *Neurology* 1988; 38:265–271.

49. Yoshioka M, Shapshak P. Expression of HIV-1 and interleukin-6 in lumbosacral dorsal root ganglia of patients with AIDS. *Neurology* 1994:1120–1130.

50. Fuller GN, Jacobs JM, Guiloff RJ. Subclinical peripheral nerve involvement in AIDS: An electrophysiological and pathological study. *Lancet* 1989; 2:937–941.

51. Kieburtz KD, Giang DW, Schiffer RB. Abnormal vitamin B12 metabolism in human immunodeficiency virus infection: Association with neurologic dysfunction. *Arch Neurol* 1991; 48:312–314.

52. Taylor WR, Wesselingh SL, Griffin JW. Unifying hypothesis for the pathogenesis of HIV-associated dementia complex, vacuolar myelopathy and sensory neuropathy. *J Acquir Immune Defic Syndr Hum Retrovirol* 1995; 9:379–388.

53. Gill P, Rarick M, Bernstein–Singer M, Harb M, Espina BM, Shaw V, Levine A. Treatment of advanced Kaposi's sarcoma using combination of bleomycin and vin-cristine. *Am J Clin Oncol* 13:316–319.

54. Figg WD. Peripheral neuropathy in HIV patients after isoniazid therapy. *Drug Intell Clin Pharmacol* 25:100–101.

55. Ochonisky S, Verroust J, Bastugi-Garin S, Gherardi R, Revuz J. Thalidomide neuropa-thy incidence and clinicoelectrophysiological findings in 42 patients. *Arch Dermatol* 130:66–69.

56. Berger AR, Arezzo JC, Schaumburg HH, Skowron G, Merigan T, Bozzette S, Richman D, Soo W. 2'3'-Dideoxycytidine (ddC) toxic neuropathy: A study of 52 patients. *Neurology* 43: 358–362.

57. Famularo G et al. Acetyl–carnitine deficiency in AIDS patients with neurotoxicity on treatment with antiretroviral nucleoside analogues. *AIDS* 11(2); 185–190.

58. Vendrell J, Heredia C, Pujol M, Vidal J, Blesa R, Graus F. Guillain–Barre syndrome associated with seroconversion for anti-HTLV–III. *Neurology* 37:544.

59. Misha BE, Sommers W, Koski CL, et al. Acute inflammatory demyelinating polyneu-ropathy in the acquired immunodeficiency syndrome. *Ann Neurol* 18:131–132.

60. Morgello S, Simpson DM. Multifocal cytomegalovirus demyelination polyneuropathy associated with AIDS. *Muscle Nerve* 17: 176–182.

61. Cornblath D, McArthur J. Predominantly sensory neuropathy in patients with AIDS and AIDS-related complex. *Neurology* 38:794,1988.

62. Cornblath D, Chaudhry V, Griffin J: Treatment of chronic inflammatory demyelination polyneuropathy with intravenous immunoglobulin. *Ann Neurol* 1991; 30:104.

63. Cliford DB, Buller RS, Mohammed S, Robison L, Storch GA. Use of polymerase chain reaction to demonstrate cytomegalovirus DNA in CSF of patients with human immunodeficiency virus infection. *Neurology* 43:75–79.

64. Kim YS, Hollander H. Polyradiculopathy due to cytomegalovirus: Report of two cases in which improvement occurred after prolonged therapy and review of the literature. *Clin Infect Dis* 17:32–37.

65. Anders HJ. Weiss N, Bogner JR, Goebel FD. Gangciclovir and foscarnet efficacy in AIDS-related CMV polyradiculopathy. *J Infect Dis* 36:29–33.

66. Griffin J, Crawford T, McArthur J. Peripheral neuropathies associated with HIV infection. In: Gendelman HE et al. (eds.), *The Neurology of AIDS.* : Chapman and Hall, 27–291.

67. Said G, Lacroix C, Chemouilli P, Goulon-Goeau C, Roullet E, Penaud D, de Broucker T, Meduri G. Cytomegalovirus neuropathy in acquired immunodeficiency syndrome: A clinical and pathological study. *Ann Neurol* 29:139–146.

68. Roullet E, Asserus V, Gozlan J, Ropert A, Said G, Baudrimont M, et Amrani M, Jacomet C. Cytomegalovirus multifocal neuropathy in AIDS: Analysis of 15 consecutive patients. *Neurology* 44:2174–2182.

69. McLeish WM, Pulido JS, Holland S, et al. The ocular manifestations of syphilis in the human immunodeficiency virus type-1 infected host. *Ophthalmology* 97:196,1990.

70. Adams RD, Victor, M. *Principles of Neurology*, 5th ed. New York: McGraw–Hill, 1993; 663.

71. Sande M, Volberding P. *The Medical Management of AIDS*, 6th ed. Philadelphia: WB Saunders, 1999; 223.

72. Navia B, Jordan B, Price R. The AIDS dementia complex. I. Clinical features. *Ann Neurol* 119:517, 1986.

73. Padgett BL, Walker DL, AuRhein GM. Cultivation of papova-like virus from human brain with progressive multifocal leukoencephalopathy. *Lancet* 971; 1:1257.

74. Cuellar ML. HIV infection-associated inflammatory musculoskeletal disorders. *Rheum Dis Clin N Am* 1998:24, Number 2.

75. Goldman . *Cecil's Textbook of Medicine*, 21st ed., 2000.

76. O'Dell MW, Levinson SF, Riggs RV. Focused review: Physiatric management of HIV-related disability. *Arch Phys Med Rehabil* 1996 Study Guide: 77, Number 3–S.

77. Wolfe F, Smythe HA, Yunus MB, et al. The American College of Rheumatology 1990 criteria for the classification of fibromyalgia: Report of the Multicenter Criteria Committee. *Arthritis Rheum* 1990; 33:160–172.

78. Ruoti RG, Morris DM, and Cole AJ. *Aquatic Rehabilitation.* Lippincott–Raven, 1997.

79. Braddom RL. *Physical Medicine & Rehabilitation, Management of Pain Disorders.* Philadelphia:WB Saunders, 1996, p. 18.

80. Bhasin SB, Storer TW, Javanbakht M, et al. Testosterone replacement and resistance exercise in HIV-infected men with weight loss and low testosterone levels. *JAMA* 2000:283, Number 6.

81. Cohen BA. HIV/AIDS management in office practice, primary care. *Clin Office Prac* September 1997:24, Number 3.

82. Levy JK, Fernandez F. Effects of methylphenidate on HIV–related memory dysfunction. Presented at the New Research Poster Session of the American Psychiatric Association Annual Meeting. Miami, May 1995, p. 20.

83. Masand PS and Tesar GE. Use of stimulants in the medically ill: Consultation–liaison psychiatry. *Psychiatric Clin N Am* 1996; 19(3):515.

84. Management of rheumatoid arthritis. In: Goroll (ed.), *Primary Care Medicine*, 4th ed. Lippincott, Williams & Wilkins, 2000.

85. Rheumatic Disease Clinics of North America, Volume 22, Number 3, August 1996. W.B. Saunders Company, p. 551. Physical Therapy for Musculoskeletal Syndromes, Andrew A. Guccione, Ph.D., PT. (see page 21 & pg. 22 of pain chapter)

86. Blanche P. Acetretin and AIDS-related Reiter's disease. *Clinical Exp Rheum* 1999, Jan–Feb; 17(1):105–6.

87. Bulbul, Williams, Schumacher. Psoriatic arthritis. *Postgraduate Med* 1995: 97, Number 4.

88. Zuckerman GR, Prakash C. Acute lower intestinal bleeding. Part II: Etiology, therapy and outcomes. *Gastrointestinal Endoscopy* 1999: 49(2):228–38.

89. Kaplan R, Conant M, Cundiff D, Maciewicz R, Ries K, Slagle S, Slywka J, Buckley B. Sustained-release morphine sulfate in the management of pain associated with acquired immune deficiency syndrome. *J Pain Symptom Manage* 1996: 12(3):150–60.

90. Kirkpatrick AF, Derasari M, Kovacs PL, Lamb BD, Miller R, Reading A. A protocol-contract for opioid use in patients with chronic pain not due to malignancy. *J Clin Anesthes* 1998: 10(5); 435–43.

91. Kimball LR, McCormick WC. The pharmacologic management of pain and discomfort in persons with AIDS near the end of life: Use of opioid analgesia in the hospice setting. *J Pain & Symptom Manage* 1996: 11(2); 88–94.

92. Breitbart W, Passik, McDonald MV, Rosenfeld B, Smith M, Kaim M, Funesti-Esch J. Patient-related barriers to pain management in ambulatory AIDS patients. *Pain* 1998: 76(1–2); 9–16.

93. Breitbart W, Kaim M, Rosenfeld B. Clinicians' perceptions of barriers to pain management in AIDS. *J Pain & Symptom Manage* 1999; 18(3): 203–12.

94. Breitbart W. Psychotropic adjuvant analgesics for pain in cancer and AIDS. *Psycho Oncology* 1998; 7(4): 333–43.

95. Zampini L et al. Pain treatment of HIV-related peripheral neuropathy. Neuroscience of HIV infection. *J Neurovirol* 1998 Jun 3–6; 4(Suppl):371.

96. Shlay JC et al. Acupuncture and amitriptyline for pain due to HIV-related peripheral neuropathy: A randomized controlled trial. *JAMA* 1998; 280:1590–1595.

97. Evans DL et al. Depression in the medical setting: Biopsychosocial interactions and treatment considerations. *J Clin Psychiatry* 1999; 60 Suppl 4:40–55; discussion 56.

98. Mellick G, MellickL. Gabapentin in the management of reflex sympathetic dystrophy. *J Pain Symptom Manage* 1995:10:265–266.

99. Neville MW. Pharmacotherapy: Gabapentin in the management of neuropathic pain. *Am J Pain Manage* 2000; 10(1):6–12 Jan.

100. Simpson DM, Olney R, McArthur J, et al. A placebo-controlled study of lamotrigene in the treatment of painful sensory polyneuropathy associated with HIV infection. *J Neurovirol* 1998; (Abstract) 4:366.

101. Scarpini E, Sacilotto G, Baron P, Cusini M, Scarlato G. Effect of acetyl-L-carnitine in the treatment of painful peripheral neuropathies in HIV+ patients. *J Periph Nerv Syst* 1997; 2(3): 250–2, 1997.

102. Simpson DM et al. Peptide T in the treatment of painful distal neuropathy associated with AIDS: Results of a placebo-controlled trial. The Peptide T Neuropathy Study Group. *Neurology* 1996; 47(5):1254–9.

103. Brose W, Gutlove D, Luther R, et al. Use of intrathecal SNX-111, a novel, N-type, voltage-sensitive, calcium-channel blocker, in the management of intractable brachial plexus avulsion pain. *Clin J Pain* 1997; 13:256–259.

104. Nadasdi L, Yamashiro D, Chung D, et al. Structure–activity analysis of a conus peptide blocker of N–type calcium channels. *Biochemistry* 1995; 26:2086–2090.

105. Rich K, Luscyndki J, Osbourne P, et al. Nerve growth factor protects adult sensory neurons from cell death and atrophy caused by nerve injury. *J Neurocytol* 1987; 16:261–268.

106. Breitbart W, Rosenfeld B, Passik S, Kaim M, Funesti-Esch J, Stein K. A comparison of pain report and adequacy of analgesic therapy in ambulatory AIDS patients with and without a history of substance abuse. *Pain* 1997; 72(1–2):235–43.

107. Kaplan R, Slywka J, Slagle S, Ries K. A titrated morphine analgesic regimen comparing substance users and nonusers with AIDS-related pain. *J Pain & Symptom Manage* 2000; 19(4):265–73.

108. Abrams DI. *Alternative Therapies*. Chapter 18.

109. Eisenberg DM, Kessler RC, Foster C, et al. Unconventional medicine in the United States: prevalence, costs and patterns of use. *N Engl J Med* 1993; 328:246.

110. Naluyange M, Ssemukasa M, Brehony E. Reflexology: A relaxation exercise for AIDS patients–Rakai district. *International Conference on AIDS Aug 7–12 1994*; 10(2):236.

111. Shlay JC, Chaloner K, Max MB. Flaws B, Reichelderfer P, Wentworth D, Hillman S, Brizz B, Cohn DL. Acupuncture and amitriptyline for pain due to HIV-related peripheral neuropathy. *JAMA* 1998; 280:1590–1596.

112. Galantino MLA, Eke-Okoro ST, Findley TW, Condolucci D. Use of noninvasive electroacupuncture for the treatment of HIV-related peripheral neuropathy: A pilot study. *J Alternative Complementary Med* 1999; 5(2):135–42.

113. Calabrese C, Wenner CA, Reeves C, Turet P, Standish LJ. Treatment of human immunodeficiency virus–positive patients with complementary and alternative medicine: A survey of practitioners. *J Alternative Complementary Med* 1998; 4(3):281–287.

114. Homsy J et al. Evaluating herbal medicine for the management of *Herpes zoster* in human immunodeficiency virus–infected patients in Kampala, Uganda. *J Alternative Complementary Med* 2000; 6(1):1–2.

115. Mowery DB. *The Scientific Validation of Herbal Medicine*. New Canaan, Conn.: Keats Publishing, 1986.

116. Smigelski C. *Eat Up! Nutrition Advice and Food Ideas for People Living With HIV and AIDS*. Tufts University.

117. Goldberg B. *Alternative Medicine: The Definitive Guide*.

118. Fishman S, Berger L. *The War on Pain*. New York:HarperCollins, 2000.

119. McCaleb RS, Leigh E, Morien K. *The Encyclopedia of Popular Herbs*. Roseville, Calif.: Prima Health Publishers, 2000.

120. Castleman M. *The Healing Herbs*. New York: Bantam Books, 1991.

121. Khan A, Dorfman D, Dalton A, Scarano A, Markarian Y, Simpson D. Treatment of painful peripheral neuropathy in HIV infection with a topical agent: Results of an open label study using 5 percent lidocaine. Neuroscience of HIV infection. *J Neurovirol* 1998 Jun 3–6; 4(Suppl):355.

122. McArthur J, Yiannoutsos C, Simpson DM, and the ACTG 291 Study Team. Trial of recombinant human nerve growth factor for HIV-associated sensory neuropathy. *J Neurovirol* 1998; (Abstract) 4:359.

123. Murray M. *The Healing Power of Herbs*. Rocklin, Calif.: Prima Publishers, 1995.

Index

Note: **Boldface** numbers indicate illustrations; italic *t* indicates a table.